PET-CT-MRI Applications of Musculoskeletal Disorders, Part I

Editors

ALI GHOLAMREZANEZHAD
ALI GUERMAZI
ALI SALAVATI
ABASS ALAVI

PET CLINICS

www.pet.theclinics.com

Consulting Editor
ABASS ALAVI

October 2018 • Volume 13 • Number 4

ELSEVIER

1600 John F. Kennedy Boulevard • Suite 1800 • Philadelphia, Pennsylvania, 19103-2899

http://www.pet.theclinics.com

PET CLINICS Volume 13, Number 4
October 2018 ISSN 1556-8598, ISBN-13: 978-0-323-64112-8

Editor: John Vassallo (j.vassallo@elsevier.com)
Developmental Editor: Casey Potter

PET Clinics (ISSN 1556-8598) is published quarterly by Elsevier Inc., 360 Park Avenue South, New York, NY 10010-1710. Months of issue are January, April, July, and October. Periodicals postage paid at New York, NY, and additional mailing offices. Subscription prices per year are $232.00 (US individuals), $396.00 (US institutions), $100.00 (US students), $263.00 (Canadian individuals), $446.00 (Canadian institutions), $140.00 (Canadian students), $268.00 (foreign individuals), $446.00 (foreign institutions), and $140.00 (foreign students). To receive student and resident rate, orders must be accompanied by name of affiliated institution, date of term, and the signature of program/residency coordinator on institution letterhead. Orders will be billed at individual rate until proof of status is received. Foreign air speed delivery is included in all Clinics subscription prices. All prices are subject to change without notice. POSTMASTER: Send address changes to PET Clinics, Elsevier Health Sciences Division, Subscription Customer Service, 3251 Riverport Lane, Maryland Heights, MO 63043. **Customer Service: 1-800-654-2452 (U.S. and Canada); 314-447-8871 (outside U.S. and Canada). Fax: 314-447-8029. E-mail: journalscustomerservice-usa@elsevier.com (for print support); journalsonlinesupport-usa@elsevier.com (for online support).**

Reprints. For copies of 100 or more of articles in this publication, please contact the Commercial Reprints Department, Elsevier Inc., 360 Park Avenue South, New York, NY 10010-1710. Tel.: 212-633-3874; Fax: 212-633-3820; E-mail: reprints@elsevier.com.

Printed in the United States of America.

PET Clinics is covered in MEDLINE/PubMed (Index Medicus).

Contributors

CONSULTING EDITOR

ABASS ALAVI, MD, MD (Hon), PhD (Hon), DSc (Hon)
Professor of Radiology and Neurology, Department of Radiology, Division of Nuclear Medicine, Hospital of the University of Pennsylvania, University of Pennsylvania Perelman School of Medicine, Philadelphia, Pennsylvania, USA

EDITORS

ALI GHOLAMREZANEZHAD, MD, DABR, FEBNM
Assistant Professor of Clinical Radiology, Keck School of Medicine of USC, University of Southern California, Los Angeles, California, USA; University Hospitals Cleveland Medical Center, Cleveland, Ohio, USA

ALI GUERMAZI, MD, PhD
Professor, Department of Radiology, Boston University School of Medicine, Boston, Massachusetts, USA

ALI SALAVATI, MD, MPH
Department of Radiology, University of Minnesota, Minneapolis, Minnesota, USA

ABASS ALAVI, MD, MD (Hon), PhD (Hon), DSc (Hon)
Professor of Radiology and Neurology, Department of Radiology, Division of Nuclear Medicine, Hospital of the University of Pennsylvania, University of Pennsylvania Perelman School of Medicine, Philadelphia, Pennsylvania, USA

AUTHORS

ALI AFSHAR-OROMIEH, MD
Department of Nuclear Medicine, Heidelberg University Hospital, Clinical Cooperation Unit Nuclear Medicine, German Cancer Research Centre, Heidelberg, Germany

HOJJAT AHMADZADEHFAR, MD, MSc
Department of Nuclear Medicine, University Hospital Bonn, Bonn, Germany

HAMZA ALIZAI, MD
Assistant Professor, Department of Radiology, NYU Langone Medical Center, New York, New York, USA

MARIET ASADOORIAN, MD
Department of Radiology, Keck School of Medicine of USC, University of Southern California, Los Angeles, California, USA

KYLE BASQUES, MD
University Hospitals of Cleveland, Case Western Reserve University, Cleveland, Ohio, USA

SANDIP BASU, MBBS (Hons), DRM, Diplomate N.B
Professor and Head, Nuclear Medicine Academic Programme, Radiation Medicine Centre (BARC), Tata Memorial Hospital Annexe, Homi Bhabha National Institute, Mumbai, India

MOHSEN BEHESHTI, MD, FEBNM, FASNC
Professor in Nuclear Medicine, Department of
Nuclear Medicine and Endocrinology, PET - CT
Center LINZ, Ordensklinikum, St Vincent's
Hospital, Linz, Austria; Department of Nuclear
Medicine and Endocrinology, Paracelsus
Medical University, Salzburg, Austria

ASHKAN HESHMATZADEH BEHZADI, MD
Department of Radiology, Weill Cornell
Medical Center, New York, New York, USA

MIKAEL BOESEN, MD, PhD
Professor, Department of Radiology, Parker
Institute, Bispebjerg and Frederiksberg
Hospital, Copenhagen, Denmark

JOHN A. CARRINO, MD, MPH
Professor of Radiology, Department of
Radiology and Imaging, Hospital for
Special Surgery, New York, New York, USA

GREGORY CHANG, MD
Section Chief of Musculoskeletal Imaging,
Associate Professor, Department of Radiology,
NYU Langone Medical Center, New York,
New York, USA

FARROKH DEHDASHTI, MD
Professor of Radiology, Mallinckrodt Institute
of Radiology, Washington University in
St. Louis, St Louis, Missouri, USA

MARKUS ESSLER, MD
Department of Nuclear Medicine, University
Hospital Bonn, Bonn, Germany

KUNIHIKO FUKUDA, MD, PhD
Honorary Professor of Radiology, The Jikei
University, Tokyo, Japan

TAKESHI FUKUDA, MD
Department of Radiology, The Jikei University
School of Medicine, Tokyo, Japan; Department
of Radiology, Stony Brook Medicine, Stony
Brook, New York

**ALI GHOLAMREZANEZHAD, MD, DABR,
FEBNM**
Assistant Professor of Clinical Radiology, Keck
School of Medicine of USC, University of
Southern California, Los Angeles, California,
USA; University Hospitals Cleveland Medical
Center, Cleveland, Ohio, USA

ALI GUERMAZI, MD, PhD
Professor, Department of Radiology, Boston
University School of Medicine, Boston,
Massachusetts, USA

PHILIP HANSEN, MD, PhD
Senior Research Consultant, Department
of Radiology, Bispebjerg and
Frederiksberg Hospital, Copenhagen,
Denmark

ROBERT HEMKE, MD, PhD
Post Doc, Departments of Radiology and
Nuclear Medicine, Faculty of Medicine,
Academic Medical Center (AMC) Amsterdam,
University of Amsterdam, Amsterdam,
The Netherlands

**HOSSEIN JADVAR, MD, PhD, MPH, MBA,
FACNM, FSNMMI**
Associate Professor of Radiology, Keck School
of Medicine of USC, Associate Professor of
Biomedical Engineering, Viterbi School of
Engineering, University of Southern California,
Los Angeles, California, USA

FRANÇOIS JAMAR, MD, PhD
Department of Nuclear Medicine, Centre du
Cancer and Institut de Recherche
Expérimentale et Clinique (IREC–IMAG),
Cliniques Universitaires Saint-Luc, Université
Catholique de Louvain (UCL), Brussels,
Belgium

JACK W. JENNINGS, MD, PhD
Associate Professor of Radiology, Mallinckrodt
Institute of Radiology, Washington University
in St. Louis, St Louis, Missouri, USA

SANAZ KATAL, MD, MPH
Tehran University of Medical Sciences (TUMS),
Tehran, Iran

MICHAEL KESSLER, MD
Case Medical Center, University Hospitals of
Cleveland, Case Western Reserve University,
Cleveland, Ohio, USA

CHRISTOS KOSMAS, MD
Assistant Professor of Radiology, University
Hospitals of Cleveland, Case Western
Reserve University, Cleveland, Ohio,
USA

OLGA KUBASSOVA, MSc, PhD
Image Analysis Group (IAG)

FREDERIC E. LECOUVET, MD, PhD
Department of Radiology, Centre du Cancer
and Institut de Recherche Expérimentale et
Clinique (IREC–IMAG), Cliniques Universitaires
Saint-Luc, Université Catholique de Louvain
(UCL), Brussels, Belgium

RENAUD LHOMMEL, MD
Department of Nuclear Medicine, Centre du
Cancer and Institut de Recherche
Expérimentale et Clinique (IREC–IMAG),
Cliniques Universitaires Saint-Luc, Université
Catholique de Louvain (UCL), Brussels, Belgium

MARIO MAAS, MD, PhD
Professor, Departments of Radiology and
Nuclear Medicine, Faculty of Medicine,
Academic Medical Center (AMC) Amsterdam,
University of Amsterdam, Amsterdam, The
Netherlands

GEORGE R. MATCUK Jr, MD
Division of Musculoskeletal Radiology,
Department of Radiology, Keck School of
Medicine of USC, University of Southern
California, Los Angeles, California, USA

JANUS DAMM NYBING, MSc
Reserch Tech, Department of Radiology,
Bispebjerg and Frederiksberg Hospital,
Copenhagen, Denmark

EDWIN H. OEI, MD, PhD
Associate Professor, Departments of
Radiology and Nuclear Medicine, Erasmus
MC, University Medical Center Rotterdam,
Rotterdam, The Netherlands

MOJTABA OLYAEI, MD
Tehran University of Medical Sciences (TUMS),
Tehran, Iran

RAHUL V. PARGHANE, MBBS, MD
Consultant Physician, Radiation Medicine
Centre (BARC), Tata Memorial Hospital Annexe,
Homi Bhabha National Institute, Mumbai, India

VASSILIKI P. PASOGLOU, MD, PhD
Department of Radiology, Centre du Cancer
and Institut de Recherche Expérimentale et
Clinique (IREC–IMAG), Cliniques Universitaires
Saint-Luc, Université Catholique de Louvain
(UCL), Brussels, Belgium

DAKSHESH B. PATEL, MD
Department of Radiology, Keck School of
Medicine of USC, University of Southern
California, Los Angeles, California,
USA

JAY PATEL, MD
Department of Radiology, Weill Cornell
Medical Center, New York, New York,
USA

KAMBIZ RAHBAR, MD
Department of Nuclear Medicine, University
Hospital Muenster, Muenster, Germany

SYED IMRAN RAZA, MBBS
Department of Radiology, Weill Cornell
Medical Center, New York, New York, USA

RAVINDER R. REGATTE, PhD
Professor, Department of Radiology, NYU
Langone Medical Center, New York, New York,
USA

IWONA SUDOŁ-SZOPIŃSKA, MD, PhD
Professor, Department of Radiology, National
Institute of Geriatrics, Rheumatology and
Rehabilitation, Department of Diagnostic
Imaging, Warsaw Medical University, Warsaw,
Poland

ANDERANIK TOMASIAN, MD
Assistant Professor of Clinical Radiology,
Department of Radiology, Keck School of
Medicine of USC, University of Southern
California, Los Angeles, California, USA

SANDY VAN NIEUWENHOVE, MD
Department of Radiology, Centre du Cancer
and Institut de Recherche Expérimentale et
Clinique (IREC–IMAG), Cliniques Universitaires
Saint-Luc, Université Catholique de Louvain
(UCL), Brussels, Belgium

HEIDI R. WASSEF, MD
Department of Radiology, Keck School of
Medicine of USC, University of Southern
California, Los Angeles, California,
USA

ERIC A. WHITE, MD
Department of Radiology, Keck School of
Medicine of USC, University of Southern
California, Los Angeles, California,
USA

Contents

In this article, the fundamentals of PET/computed tomography (CT) and PET/MRI are discussed, with their implications for evaluation of musculoskeletal disorders. This article also provides an overview of FDG and non-FDG PET tracers; the different PET, CT, and MRI protocols; and how they can be employed in an individualized manner in various disease conditions. The present role and the shortcomings of both modalities have been enumerated.

^{18}F-sodium fluoride (^{18}F-NaF) PET/computed tomography (CT) provides high sensitivity and specificity for the assessment of bone and joint diseases. It is able to accurately differentiate malignant from benign bone lesions, especially when using dynamic quantitative approaches. Its high quality, clinical accuracy, and high feasibility for patient management and greater availability of PET/CT scanners as well as decreasing trend of the cost of radiotracer all indicate the need to consider the use of ^{18}F-NaF PET/CT as standard bone imaging, particularly in malignant diseases of the skeleton.

The skeleton is a common site for cancer metastases. Bone metastases are a major cause of morbidity and mortality and associated with pain, pathologic fractures, spinal cord compression, and decreased survival. Various radionuclides have been used for pain therapy. Recently, an α-emitter has been shown to improve overall survival of patients with bone metastases from castration-resistant prostate cancer and was approved as a therapeutic agent. This article provides an overview of the state-of-the-art radionuclide therapy options for bone metastases, with focus on the role of PET imaging in therapy planning.

Whole-body MR imaging (WB-MR imaging) has become a modality of choice for detecting bone metastases in multiple cancers and bone marrow involvement by multiple myeloma or lymphoma. Combination of anatomic and functional sequences imparts an inherently hybrid dimension to this nonirradiating tool and extends the screening of malignancies outside the skeleton. WB-MR imaging outperforms bone scintigraphy and computed tomography and offers an alternative to PET in many tumors by time of lesion detection and assessment of treatment response. Much work has been done to standardize procedures, optimize sequences, validate indications, and confirm preliminary research into new applications, rendering clinical application more user-friendly.

Contrast-enhanced MR imaging (CE-MR imaging) is recommended for the diagnosis and monitoring of infectious and most inflammatory joint diseases. CE-MR imaging clearly differentiates soft and bony tissue from fluid collections and infectious debris. To improve imaging information, a dynamic CE-MR imaging (DCE-MR imaging) sequence can be applied using fast T1-weighted sequential image acquisition during contrast injection. Use of DCE-MR imaging allows robust extraction of quantitative information regarding blood flow and capillary permeability, especially when dedicated analysis methods and software are used to analyze contrast kinetics. This article describes principles of DCE-MR imaging for the assessment of infectious and inflammatory joint diseases.

MR imaging is an indispensable instrument for the diagnosis of musculoskeletal diseases. In vivo MR imaging at 7T offers many advantages, including increased signal-to-noise ratio, higher spatial resolution, improved spectral resolution for spectroscopy, improved sensitivity for X-nucleus imaging, and decreased image acquisition times. There are also, however, technical challenges of imaging at a higher field strength compared with 1.5 and 3T MR imaging systems. The authors discuss the many potential opportunities as well as challenges presented by 7T MR imaging systems and highlight recent developments in in vivo research in imaging of musculoskeletal applications in general and cartilage, skeletal muscle, and bone in particular.

Dual-energy computed tomography (DECT) enables material decomposition and virtual monochromatic images by acquiring 2 different energy X-ray data sets. DECT can detect musculoskeletal pathologic conditions that CT alone cannot, and that would otherwise require MR imaging. In this review, the authors discuss several useful techniques and applications of DECT in musculoskeletal research: virtual monochromatic images, virtual noncalcium images, gout, iodine map, and tendons.

This article discusses the role of PET-computed tomography in percutaneous minimally invasive ablation of osseous metastases, including diagnosis and preprocedural factors related to patient selection and procedure planning, intraprocedural imaging guidance, and posttreatment imaging assessment.

A wide range of musculoskeletal processes can demonstrate an increased uptake on PET-computed tomography (CT) with fluorodeoxyglucose (FDG) F 18, including reactive, benign neoplastic, inflammatory, traumatic, posttreatment, and arthritic conditions that may mimic malignancy. In addition, physiologic causes of increased FDG uptake such as asymmetric muscle use and presence of brown fat can lead to an increased FDG uptake and potential false-positive results. This article presents various case examples of nonmalignant musculoskeletal hypermetabolism on 18F-FDG PET-CT and describes useful tools to avoid the potential pitfall of misinterpreting these as malignancy.

Soft tissue sarcomas (STSs) account for less than 1% of adult solid tumors and about 7% of pediatric malignancies, causing 2% of cancer-related deaths. With the advent of PET-computed tomography (CT), the value of (18) fluorine-2-fluoro-2-deoxy-D-glucose (FDG) PET imaging to improve the management of STSs has been explored. FDG PET imaging has been found useful in restaging and treatment response assessment. This article reviews current knowledge and application of FDG PET-CT in the initial diagnosis, staging, restaging, treatment response monitoring, and prognosis, with a brief overview of the most common histologic subtypes of STS.

Primary bone malignancies are characterized with anatomic imaging. However, in recent years, there has been an increased interest in PET/computed tomography scanning and PET/MRI with fludeoxyglucose F 18 for evaluating and staging musculoskeletal neoplasms. These hybrid imaging modalities have shown promise largely owing to their high sensitivity, ability to perform more thorough staging, and ability to monitor treatment response. This article reviews the current role of PET/computed tomography scanning and PET/MRI in primary malignancies of bone, with an emphasis on imaging characteristics, clinical usefulness, and current limitations.

PET CLINICS

PROGRAM OBJECTIVE

The goal of the PET Clinics is to keep practicing radiologists and radiology residents up to date with current clinical practice in positron emission tomography by providing timely articles reviewing the state of the art in patient care.

TARGET AUDIENCE

Practicing radiologists, radiology residents, and other health care professionals who provide patient care utilizing radiologic findings.

LEARNING OBJECTIVES

Upon completion of this activity, participants will be able to:

1. Review basic principles, methodology, and imaging protocol for musculoskeletal PET/CT and PET/MRI applications.
2. Discuss novel whole-body techniques in MR imaging and future application of PET-CT-MRI in musculoskeletal disorders.
3. Recognize DCE-MRI application in joint infection and inflammation.

ACCREDITATION

The Elsevier Office of Continuing Medical Education (EOCME) is accredited by the Accreditation Council for Continuing Medical Education (ACCME) to provide continuing medical education for physicians.

The EOCME designates this enduring material for a maximum of 15 *AMA PRA Category 1 Credit*(s)™. Physicians should claim only the credit commensurate with the extent of their participation in the activity.

All other health care professionals requesting continuing education credit for this enduring material will be issued a certificate of participation.

DISCLOSURE OF CONFLICTS OF INTEREST

The EOCME assesses conflict of interest with its instructors, faculty, planners, and other individuals who are in a position to control the content of CME activities. All relevant conflicts of interest that are identified are thoroughly vetted by EOCME for fair balance, scientific objectivity, and patient care recommendations. EOCME is committed to providing its learners with CME activities that promote improvements or quality in healthcare and not a specific proprietary business or a commercial interest.

The planning committee, staff, authors and editors listed below have identified no financial relationships or relationships to products or devices they or their spouse/life partner have with commercial interest related to the content of this CME activity:

Abass Alavi, MD, MD(Hon), PhD(Hon), DSc(Hon); Hamza Alizai, MD; Mariet Asadoorian, MD; Kyle Basques, MD; Sandip Basu, MBBS(Hons), DRM, Diplomate N.B; Mohsen Beheshti, MD, FEBNM, FASNC; Ashkan Heshmatzadeh Behzadi, MD; John A. Carrino, MD, MPH; Gregory Chang, MD; Farrokh Dehdashti, MD; Markus Essler, MD; Kunihiko Fukuda, MD, PhD; Takeshi Fukuda, MD; Ali Gholamrezanezhad, MD, DABR, FEBNM; Philip Hansen, MD, PhD; Robert Hemke, MD, PhD; Hossein Jadvar, MD, PhD, MPH, MBA, FACNM, FSNMMI; François Jamar, MD, PhD; Sanaz Katal, MD, MPH; Alison Kemp; Michael Kessler, MD; Frederic E. Lecouvet, MD, PhD; Renaud Lhommel, MD; Mario Maas, MD, PhD; George R. Matcuk Jr, MD; Janus Damm Nybing, MSc; Mojtaba Olyaei, MD; Rahul V. Parghane, MBBS, MD; Vasiliki P. Pasoglou, MD, PhD; Dakshesh B. Patel, MD; Jay Patel, MD; Kambiz Rahbar, MD; Syed Imran Raza, MD; Ravinder R. Regatte, MD; Ali Salavati, MD, MPH; Iwona Sudoł-Szopińska, MD, PhD; Sandy Van Nieuwenhove, MD; John Vassallo; Vignesh Viswanathan; Heidi R. Wassef, MD; Eric A. White, MD.

The planning committee, staff, authors and editors listed below have identified financial relationships or relationships to products or devices they or their spouse/life partner have with commercial interest related to the content of this CME activity:

Mikael Boesen, MD, PhD: is a consultant/advisor for and owns stock in Image Analysis Group.
Ali Guermazi, MD, PhD: is employed by Boston Imaging Core Lab, LLC and is a consultant to EMD Serono, Inc., Kolon TissueGene, Inc., OrthoTrophix, Inc., General Electric Company, AstraZeneca, Pfizer, Inc., and Sanofi.
Jack W. Jennings, MD, PhD: is a consultant/advisor for The Advisory Board Company and participates in a speakers bureau for Medtronic and BTG International Ltd.
Christos Kosmas, MD: is a consultant/advisor for Bioclinica.
Olga Kubassova, MSc, PhD: is employed by and owns stock in Image Analysis Group.
Edwin H. Oei, MD, PhD: receives research support from General Electric Company
Anderanik Tomasian, MD: is a consultant/advisor for Medtronic.

UNAPPROVED/OFF-LABEL USE DISCLOSURE

The EOCME requires CME faculty to disclose to the participants:

1. When products or procedures being discussed are off-label, unlabelled, experimental, and/or investigational (not US Food and Drug Administration [FDA] approved); and
2. Any limitations on the information presented, such as data that are preliminary or that represent ongoing research, interim analyses, and/or unsupported opinions. Faculty may discuss information about pharmaceutical agents that is outside of

FDA-approved labelling. This information is intended solely for CME and is not intended to promote off-label use of these medications. If you have any questions, contact the medical affairs department of the manufacturer for the most recent prescribing information.

TO ENROLL

To enroll in the PET Clinics Continuing Medical Education program, call customer service at 1-800-654-2452 or sign up online at http://www.theclinics.com/home/cme. The CME program is available to subscribers for an additional annual fee of USD $235.

METHOD OF PARTICIPATION

In order to claim credit, participants must complete the following:

1. Complete enrolment as indicated above.
2. Read the activity.
3. Complete the CME Test and Evaluation. Participants must achieve a score of 70% on the test. All CME Tests and Evaluations must be completed online.

CME INQUIRIES/SPECIAL NEEDS

For all CME inquiries or special needs, please contact elsevierCME@elsevier.com.

Preface

Evolving Role of PET-Computed Tomography and PET-MR Imaging in Assessment of Musculoskeletal Disorders and Its Potential Revolutionary Impact on Day-to-Day Practice of Related Disciplines

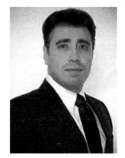 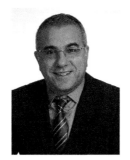 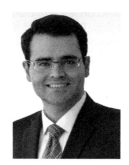 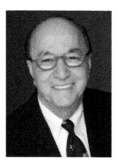

Ali Gholamrezanezhad, MD   Ali Guermazi, MD, PhD   Ali Salavati, MD, MPH   Abass Alavi, MD

Editors

With advancing technology and increasing availability of sophisticated hybrid imaging tools, there has been increasing use of PET-computed tomography (CT) and PET-MR imaging in daily clinical patient care as well as the research arena. It is therefore timely for us to bring together international experts on imaging of musculoskeletal disease using PET-CT and PET-MR imaging and provide up-to-date literature evidence on the recent development in these hybrid imaging techniques. As we all know, a major advantage of PET is its ability to depict the site of active metabolism. Therefore, foci of abnormal hypermetabolism secondary to malignancy, infection, and inflammation can be detected. By coupling this to high anatomical resolution of CT and MR imaging, we can ameliorate the major disadvantage of PET imaging. Although the main theme of this issue of *PET Clinics* is the hybrid PET-CT and PET-MR imaging, we felt it would be useful to the readers to include some articles that are dedicated to nonhybrid CT and MR imaging techniques that are novel as well as particularly relevant for musculoskeletal imaging.

This issue of *PET Clinics* has two parts. In part 1, we focus on basic concept, technical details, radiopharmaceutical agents, and perspectives related to PET-CT/PET-MR imaging application for the evaluation of musculoskeletal disorders. The article by Sandip Basu and colleagues provides a detailed overview of the basic principles and technical and methodologic considerations of the performance of PET/CT/MR imaging for musculoskeletal applications in a practical manner. This will in particular help orthopedic surgeons and rheumatologists without deep knowledge of nuclear medicine and PET technology make a foundation for successive reading and have a better understanding of the technique and the acquisition protocols. Subsequent articles cover the application of PET/CT/MR imaging with FDG and other radiopharmaceuticals in various clinical settings. These include

PET Clin 13 (2018) xiii–xiv
https://doi.org/10.1016/j.cpet.2018.07.001
1556-8598/18/© 2018 Published by Elsevier Inc.

pet.theclinics.com

applications of PET in primary soft tissue tumors of extremities and also different primary bone malignancies. The role of PET in the posttherapy setting and evaluation of response to treatment has been described in two articles. Tomasian and colleagues have discussed the role of PET in the evaluation of response to treatment by percutaneous thermal ablations. Ahmadzadehfar and colleagues also have focused on the posttreatment PET imaging in radionuclide therapy of osseous metastases. There are several articles centered around the role of PET imaging of the musculoskeletal system in the context of competing imaging modalities, including spectral and dual-energy CT, dynamic contrast-enhanced MR imaging, contrast-enhanced CT imaging (including iodine overlay image), and also quantitative MR imaging at higher magnet strengths (7 T and above). Dr Boesen and colleagues describe the utility of MR imaging for articular infection and inflammation with an emphasis on dynamic contract-enhanced MR imaging. Dr Lecouvet and colleagues explain emerging novel whole-body MR imaging technique, and Dr Regatte and colleagues provide an overview of recent developments in quantitative techniques for musculoskeletal MR imaging at 7 T. An article by Dr Fukuda focuses on the role of contrast-enhanced, spectral, and dual-energy CT applications in musculoskeletal imaging. Dr Basu and colleagues provide recent literature evidence regarding in vivo molecular imaging of inflammation and infection.

We are thankful for all the coauthors who generously donated their time and effort to the fruition of this issue of *PET Clinics*. We sincerely hope that the information we provide in this issue will be helpful to the radiologists and nonradiology colleagues who are involved in hybrid PET-CT and PET-MR imaging.

Ali Gholamrezanezhad, MD
Keck School of Medicine, University of Southern California (USC)
1520 San Pablo Street
Los Angeles, CA 90033, USA

Ali Guermazi, MD, PhD
Boston University School of Medicine
Boston Medical Centre
820 Harrison Avenue, FGH Building, 3rd Floor
Boston, MA 02118, USA

Ali Salavati, MD, MPH
Department of Radiology
University of Minnesota
420 Delaware Street Southeast
Minneapolis, MN 55455, USA

Abass Alavi, MD
Department of Radiology
Hospital of the University of Pennsylvania
3400 Spruce Street
Philadelphia, PA 19104, USA

E-mail addresses:
gholamre@med.usc.edu (A. Gholamrezanezhad)
Ali.Guermazi@bmc.or (A. Guermazi)
salavati@gmail.com (A. Salavati)
Abass.Alavi@uphs.upenn.edu (A. Alavi)

PET/Computed Tomography and PET/MR Imaging
Basic Principles, Methodology, and Imaging Protocol for Musculoskeletal Applications

Rahul V. Parghane, MBBS, MD[a,b],
Sandip Basu, MBBS (Hons), DRM, Diplomate N.B[a,b,*]

KEYWORDS
• PET/CT • PET/MRI • Musculoskeletal disorders

KEY POINTS
- Hybrid imaging with PET-CT forms a valuable tool for clinical imaging musculoskeletal disorders especially in oncological setting.
- The role and applicability of PET-MRI in musculoskeletal disorders is gradually evolving.
- Understanding of various imaging protocols would allow employing PET-CT in an individualized manner in various conditions. The appreciation of false-positive and false negative lesions on FDG-PET/CT are important for appropriate interpretation.

BASIC PHYSICS: POSITRON EMISSION AND ANNIHILATION

PET imaging provides functional and molecular information related to biological tissues and pathophysiologic processes in clinical and research practice, using radiopharmaceuticals labeled with positron emitting radioisotopes such as ^{18}F,^{11}C, ^{13}N, and ^{15}O, which are produced in a cyclotron, and ^{68}Ga and ^{82}Rb, which are produced in generators.[1–5]

In PET image acquisition, a positron-labeled pharmaceutical is injected intravenously into the patient, which is distributed throughout the body via the bloodstream, and enters the cells and tissues following specific pathophysiologic pathways. PET with fludeoxyglucose F 18 (FDG PET) is typically performed on the patient 60 minutes after intravenous (IV) injection of the positron-labeled pharmaceutical such as FDG.

As the radioisotope undergoes positron emission decay, also known as beta plus decay (β^+ decay), in which a proton inside a radionuclide nucleus is converted into a neutron while releasing a positron and a neutrino (ν_e). A positron is emitted from the nucleus and travels in tissues for a short distance before being annihilated. When the positron meets an electron, annihilation occurs, and a pair of annihilation photons moves in opposite directions at approximately 180° from each other. PET scanners are equipped with coincidence electronics to detect these pairs of photons within a narrow timing window of typically 3 to 15 nanoseconds, as these particles are emitted from the surface of the human body and hit opposite detectors nearly simultaneously in PET system.[1]

PET scanner instrument comprises a dedicated PET camera having multiple rings of detectors and these PET detectors consist of a high density of

a Radiation Medicine Centre (BARC), Tata Memorial Hospital Annexe, Parel, Mumbai 400012, India; b Homi Bhabha National Institute, Mumbai 400094, India
* Corresponding author. Radiation Medicine Centre, Bhabha Atomic Research Centre, Tata Memorial Hospital, Annexe Building, Jerbai Wadia Road, Parel, Mumbai 400 012, India.
E-mail address: drsanb@yahoo.com

PET Clin 13 (2018) 459–476
https://doi.org/10.1016/j.cpet.2018.05.003
1556-8598/18/

scintillation crystals coupled with photomultiplier tubes (PMTs). The scintillation crystals used in clinical PET imaging are either bismuth germanium oxide, gadolinium oxyorthosilicate, lutetium oxyorthosilicate, or lutetium yttrium orthosilicate that converts the energy of photons striking the detector into light. The light is converted into an amplified electric signal at a photomultiplier tube.[6]

A list-mode file is commonly used in PET systems to acquire and save data over a given time frame, where each event is tagged with a line of response position and the time point of detection. The tomographic images are reconstructed into sinograms. The tomographic image reconstruction most commonly and typically obtained by statistical iterative reconstruction methods. Every tomographic slice is reconstructed independently by only accepting a line of response within the given slice with inserting septa (thin lead or tungsten collimating rings) between scintillation crystal rings such that interring coincidences are prevented. This method of image acquisition called 2-dimensional PET, whereas 3-dimensional (3D) PET include acceptance of inter-ring coincidences resulting in high sensitivity of PET system. For this reason, 3D PET is the preferred imaging mode in all modern clinical PET systems.[1,7]

HYBRID PET/COMPUTED TOMOGRAPHY

PET imaging provides functional and molecular information of tissues, and less detailed structural information with limited spatial resolution. Computed tomography (CT) is commonly used for providing anatomic and structural details and information of tissues and organs in 3D views. The combination of a PET scanner with a CT scanner in a single hybrid PET/CT system is a highly precise and revolutionary metabolic imaging technique with detailed structural information on tissue and organs in a single setting, which has been widely applied in clinics to acquire nuclear medicine images in various oncologic and nononcologic conditions. The newer development in PET systems, such as the time-of-flight leads to (i) improvement in image contrast and (ii) a reduced noise-to-signal ratio by better localization of annihilation position on line of response. The advantage of time-of-flight in modern PET system is that it reduces the (iii) the patient dose by requirement of administering less activity and (iv) reduces the scan time in each patient with good image contrast and signal-to-noise ratio. The spiral CT scanners have evolved from 2- to 64-slice devices for attenuation correction for diagnostic CT in hybrid PET/CT system so that there is an overall improvement in the detection of lesions, less time for acquisition, and greater efficiency of the system. However, the 64-slice devices CT lead to additional radiation and low soft tissue contrast from CT also limits clinical applications of PET/CT, particularly in pediatric patients and musculoskeletal disorders, respectively.[1,6,8]

PET RADIOPHARMACEUTICALS: IN MUSCULOSKELETAL DISORDERS

Imaging is an integral part of the evaluation of musculoskeletal disorders from both diagnosis and management viewpoints and comprises primarily conventional imaging methods, such as plain film radiography, CT, and MRI, which provides high-resolution structural information. The functional and molecular information about tissue and disease characteristics is provided by the PET imaging technique through the distribution and uptake of positron-emitting radiotracers.[9]

In PET radiochemistry, ^{18}F radioisotope is the backbone for PET imaging; this is produced in a cyclotron by the nuclear reaction between oxygen 18 (^{18}O)-enriched water bombarded with protons releasing a neutron with production equation ^{18}O(p,n)^{18}F. Sodium fluoride (NaF) and ^{18}F-labeled fluorodeoxyglucose (FDG) are 2 commonly used radiotracers for PET imaging in musculoskeletal disorders.

Many studies have evaluated the role of ^{18}F-FDG PET/CT and dedicated FDG PET in musculoskeletal tumors, particularly as a potential imaging modality discriminating between high-grade sarcomas and benign tumors, and between low- and high-grade malignant tumors based on the mean standardized uptake value (SUV). Furthermore, ^{18}F-FDG PET/CT and PET scans have an added value in staging and evaluating the response to therapy in musculoskeletal tumors, thus improving patient management. However, FDG is not a specific marker for malignant musculoskeletal lesions and false-positive FDG PET findings (Table 1) have been reported with inflammation of the musculoskeletal system (eg, arthritis, osteomyelitis) and aggressive musculoskeletal benign tumors (eg, diffuse tenosynovial giant cell tumor, osteoid osteoma). The false-negative FDG PET findings were reported in certain malignant musculoskeletal tumors (eg, myxoid liposarcomas, chondrosarcoma) and, thus, it is unable to differentiate low-grade malignant lesions from the benign tumors.[10–14]

To overcome these shortcomings and to provide more precise insight into musculoskeletal tumor biology, newer and more specific radiopharmaceuticals have been investigated with a focus

Table 1
False-positive and false-negative FDG PET/PET-CT results in various musculoskeletal lesions

Primary Site	High FDG Uptake in Benign Lesions (False Positive)	Low FDG Uptake in Malignant Lesion (False Negative)
Soft tissue lesion	Pigmented villonodular synovitis Hibernoma Sarcoidosis Myositis ossificans Nonossifying fibroma Neurofibroma Schwannoma Desmoid fibromatosis Abscess Inflammatory condition	Myxoid Liposarcomas Well-differentiated liposarcomas Low-grade fibromyxoid sarcomas Spindle cell tumors
Bony lesion	Osteoid osteoma Histiocytosis X Chondroblastoma Enchondroma Giant cell tumors Fibrous dysplasia	Chondrosarcoma Chordoma

Abbreviations: CT, computed tomography; FDG, fludeoxyglucose F 18.

Reproduced from Parghane RV, Basu S. Dual-time point 18F-FDG-PET and PET/CT for differentiating benign from malignant musculoskeletal lesions: opportunities and limitations. Semin Nucl Med 2017;47:375; with permission.

on tumor grading, treatment monitoring, and determination of disease progression on an individual basis in musculoskeletal lesions. These non-FDG and more specific PET radiopharmaceuticals, for example, ^{18}F-fluoride as the bone-imaging agent, ^{18}F-fluorodeoxythymidine (FLT) as the proliferation marker, ^{11}C methionine as amino acid tracers, and ^{18}F-galacto-RGD as biomarkers of neoangiogenesis have been used in musculoskeletal lesions as shown in **Table 2**.

^{18}F-FLT PET was studied in 22 patients with suspected soft tissue or bone tumors by Buck and colleagues[15] in a prospective study, and the sensitivity of 100% for malignant lesion with a mean FLT uptake in malignant tumors (mean SUV, 4.7) was significantly higher than in benign lesions (mean SUV, 0.7; $P < .0001$) and also to differentiate between low-grade and high-grade sarcomas using ^{18}F-FLT PET at a cutoff value of 2.0 was shown in their study. The therapeutic response evaluation in soft tissue sarcoma was investigated by Benz and colleagues[16] with the help of ^{18}F-FLT PET. In their study, they found no correlation between the histopathologic response and FLT uptake and no correlation between FLT uptake and tumor proliferation index. They concluded that response assessment based on ^{18}F-FLT PET analyses do not provide an advantage over FDG PET in soft tissue sarcoma patients.

Two times higher uptake in bone, more complete, and faster excretion of the fluoride ion (^{18}F) as compared ^{99m}Tc-polyphosphonates resulted in an overall lower background activity in ^{18}F-NaF PET/CT and also the better spatial resolution of PET studies led to increasing use of ^{18}F-fluoride PET imaging in the evaluation of malignant as well as benign skeletal lesions in recent years. Gamie and El-Maghraby[17] and Lim and colleagues[18] in their studies concluded that there is a potential role for ^{18}F-NaF PET/CT in the assessment of adult patients with back pain and in identifying the underlying reasons for persistent back pain after surgical interventions of vertebrae, respectively.

In a clinical trial, PET-based radiolabeled amino acid tracers such as ^{18}F-fluoromethyltyrosine were investigated by Watanabe and colleagues[19] and Suzuki and colleagues[20]; these investigators concluded that ^{18}F-fluoromethyltyrosine PET is superior to FDG PET scanning in differentiating benign and malignant tumors, particularly between lipomas and lower malignant liposarcomas.

The longer half-life (110 minutes) of [18]fluorine, also a simple and efficient synthesis of [18]fluorine-labeled amino acids, such as fluoroethyl-L-tyrosine (FET) or L-methyltyrosine (^{18}F-fluoromethyltyrosine), makes these tracers suitable as radiopharmaceuticals for whole body PET studies and, thus, led more investigation of these tracers for their promise in clinical oncology, as compared with [11]carbon-labeled amino acids, which has short half-life (20 minutes), requiring an in-house cyclotron for the production and synthesis of radiopharmaceuticals, thus, preventing widespread use of ^{11}C-labeled amino acid and other tracers.[21,22]

Table 2
FDG and non-FDG PET tracers investigated in musculoskeletal lesions

PET Radiopharmaceuticals	Mechanism and Function at Cellular Level	Clinical Applications in Musculoskeletal Disorder
[18]F-based radiopharmaceuticals		
FDG	FDG uptake in cell through the GLUTs and glucose consumption in cell	• Staging and grading of musculoskeletal tumor[10,13] • To differentiate between benign and malignant[10,13,14] musculoskeletal lesions • Therapeutic response assessment in musculoskeletal tumor[13] • Guided biopsy from lesions[13]
NaF	Bone imaging agent, fluoride ion exchanged for a hydroxyl group in the bone crystal and forms fluoroapatite, this deposits at the bone surface where turnover is greatest	• Detection of bone metastases in oncologic cases[58,59] • Assessment of benign bone pathology- like lower back pain[17,18]
FLT	Equilibrating nucleoside transporter 1, FLT is phosphorylated to FLT monophosphate and thereby trapped in tumor cells and proliferation marker	• Staging and grading of musculoskeletal tumor[15,16] • To differentiate between benign and malignant musculoskeletal lesions[15,16] • Therapy response assessment in musculoskeletal tumor[15,16] • Guided biopsy from lesions[15,16]
FET and FMT	Uptake reflects increased active transport, protein synthesis, and amino acid metabolism in cancer cells	• Grading of musculoskeletal tumor[19–22] • To differentiate between benign and malignant musculoskeletal lesions[19–22]
[18]F galacto-RGD	Bind to αvβ3 integrin in receptor-specific manner and act as biomarker of neoangiogenesis	• Guided biopsy from lesions[58,59] • Pretherapy scan for αvβ3-targeted therapies[58,59] • Response evaluation after antiangiogenic therapies[58,59]
[18]F fluorethylcholine	An increased uptake of choline and an increased activity of choline kinase in malignant cell and is component of the membrane phospholipids	• Detection of bone metastasis[27] • Staging and restaging in prostate cancer[27]
[11]C-Based radiopharmaceuticals		
[11]C methionine	Uptake reflect amino acid metabolism in cancer cells and its incorporation into immunoglobulin of the malignant plasma cell	• TGR after neoadjuvant chemoradiotherapy in musculoskeletal tumor[58,59] • Staging and restaging in multiple myeloma[24] • To estimate tumor burden and to locate active medullary and extramedullary lesion in multiple myeloma[24]
[11]C choline	An increased uptake of choline and an increased activity of choline kinase in malignant cell and is component of the membrane phospholipids	• Detection of malignant bone and soft tissue tumors[25,26] • Detection of bone metastasis[25,26] • Staging and restaging in prostate cancer[25,26]

(continued on next page)

Table 2 (continued)		
PET Radiopharmaceuticals	Mechanism and Function at Cellular Level	Clinical Applications in Musculoskeletal Disorder
[68]Ga-based radiopharmaceuticals		
[68]Ga PSMA	PSMA is a cell surface protein that is significantly overexpressed in prostate cancer cells	• Staging and restaging in prostate cancer[28] • Detection of bone metastasis in prostate cancer[28]
DOTATATE/ DOTANOC	NETs express SSTRs on their cell membranes and radiolabeled somatostatin analogs used for disease detection in NETs	• Detection of bone/soft tissue metastases in NETs[60] • Therapy response assessment in bone/soft tissue metastases in NETs[60] • Guided biopsy from lesions[60]

Abbreviations: DOTANOC, DOTA-1-Nal3-octreotide; DOTATATE, ^{68}Ga DOTA-Tyr3 octreotate; FDG, ^{18}F fluorodeoxyglucose; FET, ^{18}F fluoroethyltyrosine; FLOT, ^{18}F fluorodeoxythymidine; FMT, ^{18}F fluoromethyltyrosine; GLUTs, glucose transporters; NaF, ^{18}F sodium fluoride; NETs, neuroendocrine tumors; PSMA, prostate-specific membrane antigen; SSTRs, somatostatin receptors; TGR, tumor grade regression.

A total of 10 patients with musculoskeletal tumors were examined by Beer and colleagues[23] by using ^{18}F galacto-RGD-PET. The uptake of ^{18}F galacto-RGD in the tumor was significantly correlated with neoangiogenesis marker, that is, the $\alpha v \beta 3$ expression level in the tumor. The low malignant tumor, such as low-grade liposarcomas, showed no an obvious uptake of ^{18}F galacto-RGD, whereas high-grade sarcomas showed a higher uptake of ^{18}F galacto-RGD in their study.

Lapa and colleagues[24] studied the usefulness of ^{11}C-methionine PET for staging and restaging of multiple myeloma and compared with FDG PET/CT. In their study, ^{11}C-methionine seemed to be superior to FDG for both staging and restaging disease at both intramedullary and extramedullary locations. ^{11}C-methionine tracer uptake was correlated with bone marrow involvement and was found to reflect a more accurate marker of tumor burden and disease activity in patients with multiple myeloma.

[11]C-choline PET was used by Tian and colleagues[25] in their research for differentiating benign and malignant tumors and comparing choline PET with FDG PET in brain tumors, head and neck tumors, bone tumors, lung tumors, and soft tissue tumors. They found that choline showed a higher contrast ratio as compared with FDG in these tumors. In conclusion, these investigators mentioned that ^{11}C-choline PET imaging may be used for differentiating malignant and benign tumors, although high uptake of choline was found in some benign tumors and tumorlike lesions.

[11]C-choline PET/CT has been mainly used for staging and restaging of bone metastases in prostate carcinoma. Fuccio and colleagues[26] investigated a patient with cancer with ^{11}C-choline PET/CT and concluded that ^{11}C-choline PET/CT had better sensitivity than bone scintigraphy for the detection of skeletal lesions in patients with prostate cancer with biochemical relapse after radical prostatectomy. Similarly, Beheshti and colleagues[27] also showed that ^{11}C-choline PET/CT detected early bone metastases in patients with prostate cancer.

[68]Gallium is a radioisotope with a half-life of 68 minutes and produced from a 68Ge-68Ga generator. [68]Gallium is labeled with Glu-NH-CO-NH-Lys prostate-specific membrane antigen (PSMA-HBED-CC) or PSMA-11, which is used for staging, restaging, and recurrence detection in patients with prostate cancer. Zacho and colleagues[28] in their review article suggested that ^{68}Ga-PSMA PET/CT detected more bony lesions than bone scintigraphy, leading to an improvement in the primary staging of patients with prostate cancer. ^{68}Ga-DOTA-Tyr3 octreotate/DOTA-1-Nal3-octreotide is commonly used for the diagnosis of neuroendocrine tumor, restaging, and recurrence detection including bony lesions, before peptide receptor radionuclide therapy for somatostatin receptor expression, and after peptide receptor radionuclide therapy for response evaluation in patients with neuroendocrine tumors.

PET/COMPUTED TOMOGRAPHY PROTOCOL FOR MUSCULOSKELETAL LESIONS

As mentioned, ^{18}F-FDG is the main and routinely used radiopharmaceutical in clinical practice for the evaluation of musculoskeletal lesions.

Patient Preparation for PET with Fludeoxyglucose F 18 and Computed Tomography Scanning

There are a few clinical factors that affect FDG biodistribution that should be considered and possibly avoided by delaying the FDG PET during the active processes. These include (i) inflammatory or infectious processes, (ii) radiation therapy (interval between therapy and FDG PET recommended is at least around 6–12 weeks), (iii) recent surgery (interval between therapy and FDG PET is around 4 weeks), (iv) recent chemotherapy (interval between therapy and FDG PET scan is 2–4 weeks), and (v) cytokines or growth factor therapy (interval between therapy and FDG PET scan is 3–4 weeks), which cause markedly increased FDG uptake in the bone marrow and that factor is important in the evaluation of musculoskeletal lesions.

Before injecting ^{18}F-FDG, patients must fast for at least 4 to 6 hours to decrease the physiologic glucose levels and reduce serum insulin levels to near basal levels. Oral hydration with water is encouraged. IV fluids containing dextrose or parenteral feedings also should be withheld for 4 to 6 hours.

In hyperglycemic states, the FDG uptake in the tumor is reduced; therefore, the blood glucose level should be checked before administrating ^{18}F-FDG. Particularly in musculoskeletal lesions, an increased blood glucose level is problematic because it causes increased insulin levels, altering the FDG biodistribution by shifting its uptake to muscle and fat, leading to difficulty in interpreting musculoskeletal lesions. Plasma glucose levels should not exceed 130 to 150 mg/dL in nondiabetic patients and not greater than 180 to 200 mg/dL in diabetic patients, so that there is no altered FDG biodistribution.

At least 24 hours before FDG PET study, all patients are advised to refrain from any strenuous activity or exercise so that the physiologic muscle FDG uptake is minimized. Benzodiazepines (5 mg) may be administered 60 minutes before FDG injection to obtain higher muscle relaxation, thus, less physiologic FDG uptake in muscles, particularly in anxious patients with higher FDG uptake in the trapezius and paraspinal muscles. After FDG injection, the patient must be seated or recumbent in a comfortable chair or bed. To prevent/reduce brown fat FDG uptake, the use of warming and low-dose beta-blockers such as oral propranolol (20 mg) 60 minutes before FDG injection may be advocated, which is important for the evaluation of musculoskeletal lesions.

Generally, the dose of FDG is 185 to 555 MBq (5–14 mCi) for adults and 3.7 to 5.2 MBq/kg (0.10–0.14 mCi/kg) for children, keeping in mind the principle of ALARA (as low as reasonably achievable). The institutional protocol is developed with consideration of patient-related factors (eg, age, weight, and body mass), and scanner-related factors (eg, crystal type lutetium oxyorthosilicate, lutetium yttrium orthosilicate, bismuth germanium oxide, gadolinium oxyorthosilicate), acquisition mode (2-dimensional, 3D), bed overlap (25%, 50%), and acquisition time per bed position. The FDG injection must be given in the contralateral arm to a primary tumor in the thorax, breast, or arm. Injection of furosemide in a dose from 2 mg/kg to 40 mg may be considered while evaluating pelvic lesions, in order to increase urinary clearance from bladder so that there is less interference from high FDG activity in the urine.

HYBRID PET/COMPUTED TOMOGRAPHY SCAN ACQUISITION

Before the era of hybrid PET/CT scans, PET studies were performed in a dedicated PET scanner 60 minutes after FDG injection in 2-dimensional and 3D modes with a total of 5 or 6 bed examinations (6 minutes emission, 4 minutes transmission), using ordered subset expectation maximization iterative reconstruction. Images were displayed in coronal, axial, and sagittal sections with 1.3-cm-thick reconstructions in inverted gray-scale maps and successive 6-mm multiplanar slices of the body. Because of the superiority and more detailed anatomic information obtained from hybrid PET/CT scans, now most of nuclear medicine departments have been adopting hybrid PET/CT scanners with standard PET and CT acquisition parameters, such as filter, reconstruction, and methods, for PET scans and helical thickness, tube current and other parameters for CT scans (PET and CT acquisition parameters are presented in **Tables 3** and **4**).

To ensure a higher tumor to background ratio, acquisition is started at 60 minutes after FDG injection and to avoid/limit involuntary motion that may lead to general or local misalignment during the hybrid PET/CT examinations. The patient must be well-supported with adequate positioning aids, for example, with knee, head and neck, and arm supports. The patient should void the urinary bladder before the acquisition of the images to obtain better quality images and limit the radiation dose to the renal collecting system and bladder. Patients must also remove metallic objects whenever possible. The emission image acquisition time is based on the administered dose of activity, patient body weight, the sensitivity and detector

Table 3
Parameters for PET scan acquisition

PET Scan Acquisition Parameters	Whole Body Acquisition	Regional Acquisition (Head and Neck)
Filter	Gaussian	Gaussian
Full width at half maximum	4.0	4.0
Zoom	1	1
Image size (pixels)	128/168	256
Reconstruction method	Iterative (cranial/caudal)	Iterative (cranial/caudal)
Interactions	2	4
Subsets	16	16
Normalization	Yes	Yes
Scatter correction	Yes	Yes
Minutes per bed	2	4

composition of the PET scanner, and acquisition method for PET/CT scan; it usually varies from 2 to 5 minutes or longer per bed position for body imaging. For imaging from the skull to the mid-thigh, the total acquisition time is ranges from 15 to 25 minutes for PET/CT scans.

POSITIONING OF PATIENT AND ANATOMIC REGION COVERAGE
Skull Base to Proximal Thigh Imaging

This is most common PET/CT acquisition for oncologic conditions. These PET/CT scans typically are acquired from the external auditory meatus to the midthigh region.

Whole Body Imaging

Images ae acquired from the top of the skull to the toes (melanoma protocol). These protocols are useful in the imaging of tumors with a high probability of involvement of the head, neck, and upper and lower limbs regions, such as osteosarcomas, rhabdomyosarcomas, liposarcomas, and malignant peripheral nerve sheath tumors, and in the evaluation of osteomyelitis.

Limited Region Imaging

Localized region acquisition include, for example, head and neck area, thoracic, and pelvic area.

Table 4
CT acquisition parameters in hybrid PET/CT

CT Scan Acquisition Parameters	Only for Attenuation Correction and Anatomic Localization	Diagnostic Parameters and Attenuation Correction
Coverage	From base of the skull to upper thighs or up to toe	From base of the skull to upper thighs or up to toe
Patient positioning	Arms up or down depending site of lesion	Arms up or down depending site of lesion
Scout	120 mV−10 mA	120 mV−10 mA
Scan type	Helical	Helical
Rotation time	0.6 s	0.5 s
Rotation length	Full	Full
Detector coverage	40 mm	40 mm
Helical thickness	3.75 mm	3.75 mm
Pitch	0.984:1	0.984:1
Table speed	39.37 mm/rotation	39.37 mm/rotation
Coverage speed	65.62 mm/s	65.62 mm/s
Tube potential	120 kV	120 kV
Tube current	Smart mA (auto mA) mA range: minimum 50−maximum 100	Smart mA (auto mA) mA range: minimum 120−maximum 650

Abbreviation: CT, computed tomography.

This acquisition is mainly used in disease that is restricted to a defined region, for example, solitary pulmonary nodule, suspicion of lung cancer, examination of hilar lymph nodes, head and neck tumors, evaluation of lower backache, giant cell tumors, and osteoid osteoma in musculoskeletal conditions.

Arms Elevated over the Head for Optimal Imaging of the Body

This protocol is commonly used in PET/CT acquisition to avoid beam-hardening artifacts over the torso produced by having the arm alongside the body, for example, in liposarcomas, leiomyosarcomas, and rhabdomyosarcomas of chest and abdominal regions.

Arms Alongside and Close to the Body Imaging

This protocol is used for the acquisition of musculoskeletal lesions involving the arm and forearm areas, for example, for sarcoma, myositis ossificans, and osteomyelitis involving upper extremities (**Fig. 1**). This protocol is also used in the evaluation of head and neck lesions and in patients not able to keep their arms elevated above the head.

COMPUTED TOMOGRAPHY PROTOCOL FOR HYBRID PET/COMPUTED TOMOGRAPHY IMAGING

Hybrid PET/CT imaging is usually performed using a protocol comprising a scanogram/scout scan/topogram and followed by a CT scan for attenuation correction and anatomic correlation. The tube current, voltage, slice thickness, rotation time and pitch, and other factors for these CT acquisition parameters should be chosen as per the objective of the CT scan for attenuation and scatter correction, and the colocalization of radiologically equivalent interpretation. Overall, CT acquisition parameters should be chosen according to the ALARA principle such that patient exposure should be minimal with an adequate dose to obtain the necessary diagnostic information. After PET and CT acquisition, sequences or protocols are used in clinical nuclear medicine for the purpose of quantification of tracer from PET imaging and diagnostic information from CT scan in hybrid PET/CT imaging (advantages and disadvantages of low-dose and diagnostic CT protocols are compared in **Table 5**).

Low-Dose Computed Tomography Protocol

CT scanning is used for attenuation correction and localization only with a low milliampere-seconds setting so that the radiation dose to the patient is low. First a CT topogram, followed by a low-dose CT scan, followed by PET acquisition comprises this protocol. No IV contrast is used in this protocol; oral contrast may or may not be used in this type of acquisition.

Diagnostic Computed Tomography with Oral and Intravenous Contrast Protocol

In this protocol, standard CT milliampere-seconds settings are used to optimize the spatial resolution

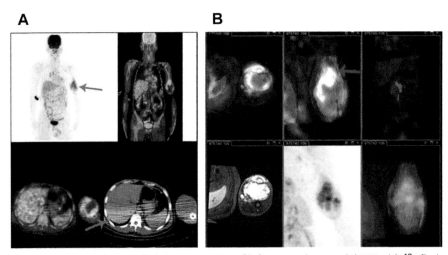

Fig. 1. A 51-year-old man with known rhabdomyosarcoma of left arm underwent (*A*) PET with ^{18}F fludeoxyglucose (FDG PET)/computed tomography (CT) acquired from skull to mid-thigh region with arm alongside of body and patient also underwent region MRI scan on different day and machine. With help of fusion software, PET data are fused with MRI data as shown in B. Beam hardening artifact develops because of arm alongside of body in PET/CT acquisition as shown in A with red arrow on the CT image. Fused PET/MRI images (*B*) shows misregistration (*blue arrow*) of PET images on MRI images, leading difficulty in the interpretation of the PET/MRI images. To avoid such misregistration and beam-hardening artifacts, an integrated whole body PET/MRI system is important.

Table 5
Variants of CT protocol in PET-CT with their advantages and disadvantages

CT Protocols	Contrast Use	Advantages	Disadvantages
Low-dose CT protocol	No use of IV contrast	Less radiation exposure dose Provides complete metabolic information	Limited structural information lead to reduces the sensitivity and specificity for detecting malignant lesions
Diagnostic CT protocol	Use of IV and oral contrast	Provide complete metabolic and anatomic information	Leads to more radiation exposure dose Requires IV contrast, may lead to side effect of contrast agents Contrast may cause error in SUV measurement Contrast agent may cause artifacts that may interfere with interpretation

Abbreviations: CT, computed tomography; IV, intravenous; SUV, standardized uptake value.

of the CT imaging with tube current modulation to minimize the radiation dose to the patient. The IV or oral contrast material is used in this protocol. First, a CT topogram is acquired followed by a whole-body diagnostic CT scan (with shallow breathing) with a 45-second delay after the thoracic CT scan (equilibrium or venous phase) if the thoracic CT scan is acquired, or with a 60-second delay after the beginning of contrast agent infusion if the thoracic CT scan is not performed. PET acquisition is acquired after whole body diagnostic CT scan is completed. An IV contrast agent is ideally given with a programmable fluid injector at a speed of 2.5 mL/s through a catheter of size 20G × 1.16″ with a location in the elbow region. The use of a multiphasic enhancement technique using IV contrast may improve the diagnostic capability of CT in characteristic enhancement patterns in malignant lesions. In addition, IV contrast agents make vessels distinct from other structures so that CT imaging specificity increases in differentiating benign from malignant FDG uptake in hybrid PET/CT studies. Oral contrast agents are used for better delineation of the gastrointestinal tract with a positive contrast agent (diluted barium); a negative or water-based contrast agent can be used for this purpose as well.[29]

Limited Area Contrast-Enhanced Diagnostic Computed Tomography Protocol

To avoid the impact of IV contrast enhancement on attenuation correction and SUV determination, first a low-dose CT protocol in hybrid PET/CT imaging is acquired, followed by an additionally limited area where an IV contrast-enhanced diagnostic CT scan is acquired involving the lesion in that region or region of interest.

Diagnostic Computed Tomography Without Oral and Intravenous Contrast Protocol

This protocol is used in cases of bony tumor (eg, osteosarcomas and chondrosarcoma) and in patients in whom use of contrast material is contraindicated (eg, allergic reaction to the iodinated contrast material, patients with nephropathy). In this protocol, the CT scan is acquired without use of oral or IV contrast agents.

Breathing Computed Tomography Protocol

To match the position of the diaphragm on the PET emission images to that of the CT transmission images, a CT transmission scan is acquired during breath holding at mid inspiration volume. Other investigators prefer the patient to continue shallow breathing during CT acquisition. Lung movement owing to respiration results in inaccurate localization of lesions at the base and periphery of the lungs, in the dome of the liver, or near any lung–soft tissue interface, and this factor may result in spurious SUV determinations. To avoid this, motion correction or respiratory gating is used in evaluation of thoracic lesions in hybrid PET/CT imaging.

In most musculoskeletal lesion evaluations involving the lower limbs and pelvic regions or multiple region involvement with a high probability of metastatic spreads to lower limbs, a whole body imaging protocol is used acquiring scan from skull to feet (eg, for osteogenic sarcoma). In contrast, lesions involving head, neck, thoracic, and upper limb regions with less of a probability of metastatic spread to the lower limbs, skull base to proximal thigh imaging or limited region imaging protocol is used (eg, evaluation of head and neck melanoma,[30] giant cell tumors, and osteoid osteoma).

For staging, restaging, and recurrence evaluation in skeletal lesions, diagnostic CT scans without an oral and IV contrast protocol is used. IV contrast is used for the evaluation muscular and soft tissue lesions (eg, liposarcomas, leiomyosarcomas, and rhabdomyosarcomas) and for the evaluation of lung lesions. Oral contrast is used for the evaluation of abdominal and pelvic lesions in the vicinity of gastrointestinal tract (eg, leiomyosarcomas and rhabdomyosarcomas).

Based on individual cases and indications, such as benign or malignant lesion, soft tissue or bony lesion, site of disease (upper or lower extremities), and for initial staging or response evaluation, the acquisition parameters must be considered before acquiring hybrid PET/CT scan so that each modality in combination will be complementary for maximum benefit. Optimizing radiation exposure to the patient is also an important consideration. The individual disease and indication and hybrid PET/CT protocol is provided in **Table 6** and a working flow chart for acquisition of PET/CT scanning is provided in **Fig. 2**.

PET WITH FLUDEOXYGLUCOSE F 18 AND COMPUTED TOMOGRAPHY SCANNING FOR MUSCULOSKELETAL APPLICATIONS: BASIC FACTS ON PERFORMANCE IN MUSCULOSKELETAL TUMORS

Musculoskeletal tumors can be divided into soft tissue tumors and bony tumors. The incidence of malignancy in soft tissue tumors is rare, accounting for 0.7% of adult and 7.0% of childhood malignancies. Soft tissue tumors can occur anywhere in the body and commonly involve the extremities and intraabdominal regions. These tumors may originate from fatty tissues (lipoma/liposarcoma), muscles (myoma/leiomyosarcoma and rhabdomyosarcoma), connective tissue (fibroma/fibrosarcoma), blood vessels (angioma, hemangioma, and angiosarcoma), and neurogenic tissue (schwannoma, malignant peripheral nerve sheath tumor, and malignant schwannoma).[31,32] Ewing sarcomas, osteosarcomas, and chondrosarcoma are common malignant bony lesions that arise from extremities, mostly from the lower limbs. Conventional imaging such as ultrasound examination is used commonly to guide biopsy from a soft tissue lesion and to establish the diagnosis of soft tissue tumor, whereas MRI is an important imaging tool for the assessment of the origin of a tumor and the evaluation of the anatomic relation to important structures such as nerves, vessels, and muscle compartments in planning the resection of musculoskeletal tumors.

One application of FDG PET/CT scanning in the musculoskeletal system is to differentiate benign lesions from malignant lesions based on quantitative measure of FDG uptake. Generally, the SUV, ranging between 0.70 and 1.35 in benign and between 3.20 and 6.90 in malignant soft tissue lesion, has been reported with some exception with high uptake in benign lesions and low uptake in malignant lesions. To clearly define the lesion, it is recommended that additional clinical and imaging information such as ultrasound examination and MRI used to distinguish between benign and malignant musculoskeletal lesions. PET cannot replace a biopsy; histopathologic confirmation in unclear cases is crucial in evaluating tumors of the musculoskeletal system.

FDG PET/CT scanning is a sensitive investigation in the detection of musculoskeletal lesions. Bastiaannet and colleagues[33] in their metaanalysis showed a pooled sensitivity of 0.88 (0.83–0.93), specificity of 0.86 (0.81–0.91), and accuracy of 0.87 (0.83–0.90) for the detection of soft tissue tumors.

Grading is an important factor in the evaluation of musculoskeletal tumors. Several studies showed a positive correlation between FDG uptake and the histopathologic grade of musculoskeletal tumors. PET may help to ensure accurate grading and prognostication in sarcomas by guiding the biopsy to the most biologically significant region as shown by Folpe and colleagues,[34] with a positive correlation between the SUV and histopathologic grade.

For therapy planning and prognostic stratification in musculoskeletal tumors, accurate staging is very important. Metastatic spread from musculoskeletal tumors occurs anywhere in the body, but most typically in the lung, soft tissue, and lymph nodes. FDG PET/CT scanning is superior to conventional imaging for the detection of lymph node metastases in musculoskeletal tumors as shown by Volker and colleagues[35] and Tateishi and colleagues[36] in their studies.

Various studies have shown that FDG PET alone is not a sensitive imaging modality for the detection of lung metastases; PET alone may fail to show FDG uptake in lung lesions smaller than 6 mm. The thin-slice full inspiration diagnostic CT scan in the hybrid PET/CT scan provide CT images that are highly sensitive for the detection of pulmonary metastases.

Neoadjuvant chemotherapy or radiotherapy before resection is usually done in large size, intermediate to high-grade musculoskeletal tumors. Accurate noninvasive assessment of the response to therapy is valuable to guide therapeutic decisions and to avoid ineffective chemotherapy or

Table 6
Disease-specific recommendations for PET and CT Protocol

Malignant Musculoskeletal Tumors			
Malignant Lesion	**Sites (Most Common)**	**PET Coverage[a]**	**CT Protocol[b]**
Osteosarcomas	Distal end of the femur and the proximal ends of the tibia and humerus sites	Whole body imaging	Diagnostic CT without oral and IV contrast protocol
Ewing sarcoma	Femur, pelvis and upper limb regions	Whole body imaging	Diagnostic CT without oral and IV contrast protocol
Chordomas	Sacrococcygeal region	Skull to proximal thigh imaging	Diagnostic CT without oral and IV contrast protocol
Chondrosarcomas	Pelvis and femur sites	Whole body imaging	Diagnostic CT without oral and IV contrast protocol
Rhabdomyosarcomas	Head and neck regions	Whole body imaging	Diagnostic CT with oral and IV contrast protocol
Liposarcomas	Buttocks, thighs, lower extremities, and retroperitoneal regions	Whole body imaging	Diagnostic CT with oral and IV contrast protocol
Leiomyosarcomas	Retroperitoneal and proximal extremities regions	Whole body imaging	Diagnostic CT with oral and IV contrast protocol
Malignant peripheral nerve sheath tumors	Extremities region	Whole body imaging	Diagnostic CT with oral and IV contrast protocol
Benign Musculoskeletal Tumors and Lesions			
Benign Lesion	**Sites (Most Common)**	**PET Coverage[a]**	**CT Protocol[b]**
Osteoid osteoma	Limbs regions	Limited-region imaging	Diagnostic CT without oral and IV contrast protocol
Intraosseous hemangioma	Vertebral (thoracic vertebra)and skull regions	Skull to proximal thigh imaging Limited region imaging	Diagnostic CT without oral and IV contrast protocol
Enchondromas and enchondromatosis	Small bones of the hands and feet regions Multiple bony sites	Whole body imaging— multiple sites Limited region imaging—single site	Diagnostic CT without oral and IV contrast protocol
Giant cell tumors	Lower end of the femur or upper end of the tibia regions	Whole body imaging Limited-region imaging	Diagnostic CT without oral and IV contrast protocol
Osteomyelitis	Lower limbs and vertebrae regions	Whole body imaging Limited-region imaging	Diagnostic CT with IV contrast protocol

Abbreviations: CT, computed tomography; IV, intravenous.

[a] Skull to proximal thigh imaging protocol is used for lesion involving head, neck, thoracic, and upper limbs regions with less chance of metastatic spread to lower extremity.

[b] Low-dose CT scan protocol is used instead of diagnostic CT for treatment response evaluation, in which CT is used for attenuation correction and localization only. Oral contrast is used in abdominal and pelvic lesions particularly in the vicinity of gastrointestinal tract.

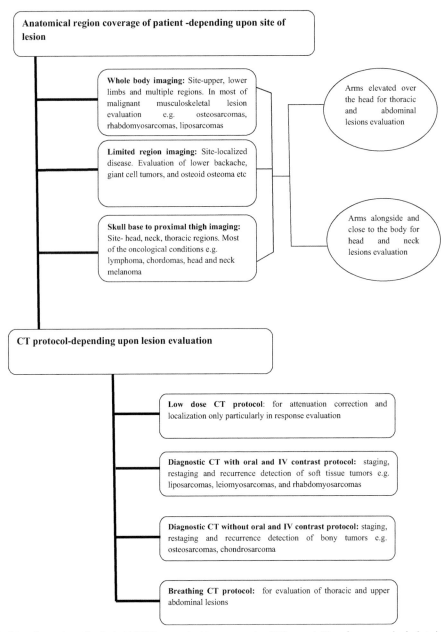

Fig. 2. Working flow chart for hybrid PET/computed tomography (CT) acquisition for musculoskeletal lesion evaluation. IV, intravenous.

radiation therapy. FDG PET/CT scanning is superior to morphologic imaging in assessing the response to therapy in musculoskeletal tumors, as shown in various studies.[37]

FDG PET scans show a high sensitivity for the detection of local recurrence in high-grade musculoskeletal tumor as shown in various studies.[38] The detection of recurrence of musculoskeletal tumors is challenging owing to the anatomic alterations caused by prior treatment. The use of a metallic prosthesis in limb salvage therapy can cause beam-hardening artifacts in CT scans and

susceptibility artifacts in MRI, which lead to inferior imaging quality in these conditions.

BASICS OF PET/MR IMAGING

Newer research has been directed toward combining and developing PET/MRI as an imaging modality without compromising the imaging quality of PET or MRI individually. Whole-body PET/MRI systems are now available for clinical deployment.

In MRI acquisition, a strong magnetic field is produced that causes an interaction with the PET system, which can lead to quality degradation of both modalities. To solve this issue, 2 major design concepts of whole body PET/MRI have been developed: sequential scanning systems and simultaneous scanning systems. In the sequential PET/MRI system, PET and MRI images are acquired sequentially on 2 distinct devices as part of a single examination. Because there is little interaction between the PET and MRI devices in the sequential system, this leads to easy establishment of sequential system.[39]

Scans obtained by the PET and MRI modalities are registered by software according to the sensor-coded bed position. The advantage of this system is that PET and MRI can operate separately when the patient does not need dual modality information. It is flexible according to the application and workload in hospital and clinical practices, but because the 2 modalities are acquired at different time points, it is difficult to guarantee that the position, posture, and metabolic state of the patient are the same. This factor leads to difficulties in the registration of 2 modalities under certain conditions and results in the degradation of image quality of the PET/MRI system.[40–42]

To overcome the disadvantages of the sequential system, simultaneous PET/MRI systems have been developed. In simultaneous PET/MRI systems, PET and MRI images are acquired at the same time. To solve the interaction problem in PET/MRI system, totally redesigning the structures of the PET and MRI devices were done in simultaneous PET/MRI systems. In the initial phases of development, there were many practical problems in simultaneous PET/MRI acquisition: (i) the photomultiplier tube in the PET system cannot work properly in the magnetic field of the MRI system, (ii) the PET photodetector may interfere with the radiofrequency and gradient coils, resulting in a nonuniform magnetic field, and (iii) an eddy current may occur if metallic shielding is adopted.[43] Many prototype PET/MRI systems were designed and developed to overcome these problems. These include magnetically immune photomultiplier tube (eg, avalanche photodiodes and silicon photomultipliers) as substitutes for PMTs. An avalanche photodiode not only has higher quantum efficiency, but also requires a lower supply voltage and are small in size, making the PET detector easy to integrate with an MRI device. All those characteristics made avalanche photodiodes very suitable for simultaneous PET/MRI equipment. Adoption of time-of-flight technology in the PET/MRI system led to significant improvement in the spatial resolution, reduced the dose of radiation to patient,

and enhanced the precision of attenuation correction in PET/MRI images.

The loss of signal proportional to the depth of the annihilation event from the surface and the regional tissue density required attenuation correction in a PET system. Attenuation correction is a postprocessing step and essential in producing PET images of diagnostic quality and quantitative accuracy. The present solution of a CT-based transmission a system is used in PET/CT attenuation correction; this process is not possible in a PET/MRI system. The CT scan measures photon attenuation and, being similar in principle to PET, allows attenuation correction of the higher energy (511 keV) gamma photons. Because MRI measures signals based on proton density, an MRI is unable to provide an analogous attenuation correction with a CT scan. Software-based algorithms (eg, artificial intelligence algorithms or template datasets) are used to derive attenuation correction maps or dedicated attenuation correction sequences such as 2-point Dixon volume-interpolated breath-hold examination sequences are used for attenuation correction in PET/MRI systems.[44]

PET/MR IMAGING PROTOCOL

Sequential PET/MRI requires longer acquisition times compared with simultaneous PET/MRI, because in sequential PET/MRI, the patient is imaged twice, once with PET and once with MRI.

As in FDG PET/CT, the requirement before image acquisition is 4 to 6 hours of fasting, control of blood glucose level, and the need for rest after FDG injection to minimize muscle uptake is also valid for PET/MRI acquisition. Contraindications to PET/MRI are the same as for MRI (eg, metallic implants and pacemakers) and for PET (eg, pregnancy and breast feeding).

Patient positioning for PET/MRI is more important and precise, especially with regard to patient centering on the imaging couch and positioning of the surface coils, to optimize the MRI image signal and avoid artifacts. Once the patient is positioned, an MRI localizer sequence (analogous to a scout scan in CT) is acquired to determine the scan range. Thereafter, PET acquisition is straightforward, requiring input of the number of bed positions and time at each bed position (typically 3–4 minutes). Concurrent with PET acquisition, an MRI attenuation correction sequence (2-point Dixon volume-interpolated breath-hold examination) is acquired, followed by the diagnostic MRI sequences for the current bed position. Various diagnostic MRI sequences may be selected and can be varied flexibly according to body region and clinical question, but usually at a minimum include a T1-weighted and a T2-weighted sequence. A minimalist PET/MRI protocol including only 2-point Dixon volume-interpolated breath-hold examination for both attenuation correction and anatomic localization takes less than 20 minutes to perform.[45] In contrast, a typical whole body study including organ-targeted sequences can easily take 60 minutes or more, compared with about the 15 to 30 minutes typical for PET/CT scanning.

For musculoskeletal tumors, basic MRI acquisition guidelines are given by the Scandinavian Sarcoma Group,[46] in which the MRI protocol is simple, robust, and relatively short. There are 5 MRI pulse sequences. They recommended MRI of suspected musculoskeletal tumors on a high-field system (minimum 1.0 T) MRI device with following sequences:

1. Coronal short tau inversion recovery sequence with a large field of view for bone tumors, preferably covering 2 adjacent joints;
2. Axial T1-weighted spin echo sequence (without fat suppression); and
3. Axial T2-weighted fast/turbo spin echo sequence (without fat suppression) with identical slice thickness and coverage, as for the T1-weighted sequence.

In their guidelines, they mentioned that this protocol is sufficient for the evaluation of musculoskeletal tumor in most cases. The short tau inversion recovery sequence is used for the detection of high signaling changes, such as tumors, inflammation, and hemorrhage. The T1-weighted sequence is important for the characterization of lipomatous lesions. The T2-weighted sequence is used in conjunction with the T1-weighted sequence for tumor characterization and to evaluate fascia planes important for surgery.

The Scandinavian Sarcoma Group recommended the use of IV gadolinium contrast medium in uncertain cases with a lesion of myxomatous or purely cystic nature, in hemorrhage where an underlying soft tissue tumor may be suspected, and equivocal findings on imaging with the following imaging protocol.

1. Axial spin echo T1-weighted sequence, with identical imaging parameters as a precontrast sequence. If fat saturation is used, a precontrast fat-saturated sequence is needed.
2. If further anatomic evaluation needed, a sagittal spin echo T1-weighted sequence with fat saturation may be performed.

ADVANTAGES OF PET/MR IMAGING

In PET/CT imaging, CT examination causes additional radiation exposure to the patient, whereas in PET/MRI imaging, MRI does not cause ionizing radiation exposure, which is an important consideration for pediatric patients where the radiation dose is strictly controlled and in cases where continuous monitoring of treatment progress is necessary. This factor has implications for musculoskeletal tumor evaluations, because these tumors are common in the pediatric population and require continuous monitoring.

MRI has excellent soft tissue contrast and the variety of imaging sequences result in better imaging than with CT scanning in a complicated heterogeneous tissue environment without using a contrast medium. This factor is particularly relevant for the musculoskeletal system. In the state-of-the-art PET/MRI system, MRI and PET can acquire data simultaneously. This process results in anatomic, metabolic, and molecular information being provided at the same time for musculoskeletal lesions. Other advantages of PET/MRI include advanced MRI sequences suited for multiparametric lesion characterization; cross-validation of PET and MRI data, which may provide additional valuable information; PET/MRI may decrease the need for additional imaging; and it provides more accurate coregistration of PET/MRI data.[47–49]

PET/MR IMAGING MUSCULOSKELETAL APPLICATIONS
PET/MR Imaging in Musculoskeletal Tumors

In soft tissue tumors and sarcomas, MRI and FDG PET/CT scanning are commonly used. For the characterization of bony tumors and soft tissue tumors, gadolinium-enhanced MRI is the current reference standard, which provides superior soft tissue contrast, tumor involvement of soft tissue and neurovascular structures, and extent of marrow changes on MRI.

The role of MRI in the identification, treatment planning (especially presurgical planning), and follow-up in patients of sarcoma is unique. FDG PET provides a quantitative estimation of metabolism, which provides important information about tumor regarding the nature, histopathologic characteristics, response to neoadjuvant therapy, and clinical outcomes in musculoskeletal tumors. PET can provide more sophisticated quantitative FDG PET imaging markers in terms of metabolic tumor volume and total lesion glycolysis, which takes into account tumor burden and tumor heterogeneity. Thus, FDG

PET imaging may add further knowledge for prognostication and evaluation of the response to therapy in musculoskeletal tumors. The treatment of musculoskeletal tumor includes radiation therapy; therefore, improved tumor delineation by hybrid PET/MRI may be of importance owing to the increasing tendency of image-guided intensity-modulated radiotherapy with accurate margins.

PET/MR Imaging in Metastatic Disease of the Musculoskeletal System

Bone scintigraphy has been the method of choice for many years for detecting bony metastases, especially in cases with increased local bone turnover. However, bone scans have a low spatial resolution, and some tumors, such as lymphoma, neuroendocrine tumors, and renal cell carcinomas, cause isolated bone marrow infiltration or osteolytic metastases without any or only very little activation of normal bone turnover.[50,51]

MRI has the capability to reveal with high spatial and soft tissue resolution intramedullary metastases before further cortical destruction occurs.[52,53] Beiderwellen and colleagues[54] in their study compared FDG PET/MRI with FDG PET/CT scans in 67 oncology patients with various primary tumors to assess osseous metastases. They concluded PET/MRI provide superior lesion conspicuity for osseous metastases and enables the delineation of more malignant lesions than PET/CT scanning, especially for small metastases.

PET/MR Imaging in Inflammatory and Infectious Musculoskeletal Disorders

Contrast-enhanced MRI is the current reference standard in the diagnosis and follow-up of inflammatory and infectious musculoskeletal disease conditions. The high resolution provided by MRI delineates the extent of tissue inflammation. FDG accumulation occurs in inflammatory and infectious tissues. This factor leads to a strong correlation between FDG PET and MRI in the evaluation of patients with rheumatoid arthritis and permits actual quantification of synovial joint inflammation as well as detection of disease activity.[55,56]

Musculoskeletal soft tissue infection usually manifests as hematogenous cellulitis/myositis or a wound infection. Early recognition of this condition may be delayed by the nonspecific nature of the initial clinical signs and symptoms. MRI is the most useful imaging modality in the diagnosis and delineation of necrotizing fasciitis. PET/MRI may provide differentiating features from nonnecrotizing soft tissue infections and inflammatory conditions, which is clinically difficult to differentiate from necrotizing fasciitis.

Limitations of PET/MR Imaging

Owing to cost and time constraints, PET/MRI protocols will be a compromise between time effectiveness and the use of a high-resolution imaging device. Time-consuming acquisition protocols associated with PET/MRI lead to potential motion artifacts, changes in the biodistribution of radiotracers, and patient discomfort. Discrepancy in the SUV occurred when same lesion measured on PET/MRI and PET/CT. Wiesmüller and colleagues[57] in their study showed that the differences in SUV value between PET/CT and PET/MRI with less mean value of SUV by PET/MRI. Smooth operation of PET/MRI required training of medical and technical staffs from radiology and nuclear medicine department.

SUMMARY

Hybrid PET/CT scanning and PET/MRI with FDG and other radiotracers is based on a complex set of basic physiologic and pathophysiologic, chemical and radiochemical, physical and radiophysical, and technical concepts and processes, probably make these imaging methods more difficult to understand and handle than the more common and more widespread structural imaging modalities as conventional radiography and CT scanning.

At present, PET/CT scanning remains a popular and valuable tool in oncology and in the evaluation of the musculoskeletal system, particularly in malignant musculoskeletal lesions, infection, and inflammatory conditions for the detection, characterization, and monitoring of other musculoskeletal disorders. Specific PET/CT protocols are used in the musculoskeletal system, depending on the individual case, site of lesions, and other parameters under evaluation.

With the availability of integrated whole body PET/MRI scanners, true simultaneous PET and MRI has been possible, which has led to new developments in hybrid imaging in oncologic and various conditions. This factor is particularly important in the musculoskeletal system, because combining PET molecular and functional information with MRI structural information and multiparametric lesion evaluation is possible in single device with a one-stop shop. The PET/MRI protocol if convenient, and would solve the major problem faced during musculoskeletal system evaluation. In addition, the use of a specific radiotracer other than FDG can potentially provide molecular information that is complementary to MRI in hybrid PET/MRI.

REFERENCES

1. Basu S, Hess S, Nielsen Braad PE, et al. The basic principles of FDG-PET/CT imaging. PET Clin 2014;9: 355–70.
2. Phelps ME. The merging of biology and imaging into molecular imaging. J Nucl Med 2000;41:661–81.
3. Ruth T. Accelerating production of medical isotopes. Nature 2009;457:536–7.
4. Miller G. Alzheimer's biomarker initiative hits its stride. Science 2009;326:386–9.
5. Friston KJ. Modalities, modes, and models in functional neuroimaging. Science 2009;326:399–403.
6. Hu Z, Yang W, Liu H. From PET/CT to PET/MRI: advances in instrumentation and clinical applications. Mol Pharm 2014;11:3798–809.
7. Hudson HM, Larkin RS. Accelerated image reconstruction using ordered subsets of projection data. IEEE Trans Med Imaging 1994;13:601–9.
8. Schwaiger M, Ziegler S, Nekolla SG. PET/CT: challenge for nuclear cardiology. J Nucl Med 2005;46: 8–9.
9. Chen K, Blebea J, Laredo JD, et al. Evaluation of musculoskeletal disorders with PET, PET/CT, and PET/MR imaging. PET Clin 2008;3:451–65.
10. Aoki J, Watanabe H, Shinozaki T, et al. FDG PET of primary benign and malignant bone tumors: standardized uptake value in 52 lesions. Radiology 2001;219:774–7.
11. Kubota R, Kubota K, Yamada S, et al. Microautoradiographic study for the differentiation of intratumoral macrophages, granulation tissues and cancer cells by the dynamics of fluorine-18-fluorodeoxyglucose uptake. J Nucl Med 1994;35:104–12.
12. Shreve PD, Anzai Y, Wahl RL. Pitfalls in oncologic diagnosis with FDG PET imaging: physiologic and benign variants. Radiographics 1999;19:61–77.
13. Nieweg OE, Pruim J, van Ginkel RJ, et al. Fluorine-18-fluorodeoxyglucose PET imaging of soft-tissue sarcoma. J Nucl Med 1996;37:257–61.
14. Parghane RV, Basu S. Dual-time point 18F-FDG-PET and PET/CT for differentiating benign from malignant musculoskeletal lesions: opportunities and limitations. Semin Nucl Med 2017;47:373–91.
15. Buck AK, Herrmann K, Büschenfelde CM, et al. Imaging bone and soft tissue tumors with the proliferation marker [18F]fluorodeoxythymidine. Clin Cancer Res 2008;14:2970–7.
16. Benz MR, Czernin J, Allen-Auerbach MS, et al. 3'-deoxy-3'-[18F] fluorothymidine positron emission tomography for response assessment in soft tissue sarcoma: a pilot study to correlate imaging findings with tissue thymidine kinase 1 and Ki-67 activity and histopathologic response. Cancer 2012;118: 3135–44.
17. Gamie S, El-Maghraby T. The role of PET/CT in evaluation of facet and disc abnormalities in patients with low back pain using (18)F Fluoride. Nucl Med Rev Cent East Eur 2008;11:17–21.
18. Lim R, Fahey FH, Drubach LA, et al. Early experience with fluorine-18 sodium fluoride bone PET in young patients with back pain. J Pediatr Orthop 2007;27:277–82.
19. Watanabe H, Inoue T, Shinozaki T, et al. PET imaging of musculoskeletal tumours with fluorine-18 alpha-methyltyrosine: comparison with fluorine-18 fluorodeoxyglucose PET. Eur J Nucl Med 2000;27: 1509–17.
20. Suzuki R, Watanabe H, Yanagawa T, et al. PET evaluation of fatty tumors in the extremity: possibility of using the standardized uptake value (SUV) to differentiate benign tumors from liposarcoma. Ann Nucl Med 2005;19:661–70.
21. Weber WA, Wester HJ, Grosu AL, et al. O-(2-[18F]fluoroethyl)-Ltyrosine and L-[methyl-11C]methionine uptake in brain tumours: initial results of a comparative study. Eur J Nucl Med 2000;27:542–9.
22. Inoue T, Tomiyoshi K, Higuichi T, et al. Biodistribution studies on L-3-[fluorine-18]fluoro-alpha-methyl tyrosine: a potential tumor detecting agent. J Nucl Med 1998;39:663–7.
23. Beer AJ, Haubner R, Sarbia M, et al. Positron emission tomography using [18F]Galacto-RGD identifies the level of integrin alpha(v) beta3 expression in man. Clin Cancer Res 2006;12:3942–9.
24. Lapa C, Knop S, Schreder M, et al. 11C-Methionine-PET in multiple myeloma: correlation with clinical parameters and bone marrow involvement. Theranostics 2016;6:254–61.
25. Tian M, Zhang H, Oriuchi N, et al. Comparison of 11C-choline PET and FDG PET for the differential diagnosis of malignant tumors. Eur J Nucl Med Mol Imaging 2004;31:1064–72.
26. Fuccio C, Castellucci P, Schiavina R, et al. Role of 11C-choline PET/CT in the re-staging of prostate cancer patients with biochemical relapse and negative results at bone scintigraphy. Eur J Radiol 2012; 81:893–6.
27. Beheshti M, Vali R, Waldenberger P, et al. The use of F-18 choline PET in the assessment of bone metastases in prostate cancer: correlation with morphological changes on CT. Mol Imaging Biol 2009;11: 446–54.
28. Zacho HD, Nielsen JB, Haberkorn U, et al. 68 Ga-PSMA PET/CT for the detection of bone metastases in prostate cancer: a systematic review of the published literature. Clin Physiol Funct Imaging 2017. [Epub ahead of print].
29. Antoch G, Kuehl H, Kanja J, et al. Dual-modality PET/CT scanning with negative oral contrast agent

to avoid artifacts: introduction and evaluation. Radiol 2004;230:879–85.

30. Querellou S, Keromnes N, Abgral R, et al. Clinical and therapeutic impact of 18F-FDG PET/CT whole-body acquisition including lower limbs in patients with malignant melanoma. Nucl Med Commun 2010;31:766–72.

31. Mendenhall WM, Indelicato DJ, Scarborough MT, et al. The management of adult soft tissue sarcomas. Am J Clin Oncol 2009;32:436–42.

32. Komdeur R, Hoekstra HJ, van den Berg E, et al. Metastasis in soft tissue sarcomas: prognostic criteria and treatment perspectives. Cancer Metastasis Rev 2002;21:167–83.

33. Bastiaannet E, Groen H, Jager PL, et al. The value of FDG-PET in the detection, grading and response to therapy of soft tissue and bone sarcomas; a systematic review and meta-analysis. Cancer Treat Rev 2004;30:83–101.

34. Folpe AL, Lyles RH, Sprouse JT, et al. (F-18) fluorodeoxyglucose positron emission tomography as a predictor of pathologic grade and other prognostic variables in bone and soft tissue sarcoma. Clin Cancer Res 2000;6:1279–87.

35. Volker T, Denecke T, Steffen I, et al. Positron emission tomography for staging of pediatric sarcoma patients: results of a prospective multicenter trial. J Clin Oncol 2007;25:5435–41.

36. Tateishi U, Hosono A, Makimoto A, et al. Comparative study of FDG PET/CT and conventional imaging in the staging of rhabdomyosarcoma. Ann Nucl Med 2009;23:155–61.

37. Evilevitch V, Weber WA, Tap WD, et al. Reduction of glucose metabolic activity is more accurate than change in size at predicting histopathologic response to neoadjuvant therapy in high-grade soft-tissue sarcomas. Clin Cancer Res 2008;14: 715–20.

38. Arush MW, Israel O, Postovsky S, et al. Positron emission tomography/computed tomography with 18fluoro-deoxyglucose in the detection of local recurrence and distant metastases of pediatric sarcoma. Pediatr Blood Cancer 2007;49: 901–5.

39. Kalemis A, Delattre BM, Heinzer S. Sequential whole-body PET/MR scanner: concept, clinical use, and optimization after two years in the clinic. The manufacturer's perspective. MAGMA 2013;26: 5–23.

40. Zaidi H, Ojha N, Morich M, et al. Design and performance evaluation of a whole-body Ingenuity TF PET/MRI system. Phys Med Biol 2011;56: 3091–106.

41. Veit-Haibach P, Kuhn FP, Wiesinger F, et al. PET-MR imaging using a tri-modality PET/CT-MR system with a dedicated shuttle in clinical routine. MAGMA 2013; 26:25–35.

42. Queiroz MA, Hüllner M, Kuhn F, et al. PET/MRI and PET/CT in follow-up of head and neck cancer patients. Eur J Nucl Med Mol Imaging 2014;41: 1066–75.

43. Peng BJ, Wu Y, Cherry SR, et al. New shielding configurations for a simultaneous PET/MRI scanner at 7 T. J Magn Reson 2014;239:50–6.

44. Wagenknecht G, Kaiser HJ, Mottaghy FM, et al. MRI for attenuation correction in PET: methods and challenges. MAGMA 2013;26:99–113.

45. Drzezga A, Souvatzoglou M, Eiber M, et al. First clinical experience with integrated whole-body PET/MR: comparison to PET/CT in patients with oncologic diagnoses. J Nucl Med 2012;53:845–55.

46. The Scandinavian Sarcoma group guidelines for basic MRI of suspected bone and soft tissue tumours. 2012. Available at: http://www.ssg-org.net/wp-con tent/uploads/2011/05/Guidelines-for-basic-MRI-examination-of-suspected-bone-and-soft-tissue-tumors. pdf. Accessed March 31, 2016.

47. Jadvar H, Colletti PM. Competitive advantage of PET/MRI. Eur J Radiol 2014;83:84–94.

48. Bashir U, Mallia A, Stirling J, et al. PET/MRI in oncological imaging: state of the art. Diagnostics (Basel) 2015;5:333–7.

49. Fraum TJ, Fowler KJ, McConathy J. PET/MRI: emerging clinical applications in oncology. Acad Radiol 2016;23:220–36.

50. Talbot JN, Paycha F, Balogova S. Diagnosis of bone metastasis: recent comparative studies of imaging modalities. Q J Nucl Med Mol Imaging 2011;55: 374–410.

51. Yang HL, Liu T, Wang XM, et al. Diagnosis of bone metastases: a meta-analysis comparing [18]FDG PET, CT, MRI and bone scintigraphy. Eur Radiol 2011;21:2604–17.

52. Heindel W, Gubitz R, Vieth V, et al. The diagnostic imaging of bone metastases. Dtsch Arztebl Int 2014;111:741–7.

53. O'Sullivan GJ, Carty FL, Cronin CG. Imaging of bone metastasis: an update. World J Radiol 2015;7: 202–11.

54. Beiderwellen K, Huebner M, Heusch P, et al. Whole-body [18F] FDG PET/MRI vs. PET/CT in the assessment of bone lesions in oncological patients: initial results. Eur Radiol 2014;24:2023–30.

55. Goerres GW, Forster A, Uebelhart D, et al. F-18 FDG whole-body PET for the assessment of disease activity in patients with rheumatoid arthritis. Clin Nucl Med 2006;31:386–90.

56. Palmer WE, Rosenthal DI, Schoenberg OI, et al. Quantification of inflammation in the wrist with gadolinium-enhanced MR imaging and PET with 2-[F-18]-fluoro-2-deoxy-D-glucose. Radiology 1995; 196:647–55.

57. Wiesmüller M, Quick HH, Navalpakkam B, et al. Comparison of lesion detection and quantitation of

tracer uptake between PET from a simultaneously acquiring whole-body PET/MR hybrid scanner and PET from PET/CT. Eur J Nucl Med Mol Imaging 2013;40:12–21.

58. Wieder HA, Pomykala KL, Benz MR, et al. PET tracers in musculoskeletal disease beyond FDG. Semin Musculoskelet Radiol 2014; 18:123–32.

59. Al-Ibraheem A, Buck AK, Beer AJ, et al. Alternative PET tracers in musculoskeletal disease. PET Clin 2010;5:363–74.

60. Tirosh A, Kebebew E. The utility of 68Ga-DOTATATE positron-emission tomography/computed tomography in the diagnosis, management, follow-up and prognosis of neuroendocrine tumors. Future Oncol 2018;14:111–22.

^{18}F-Sodium Fluoride PET/ CT and PET/MR Imaging of Bone and Joint Disorders

Mohsen Beheshti, MD, FEBNM, FASNC[a,b,*]

KEYWORDS

- ^{18}F-NaF • PET/CT • PET/MR imaging • Malignant bone disease • Benign bone disease

KEY POINTS

- The most common auspicious indications of Sodium Fluoride F 18 (^{18}F-NaF) PET/CT in benign bone diseases are insufficiency fractures, occult fractures, osteoarthritis, osteoid osteoma, failed back surgery, child abuse, and evaluation of joint prosthesis as well as metabolic bone diseases.
- ^{18}F-NaF PET/CT is highly accurate modality clearly superior to ^{99m}Tc–methylene diphosphonate planar imaging or single-photon emission CT/CT for staging and restaging of malignant bone disease.
- ^{18}F-NaF PET/CT seems to be promising in differentiating benign from malignant bone lesions, particularly when using dynamic quantitative approaches.
- There are currently no available data supporting the superiority of ^{18}F-NaF PET/MR imaging to ^{18}F-NaF PET/CT for the assessment of bone diseases in the routine clinical practice. With the development and more availability of PET/MR imaging, however, this modality may yield new applications for the widespread use of ^{18}F-NaF in clinical management of malignant diseases, particularly in prostate and breast cancer patients.

INTRODUCTION

Sodium Fluoride F 18 (^{18}F-NaF) is a positron-emitting radiotracer that was first introduced in 1962 for skeletal scintigraphy. Its clinical use was limited, however, at that time mainly due to a short half-life of 109.74 minutes and tracer characteristics that were less ideal for conventional gamma cameras. Thus, it had been largely replaced in the late 1970s by ^{99m}Tc-labeled diphosphonates, which showed optimal characteristics for conventional gamma-based scintigraphy.

With the improvements of PET/CT scanners, high-resolution imaging of bone became a reality; therefore, ^{18}F-NaF was reintroduced for clinical and research investigations in assessment of benign and malignant bone diseases.

^{18}F-NaF is a bone-seeking agent that directly incorporates into the bone matrix, converting hydroxyapatite to fluoroapatite.[1] ^{18}F-NaF is rapidly cleared from the plasma due to small protein-bound proportion with a first-pass extraction rate of 100%, with only 10% remaining in plasma 1 hour after injection.[2,3] Thus, it provides desirable characteristics of high and rapid bone uptake, accompanied by very rapid blood clearance, resulting in a high bone-to-background ratio and

Conflict of Interest: This is study received no funding and the author declares that he has no conflict of interest.
[a] Department of Nuclear Medicine and Endocrinology, PET - CT Center LINZ, Ordensklinikum, St Vincent's Hospital, Seilerstaette 4, Linz A-4020, Austria; [b] Department of Nuclear Medicine and Endocrinology, Paracelsus Medical University, Muellner Hauptstrasse 48, Salzburg A-5020, Austria
* Corresponding author. Department of Nuclear Medicine and Endocrinology, PET - CT Center LINZ, Ordensklinikum, St Vincent's Hospital, Seilerstaette 4, Linz A-4020, Austria.
E-mail address: mohsen.beheshti@ordensklinikum.at

PET Clin 13 (2018) 477–490
https://doi.org/10.1016/j.cpet.2018.05.004
1556-8598/18/© 2018 Elsevier Inc. All rights reserved.

pet.theclinics.com

high-quality images of the skeleton in less than 1 hour after tracer intravenous administration.

Although only a few studies have compared ^{18}F-NaF with ^{99m}Tc–methylene diphosphonate (MDP) for evaluation of bone and joint disorders, ^{18}F-NaF PET seems more sensitive than conventional bone scanning, showing a higher contrast between normal and abnormal tissue and with the potential for the assessment of small bony structures especially in the spine.[4–11]

This article reviews the available literature and summarizes the clinical experience with ^{18}F-NaF PET/CT in benign and malignant bone diseases.

^{18}F–SODIUM FLUORIDE PET/COMPUTED TOMOGRAPHY IN BENIGN BONE DISEASE
Metabolic Bone Disease

[18]F-NaF PET/CT provides a novel tool for assessing bone metabolism that complements the conventional methods. Unlike biochemical markers, which globally measure the integrated response to therapy in the whole skeleton, ^{18}F-NaF PET can differentiate the changes occurring at sites of clinically relevant osteoporotic fractures, such as the spine and hip. Effective bone plasma flow (K_1), from which bone blood flow can be estimated, can be obtained by measuring the fluoride plasma clearance to bone mineral (K_i) using dynamic PET acquisitions at the specific anatomic sites within the field of view of the PET scanner. After the dynamic images, static acquisitions can be performed to estimate Ki at additional bony sites by taking 2 and 4 venous blood samples to derive the input function.[12] In addition, standardized uptake value (SUV) can be used for semiquantitative analysis. Measurements of K_i, however, are more complicated to perform than SUV. Nevertheless, they have the advantage that they are specific to the bone metabolic activity at the site of measurement whereas SUV might be influenced by multiple biological and technical factors.

Using the quantitative and semiquantitative approaches, ^{18}F-NaF PET/CT has been used in different metabolic bone diseases. In author's experience, ^{18}F-NaF PET/CT can be helpful for the evaluation of bone involvement in hyperparathyroidism. It is also a sensitive modality for detecting the areas of increased bone remodeling or insufficiency fractures. Moreover, the CT part provides useful information regarding the extension of brown tumors and bone stability.

In an experimental trial, ^{18}F-NaF PET/CT was used for noninvasive measurement of bone turnover.[13] The investigators reported that ^{18}F-NaF PET/CT provides quantitative estimates of bone blood flow and metabolic activity that correlate with histomorphometric indices of bone formation in the normal bone tissue of the mini pigs (baby or small pigs). They concluded that ^{18}F-NaF PET/CT may facilitate follow-up of patients with metabolic bone diseases and reduce the number of invasive bone biopsies.[13]

In another study, researchers described a good correlation between ^{18}F-NaF metabolism and serum markers like alkaline phosphatase and parathormone levels in patients with renal osteodystrophy.[14] ^{18}F-NaF PET/CT study was useful to differentiate lesions with low versus high turnover in renal osteodystrophy and provided quantitative estimates of bone cell activity.

Furthermore, ^{18}F-NaF PET/CT was shown promising for quantitative assessment of the effects of bisphosphonate treatment on bone remodeling and metabolism in patients with glucocorticoid-induced osteoporosis.[15]

In a research study by the author's group, a significant correlation was found between semiquantitative ^{18}F-NaF PET analysis and T and Z scores on dual-energy x-ray bone-absorptiometry in lumbar spine of osteoporotic patients.[16] The potential of ^{18}F-NaF PET for prediction of bone mineral deficit, however, should be evaluated in future prospective studies.[16]

Inflammatory Bone and Joint Disease

Inflammatory and rheumatologic diseases involving bones and joints like rheumatoid arthritis and spondyloarthropathy are among the most common indications for conventional bone scintigraphy (BS). Tracer perfusion on early-phase images and distribution pattern of involved joints as well as intensity of tracer uptake on BS are useful for the detection and characterization of various inflammatory diseases and help guide treatment.

BS has important limitations, however, in assessment of inflammatory bone diseases despite its established indication. In a systematic literature review, BS was positive in only 52% of the patients with established ankylosing spondylitis (AS) and in 49.4% of the patients with probable sacroiliitis.[17] This low sensitivity might be one of the reasons that in many institutions MR imaging has replaced BS as the first-line imaging tool in patients with suspected AS or other spondyloarthropathies. MR imaging is more sensitive and has superior performance than BS in detecting sacroiliitis in the early stage.[18]

There are few publications assessing the impact of ^{18}F-NaF PET/CT in patients with rheumatologic disease. In a study, Strobel and colleagues[19] compared the value of ^{18}F-NaF PET/CT in detection of sacroiliitis compared with BS. They examined 15 patients with AS fulfilling the modified New York criteria, and 13 patients with mechanical back pain served as the control group. The investigators implemented a ratio between uptake in the sacroiliac joints (SIJs) and the sacrum (S) similar to the measurement established for BS. Using a SIJ/S ratio of greater than 1.3 as the threshold for sacroiliitis, ^{18}F-NaF PET/CT showed, in patient-based analysis, significantly superior sensitivity of 80% compared with 47% for BS. In addition, ^{18}F-NaF PET/CT imaging had the advantage of morphologic information about the joints with CT. The investigators reported that the morphologic information of the low-dose CT led to the correct diagnosis in patients with advanced ankylosis because the scintigraphic activity of the involved joint decreased with the time. This issue may not be currently relevant, however, with the development of dedicated single-photon emission CT/CT (SPECT/CT) cameras.

Moreover, patients with spondyloarthropathies also may suffer from enthesopathies and arthritis. Although ^{18}F-NaF PET/CT seems to be a sensitive tool to identify sites of enthesitis, it is difficult to obtain sufficient information from early-phase images—similar to those familiar on 3-phase BS—due to rapid blood clearance and first-pass extraction of ^{18}F-NaF.[3] This might be a limitation in patients with active inflammatory process in bone and joints, because the important information of early uptake in the periarticular soft tissue as an indicator for active arthritis might be missed on ^{18}F-NaF PET/CT. Another study found that early-phase images (ie, 2 minutes after injection) may show increased regional blood flow in the inflammatory or infectious bone diseases.[20]

MR imaging seems also play an evolving role in imaging of inflammatory bone diseases. With increasing implementation and velocity of whole-body MR imaging, it may become a competitor of multiphase BS for this indication.[21] The feasibility of performing whole-body acquisition, however, is still an important advantage of BS compared with MR imaging. In addition, most of the so-called whole-body MR imaging protocols only include the axial skeleton sparing the peripheral bony structures. In a preliminary study, Fischer and colleagues[22] compared whole-body MR imaging and ^{18}F-NaF PET/CT in 10 patients with AS. They showed that increased ^{18}F-NaF uptake on PET correlated only modestly with bone marrow edema on MR imaging in the spine (kappa = 0.25) whereas there was a better correlation in the SIJ (kappa = 0.64). These initial data may indicate that bone marrow edema on MR imaging and increased uptake on ^{18}F-NaF PET/CT

do not represent the same pathology. Functional imaging using bone-seeking agents in nuclear medicine imaging (eg, ^{18}F-NaF PET/CT) may detect increased bone remodeling caused not only by inflammation but also mainly by osteoproliferative reparative changes in the chronic phase of the disease.

Furthermore, ^{18}F-NaF PET/CT seems to provide better information comparing anatomic imaging for the evaluation of the disease progression and response to therapy in inflammatory bone diseases. A recent study evaluated the value of ^{18}F-NaF PET in treatment monitoring of 12 patients with clinically active AS during anti–tumor necrosis factor therapy. The investigators reported significant decrease of ^{18}F-NaF uptake in clinical responders in the costovertebral (mean SUV area under the curve −1.0; P<.001) and SIJ (mean SUV area under the curve −1.2; P = .03) in contrast to nonresponders.[23] Therefore, ^{18}F-NaF PET/CT might be an interesting tool for the monitoring of therapy response, in particular in patients with metabolic or inflammatory bone diseases.

Trauma

Conventional radiograph is established as the first-line imaging modality for assessment of traumatic fractures, especially in the extremities. Occult or complex involving fractures, however, which are not visible on standard radiographs, are usually imaged with CT because of its high sensitivity, short acquisition time, and wide availability. The impact of ^{18}F-NaF PET/CT in trauma has been discussed in published studies. The results are promising in child abuse, in which highly sensitive modalities are required to assess the whole skeleton and to determine new and old fractures. Drubach and colleagues[24] compared the value of ^{18}F-NaF PET with standard high-detail skeletal survey in 22 pediatric cases (<2 years) suspected of child abuse. ^{18}F-NaF PET was able to detect more lesions compared with radiographs (200 vs 156). ^{18}F-NaF PET was especially sensitive in the detection of thoracic fractures (ie, ribs, sternum, clavicle, and scapula) but inferior regarding the detection of metaphyseal fractures, the typical presentation of child abuse. A review article presented that ^{18}F-NaF PET/CT has been used for a wide variety of indications in children and young adults.[25] Almost all pediatric ^{18}F-NaF PET/CT scans are performed to assess benign bone diseases, most commonly back pain, in a wide variety of circumstances, including patients with sports injuries, scoliosis, trauma, and back pain after surgery.[25]

Furthermore, ^{18}F-NaF PET/MR imaging has been used for assessment of patients with foot pain suspicious for stress fracture.[26,27] The investigators reported that ^{18}F-NaF PET/MR imaging seems to be a useful modality to diagnose stress fractures and stress reactions of the foot and ankle area, especially when conventional modalities, such as plain radiographs, fail. Review of current publications shows that ^{18}F-NaF PET/CT seems superior to conventional imaging modalities in the detection of all kinds of fractures, including occult fractures in complex anatomic regions, insufficiency fractures, and pathologic fractures.[28–31] Currently, most of literature regarding this topic is limited to case reports, and the additional value of ^{18}F-NaF PET/CT in comparison with the other established imaging methods should be evaluated in future studies.

Evaluation of Joint Prosthesis

Prosthetic joint replacement surgeries are becoming more widespread with increasing life expectancy. Postsurgical complications, however, such as loosening, infection, and fracture, still occur in a considerable number of patients despite advances in orthopedic techniques. Therefore, accurate noninvasive diagnosis of the complications is pivotal for optimal patient management. In particular, differentiation of situation with similar clinical presentations (eg, infection vs aseptic loosing) is of great importance.

Radiography is considered as first-line imaging modality for the assessment of the patients after hip or knee arthroplasties. It provides useful information, however, when relevant abnormalities, such as remarkable prosthetic dislocation, fractures, and wide radiolucency, are seen. Three-phase BS is established as one of the standard diagnostic methods for assessment of complications after joint replacement. Three-phase BS has a high negative predictive value to rule out common postarthroplasty complications like loosening or infection. It suffers, however, from sufficient specificity. Additional SPECT/CT technique to 3-phase BS provides anatomic information and consequently improves specificity.[32] Metal artifacts causing by prosthetic devices, however, may affect the quality of CT. In a study by Hirschmann and colleagues,[32] ^{99m}Tc-hydroxydiphosphonate-SPECT/CT imaging changed the suspected diagnosis and the proposed treatment in 19 of 23 (83%) painful knees after arthroplasty.

In addition, correlative specific nuclear medicine scans using gallium Ga 67 (^{67}Ga), ^{111}In-labeled white blood cell, ^{99m}Tc–sulfur colloid bone, ^{111}In-labelled polyclonal immunoglobulin G (IgG), and ^{99m}Tc-antigranulocyte monoclonal antibody scans have been additionally performed to increase the specificity of 3-phase BS.[33] ^{111}In-labeled WBS scintigraphy is one of the common methods for imaging of infection. It has its own limitations, however, such as problems with in vitro labeling process, availability, and the need for a correlative bone marrow imaging, to be done routinely.

[18]F-NaF PET/CT showed promising in the primary studies assessing complications after joint replacements. Kobayashi and colleagues[34] performed a prospective study, including 65 joints with total hip arthroplasty. They proposed 3 different patterns of uptake in the evaluation of the joints: type 1: no uptake; type 2: minor uptake limited to within one-half of the bone-implant interface, and type 3: major uptake that extends over one-half of the bone-implant interface. Maximum SUV (SUVmax) was also analyzed at all sites of increased uptake. There was a significant difference between the SUVmax values in the knees with aseptic compared with that with septic loosening. Sensitivity and specificity were 95% and 98%, respectively, for the diagnosis of infection using type 3 pattern.[34] The investigators claimed that the classification of proposed uptake pattern can be performed relatively simpley.[34] They concluded that ^{18}F-NaF PET/CT is promising in the differentiation of aseptic loosening from infection. Another study by the same group of researchers evaluated the use of ^{18}F-NaF PET/CT to determine the appropriate tissue sampling region in cases of suspected periprosthetic infection after total hip arthroplasty.[35] They enrolled 23 hips suspicious of septic loosening scheduled for revision and 23 asymptomatic hips as a control group. Findings suggested that preoperative assessment of major ^{18}F-NaF uptake markedly improves the accuracy of tissue sampling and the sensitivity of tissue examinations.[35]

In another study, the investigators evaluated the value of ^{18}F-NaF PET in the early diagnosis of aseptic loosening after total knee arthroplasty.[36] They prospectively evaluated 14 patients with suspected aseptic loosening diagnosed by intraoperative findings or by long-term clinical evaluation. The sensitivity, specificity, and accuracy of ^{18}F-NaF PET were 100%, 56%, and 71%, respectively, in the early diagnosis of painful knees after arthroplasty.[36] Moreover, no false-negative results were reported in this study.

In a comparative study, the accuracy of 3-phase BS, ^{18}F-NaF PET/CT, and fluorodeoxyglucose F 18 (^{18}F-FDG) PET/CT was evaluated in 46 patients with painful hip prosthesis.[37] The accuracy rates of 3-phase BS, ^{18}F-NaF PET/CT, and ^{18}F-FDG PET/CT were 84%, 91%, and 94%, respectively. No significant difference was observed between

SUVmax in the PET/CT modalities on the loosened prostheses and those that were infected. Despite the high reported accuracy of ^{18}F-FDG PET/CT in postarthroplasty assessment of the painful joints in the former study, its value contradicts other publications, with an accuracy between 67% and 95%.[38]

Although, ^{18}F-NaF PET/CT seems to be promising in assessment of painful joints after arthroplasty, there current available data do not support its value as standard imaging. More availability of PET/CT systems and development of dynamic and quantitative approaches, however, will probably play a major role in future. In the meantime, 3-phase conventional BS including SPECT or SPECT/CT continues to have its position for evaluation of painful joint prostheses.

Benign Bone Tumors

There are few studies regarding the impact of ^{18}F-NaF PET/CT in benign bone tumors. The high image quality of ^{18}F-NaF PET/CT, however, can make it a useful alternative to ^{99m}Tc-MDP SPECT/CT for evaluating benign skeletal lesions, such as osteoid osteoma and Langerhans cell histiocytosis, especially in complex anatomic regions like vertebral spines or wrist and feet.[25,29] Also, it seems superior to MR imaging in individual cases because MR imaging might be misleading in the detection of osteoid osteoma. The combination of increased scintigraphic focal uptake and corresponding nidus on CT part of the ^{18}F-NaF PET/CT or ^{99m}Tc-MDP SPECT/CT study makes it feasible for correct diagnosis of osteoid osteoma.[39] To the author's knowledge, ^{18}F-NaF PET/CT might be misleading in some incidentally diagnosed benign tumors like enchondroma due to its high uptake in such tumors. Therefore, such incidental findings should be interpreted with caution concerning the morphologic findings on CT.

Miscellaneous Indications

Primary studies showed promising results of ^{18}F-NaF PET/CT in assessment of patients with back pain.[40,41] A study by Ovadia and colleagues[41] found a high diagnostic accuracy of ^{18}F-NaF PET/CT in 15 adolescents with unclear back pain and inconclusive conventional imaging. The predominant pathologies included spondylolysis, fractures and osteoid osteoma.

In addition, ^{18}F-NaF PET/CT seems to provide useful information in patients suspicious for failed back surgery. Metal loosening, fracture, nonunion or pseudoarthrosis, suprafusional or infrafusional degeneration, and infection are the common possible complications after vertebral surgery

(**Fig. 1**).[29] In the author's experience, hybrid imaging modalities, providing appropriate metabolic information of bone turnover with anatomic correlation, can better identify complications in many cases.

^{18}F-NaF showed also promising for the evaluation of osteonecrosis, bone graft healing and viability, condylar hyperplasia, and degenerative diseases.[42–46] Further research is warranted, however, due to few data for these clinical indications.

^{18}F–SODIUM FLUORIDE PET/COMPUTED TOMOGRAPHY IN THE ASSESSMENT OF MALIGNANT BONE DISEASE

The results of a prospective multicenter randomized trial are under way comparing the value of ^{18}F-NaF PET/CT with ^{99m}Tc-MDP BS in 488 patients with breast, prostate, and lung cancers.[47] The Centers for Medicare and Medicaid Services agreed on a decision memorandum regarding the use of ^{18}F-NaF PET for assessment of metastatic bone disease in February 2010, concluding that the available data were sufficient to allow for ^{18}F-NaF PET coverage under coverage with evidence development.[48] This led to the creation of the National Oncologic PET Registry for ^{18}F-NaF.[49] ^{99m}Tc-MDP BS has been the standard method for initial staging, therapy monitoring, and detection of areas at risk for pathologic fracture in patients with suspicious bone metastases in various cancers. Despite high sensitivity of conventional ^{99m}Tc-MDP BS for the detection of advanced skeletal metastases, it may suffer in accurately detecting early involvement, particularly in complex bone structures. Moreover, this modality relies on the identification of the osteoblastic reaction of the involved bone and regional blood flow rather than the detection of the tumor itself.[48,50]

^{18}F-NaF PET proved more accurate than ^{99m}Tc-MDP planar imaging or SPECT for localizing and characterizing malignant bone lesions.[6,51–54] This high-quality technique has increase clinical accuracy and provided greater convenience to patientss and referring physician.[55,56] These all indicate the need to reconsider the use of ^{18}F-NaF PET/CT for imaging of malignant bone diseases.[56] Despite the high performance of ^{18}F-NaF PET/CT, its clinical utilization remains limited due to the fact of its higher cost and less availability of PET/CT scanners comparing gamma cameras.

Primary Bone Tumors

Primary bone tumors are rare malignancies that occur primarily in pediatric patients and young adults, accounting for approximately 5% of

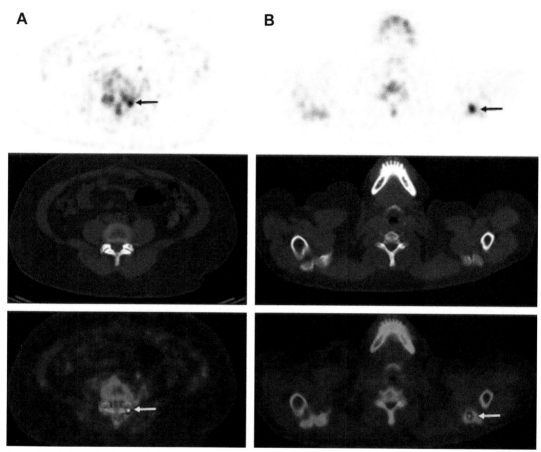

Fig. 1. ^{18}F-NaF PET/CT (transaxial views, *upper*: PET, *mid*: CT, *lower*: fusion PET/CT): focal increased tracer uptake on a facet joint (*A*) and in the left acromioclavicular joint (*B*), suggestive of chronic arthritis (*arrows*).

childhood malignancies and 0.2% of all primary cancers in adults.[57] In 2012, an estimated 2890 new cases have been diagnosed in the United States and 1410 people died from primary bone cancers.[58] Genetic factors and radiation therapy have been introduced as possible causes; however, the etiology remains unclear.[59] The development of new diagnostic modalities and treatment approaches, particularly for early-stage disease, led to improvements in survival. Primary bone cancers present usually a poor prognostic. Therefore, it early diagnosis and appropriate treatment is crucial for optimal management of the disease.

Osteosarcoma is the most common malignant primary bone tumor, accounting for 35% of bone tumors.[60] Accurate staging of osteosarcoma is important because it provides necessary information for clinical staging and monitoring response to therapy as well as prognosis. Significant prognostic factors are tumor size and site, presence and location of metastases, and response to chemotherapy. Plain radiographs and MR imaging are routinely performed for the evaluation of the primary tumor. ^{99m}Tc-MDP BS is known as standard imaging for assessment of distant metastases.[59]

The impact of ^{18}F-NaF PET/CT in the diagnosis of osteosarcoma has been reported in preliminary studies mostly with small number of cases. Hoh and colleagues[61] evaluated the use of ^{18}F-NaF for PET imaging of the skeleton. Osteosarcoma was detected in 4 of 13 patients with documented malignant bone tumors. They reported that osteosarcoma had the highest tumor–to–normal bone activity ratios compared with other bone neoplasms. In 1 patient, the tumor activity was notably reduced after treatment with chemotherapy and immunotherapy, which may suggest the usefulness of the quantitative ^{18}F-NaF PET/CT for assessing the treatment response, especially in a neoadjuvant setting before surgery. In addition, high ^{18}F-NaF uptake has been reported in patients with proved lung metastases from osteosarcoma similar to the findings on ^{99m}Tc-MDP BS.[62] This is of great importance given that several studies demonstrated that ^{18}F-FDG PET/CT seems to have limited value in detection of pulmonary metastases from osteosarcomas and Ewing sarcomas, even in large lesions.[63–65]

Ewing sarcoma is the third most common bone neoplasm, accounting for approximately 16% of malignant bone tumors.[59] The pathogenesis and etiology may be related to genetic factors.[59] Locoregional lymph node metastases are rare. Distant metastases are detectable in 25% of cases most commonly in the lung, bone and bone marrow.[66]

Thorax CT scan and ^{99m}Tc-MDP BS are the standard imaging for the assessment of distant metastases. To the author's knowledge, there is no published study, so far, evaluating the impact of ^{18}F-NaF PET/CT in Ewing sarcoma, given its low incidence. It is assumed, however, that Ewing sarcoma lesions tend to demonstrate intense ^{18}F-NaF.[48]

Multiple myeloma is a neoplastic proliferation of plasma cells within the bone marrow. The characteristic bone lesions are sharply defined small osteolytic formations with no relevant reactive bone remodeling.[67] Thus, ^{99m}Tc MDP BS has a limited role in staging of multiple myeloma, with a sensitivity of 40% to 60% mainly due to the lack of radiotracer uptake in the lytic lesions.[68] The standard skeletal survey includes a series of plain films of the chest, skull, humerus, femur, pelvis, and spine or whole-body MR imaging.

The role of ^{18}F-NaF PET/CT in multiple myeloma is currently being investigated in several ongoing research trials. The preliminary reports indicate that the potential for quantitation makes ^{18}F-NaF PET/CT more attractive comparing to conventional bone scanning.[69–71] An early report of a recent comparative prospective study in 14 patients with multiple myeloma showed that whole-body MR imaging detects on average significantly more malignant bone lesions suggestive of multiple myeloma compared with whole-body skeletal x-ray survey, ^{18}F-FDG PET/CT, and ^{18}F-NaF PET/CT.[72] The results of Imaging Young Myelome - IMAgerie JEune Myélome (IMAJEM) prospective trial, however, showed that there is no difference in the detection of bone lesions at diagnosis of multiple myeloma when comparing ^{18}F-FDG PET/CT and MR imaging. The investigators concluded that ^{18}F-FDG PET/CT is a powerful tool to evaluate the prognosis of de novo myeloma.[73]

Metastatic Bone Disease

Several imaging modalities, such as ^{99m}Tc-MDP BS, CT, MR imaging, PET/CT, and PET/MR imaging, have been investigated for the evaluation of patients with suspected bone metastases.

PET/CT and PET/MR imaging assessment of the skeleton can be mainly performed with ^{18}F-NaF, ^{18}F-FDG, and ^{68}Ga-PSMA.

In an initial experience, Even-Sapir and colleagues.[74] evaluated ^{18}F-NaF PET/CT in 44 patients with breast, prostate, lung, colon, nasopharynx, testes, gastrointestinal, lymphoma, melanoma, multiple myeloma, sarcoma, giant cell tumor and carcinoid neoplasms. The investigators reported sensitivity and specificity of 88% and 56%, respectively, for ^{18}F-NaF PET alone and 100% and 88% for PET/CT, respectively, in patient-based analysis. They concluded that ^{18}F-NaF PET/CT is able to accurately differentiate malignant from benign bone lesions.

Another study compared the impact of ^{18}F-NaF PET/CT and ^{18}F-FDG PET/CT for the assessment of bone metastases in a heterogeneous population of patients with sarcoma, prostate cancer, breast cancer, colon cancer, bladder cancer, lung cancer, paraganglioma, lymphoma, gastrointestinal cancer, renal cancer, and salivary gland cancer.[53] The investigators reported sensitivity and specificity of 87.5% and 92.9%, respectively, for ^{99m}Tc-MDP BS; 95.8% and 92.9%, respectively, for ^{18}F-NaF PET/CT; and 66.7% and 96.4%, respectively for ^{18}F-FDG PET/CT.

Prostate, breast, and lung cancers are the most common malignancies in which ^{18}F-NaF PET/CT has been examined. Due to a predominantly sclerotic pattern of bone metastases in prostate cancer, ^{99m}Tc-MDP BS have routinely been performed in the assessment of high-risk patients. ^{18}F-FDG PET suffers from low sensitivity for the detection of prostate cancer lesions. PET/CT using ^{18}F-choline and ^{11}C-choline showed an accurate modality in prostate cancer recurrence for detecting local recurrence, regional lymph node, and distant metastases after radical prostatectomy and radiation therapy.[75–77] ^{18}F-NaF PET/CT seems to have an important role in the assessment of bone metastases in both staging and restaging of prostate cancer patients.[78–81]

A published study evaluated the value of ^{99m}Tc-MDP planar BS, multi–field-of-view SPECT, ^{18}F-NaF PET, and ^{18}F-NaF PET/CT, compared in the detection of bone metastases in 44 high-risk prostate cancer patients.[51] In a patient-based analysis, the sensitivity, specificity, positive predictive value, and negative predictive value were 70%, 57%, 64%, and 55%, respectively, of ^{99m}Tc-MDP planar BS; 92%, 82%, 86%, and 90%, respectively, of multi–field-of-view SPECT; 100%, 62%, 74%, and 100%, respectively, of ^{18}F-NaF PET; and 100% for all parameters of ^{18}F-NaF PET/CT.[51]

Another comparative study by the author's group attempts to determine the potential of

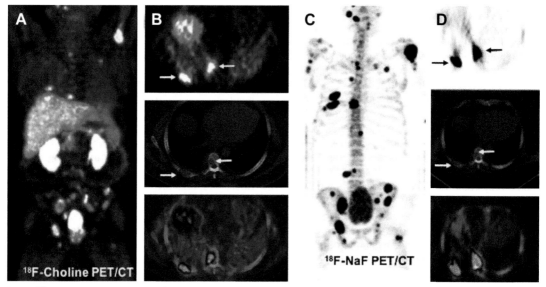

Fig. 2. ^{18}F-NaF PET/CT in staging of a prostate cancer patient with a PSA level of 141 ng/mL and Gleason score of 9 (5 + 4). (A) ^{18}F-choline PET MIP (maximum intensity projection) image shows pathologic increased tracer uptake on both prostate lobes (*white arrow*) with multiple ^{18}F-choline positive bone and lymph node metastases. (B) ^{18}F-choline PET/CT (transaxial, *upper*: PET, *middle*: CT, *lower*: fusion PET/CT) is able to better verify the localization of the pathologic uptakes on the skeleton (*upper panel [arrows]*) with corresponding osteolytic changes on CT (*middle [C, D]*). (C) ^{18}F-NaF PET/CT image (maximum intensity projection and transaxial) shows multiple bone metastases corresponding with ^{18}F-choline PET/CT findings. (D) 18F-NaF PET/CT (transaxial, *upper*: PET, middle: CT, *lower*: fusion PET/CT) images show marked increased 18F-NaF uptake (*upper-arrows*) in the osteolytic metastases (*mid-arrows*).

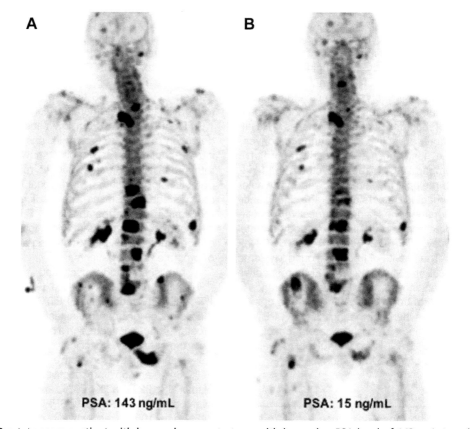

Fig. 3. Prostate cancer patient with known bone metastases with increasing PSA level of 143 ng/mL under hormone therapy and bisphosphonate supportive care. (A) ^{18}F-NaF PET maximum intensity projection shows multiple bone metastases on the skeleton. (B) ^{18}F-NaF PET (maximum intensity projection): restaging after chemotherapy shows partial remission of the disease correlation with clinical findings.

^{18}F-NaF PET/CT and ^{18}F-choline PET/CT for assessment of bone metastases in 38 prostate cancer patients.[81] In a lesion-based analysis, the sensitivity and specificity of PET/CT in detection of bone metastasis were 81% and 93%, respectively, for ^{18}F-NaF PET/CT and 74% and 99%, respectively, for ^{18}F-choline PET/CT. In a patient-based analysis, there was good agreement between ^{18}F-choline and ^{18}F-NaF PET/CT (kappa = 0.76). ^{18}F-NaF PET/CT demonstrated higher sensitivity than ^{18}F-choline PET/CT in the detection of bone metastases; however, it was not statistically significant (**Fig. 2**).

^{18}F-NaF PET/CT may also play an important role in therapy monitoring in prostate cancer (**Fig. 3**). Due to the similarity in the uptake mechanism between ^{223}Ra-chloride and ^{18}F-NaF, it seems an ideal tracer for staging and restaging of patients who undergo ^{223}Ra-chloride or ^{177}Lu-PSMA therapy (**Fig. 4**).

In a study comparing the qualitative ^{99m}Tc-MDP BS with the semiquantitative ^{18}F-NaF PET for assessment of treatment response with ^{223}Ra-chloride, the investigators concluded that ^{18}F-NaF PET is more accurate than the ^{99m}Tc-MDP BS.[82]

The most common site of metastases from breast cancer is the skeleton. These are predominantly osteolytic lesions; however, 15% to 20% of patients can present osteoblastic lesions.[83] ^{18}F-NaF PET seems to play an important prognostic role in breast cancer patients.[84]

In a study by Petrén-Mallmin and colleagues,[5] pathologic bony uptakes on ^{18}F-NaF PET were correlated with morphologic findings on CT in breast cancer patients with bone metastases (**Fig. 5**). The investigators found that all lytic, sclerotic, and mixed lesions on CT showed increased uptake of ^{18}F-NaF on PET (see **Fig. 2**). Small lytic lesions with 2 mm to 3 mm in size were not detected on ^{18}F-NaF PET. Moreover, there was no remarkable difference in the uptake of ^{18}F-NaF between lytic and sclerotic lesions. Both lytic and sclerotic lesions showed 5 times to 10 times higher uptake than normal bone.

Furthermore, ^{18}F-NaF PET seems more accurate for assessing response to therapy compared with conventional imaging modalities. Doot and

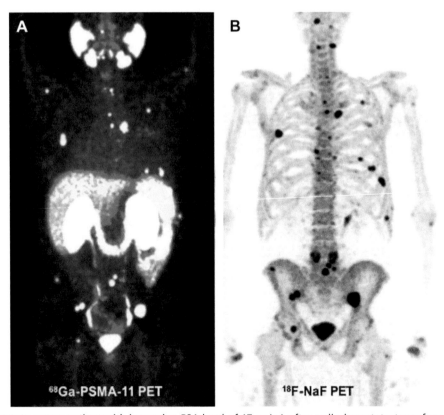

Fig. 4. Prostate cancer patient with increasing PSA level of 17 ng/mL after radical prostatectomy for planning of the radionuclide therapy with ^{223}Ra-chloride or ^{177}Lu-PSMA. (*A*) ^{68}Ga-PSMA-11 PET: maximum image projection shows also multiple metastases in the skeleton. (*B*) ^{18}F-NaF PET (maximum intensity projection): in 2 weeks interval shows multiple bone metastases corresponding to ^{68}Ga-PSMA PET/CT as a highly specific method.

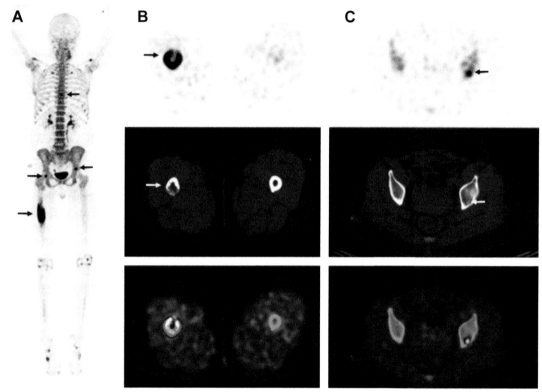

Fig. 5. Staging in a breast cancer patient. (*A*) ^{18}F-NaF PET: maximum intensity projection (MIP) with multiple lesions in the skeleton (*arrows*) suggestive of bone metastases. (*B, C*) ^{18}F-NaF PET/CT: transaxial views; atypical metastases in the middle part of right femur, which is verified by histopathology. Correlation of PET findings (*upper-arrows [B, C]*) with morphologic changes on CT (*middle-arrows [B, C]*) and fusion PET/CT (*lower*) allows better interpretation of the lesions.

colleagues[85] performed dynamic ^{18}F-NaF PET to define the fluoride kinetics of bone metastases in breast cancer patients. They found that ^{18}F-NaF transport (K1) and flux (Ki) were significantly different in metastases and normal bone. The investigators also concluded that ^{18}F-NaF PET not only is suitable for detecting bone metastases but also seems to play an important role for the evaluation of bone turnover in response to therapy by suggested quantitative approach.

Lung cancer is the second most common malignancy, accounting for 14% of all malignancies.[58] Bone metastases were detected in 20% to 30% of patients at initial diagnosis and in 35% to 60% at autopsy.[86–88] Thus, accurate staging is crucial in patients with lung cancer to rule out distant metastases and to select proper treatment. In a prospective study with 53 lung cancer patients, Schirrmeister and colleagues[89] compared the diagnostic accuracy of ^{18}F-NaF PET and ^{99m}Tc-MDP BS with and without SPECT at the initial staging. In 12 patients with bone metastases, there were 6 false-negative results on the ^{99m}Tc-MDP BS, 1 on SPECT, and none on

[18]F-NaF PET. ^{99m}Tc-MDP SPECT and ^{18}F-NaF PET changed clinical management in 5 patients (9%) and 6 patients (11%), respectively. The investigators concluded that ^{18}F-NaF PET is the most accurate whole-body imaging modality for screening for bone metastasis. Similar results were reported by another group in initial staging of 103 patients with lung cancer.[90] Another study examined the diagnostic accuracy of ^{18}F-FDG PET/CT and ^{18}F-NaF PET/CT for the detection of bone metastases in 126 patients with NSCLC.[52] The investigators reported that integrated ^{18}F-FDG PET/CT is superior to ^{99m}Tc-MDP BS for the detection of osteolytic metastases in NSCLC. They also claimed that ^{18}F-NaF PET seems to be at least as sensitive for the detection of bone metastasis compared with ^{18}F-FDG PET/CT. ^{18}F-FDG PET/CT was able, however, to determine higher number of patients with bone metastases.

In addition, some studies performed both ^{18}F-NaF and ^{18}F-FDG in a single PET/CT scan for assessment of bone metastases,[91–93] concluding that this dual-tracer approach may result in a more convenient schedule for the patient, less radiation, and potential savings in health care costs. With the development and more availability of PET/MR imaging, this modality may yield new applications for the widespread use of 18F-NaF in clinical management of breast cancer patients in the near future with PET/MR imaging.

REFERENCES

1. Bridges RL, Wiley CR, Christian JC, et al. An introduction to Na(18)F bone scintigraphy: basic principles, advanced imaging concepts, and case examples. J Nucl Med Technol 2007;35(2):64–76 [quiz: 78–9].
2. Cook GJR. PET and PET/CT imaging of skeletal metastases. Cancer imaging 2010;10:1–8.
3. Czernin J, Satyamurthy N, Schiepers C. Molecular mechanisms of bone 18F-NaF deposition. J Nucl Med 2010;51(12):1826–9.
4. Fogelman I, Cook G, Israe O, et al. Positron emission tomography and bone metastases. Semin Nucl Med 2005;35(2):135–42.
5. Petrén-Mallmin M, Andreasson I, Ljunggren O, et al. Skeletal metastases from breast cancer: uptake of 18F-fluoride measured with positron emission tomography in correlation with CT. Skeletal Radiol 1998;27(2):72–6.
6. Schirrmeister H, Guhlmann A, Elsner K, et al. Sensitivity in detecting osseous lesions depends on anatomic localization: planar bone scintigraphy versus 18F PET. J Nucl Med 1999;40(10):1623–9.
7. Hawkins RA, Choi Y, Huang SC, et al. Evaluation of the skeletal kinetics of fluorine-18-fluoride ion with PET. J Nucl Med 1992;33(5):633–42.
8. Schirrmeister H, Guhlmann A, Kotzerke J, et al. Early detection and accurate description of extent of metastatic bone disease in breast cancer with fluoride ion and positron emission tomography. J Clin Oncol 1999;17(8):2381–9.
9. Langsteger W, Heinisch M, Fogelman I. The role of fluorodeoxyglucose, 18F-dihydroxyphenylalanine, 18F-choline, and 18F-fluoride in bone imaging with emphasis on prostate and breast. Semin Nucl Med 2006;36(1):73–92.
10. Beheshti M, Langsteger W, Fogelman I. Prostate cancer: role of SPECT and PET in imaging bone metastases. Semin Nucl Med 2009;39(6):396–407.
11. Schirrmeister H. Detection of bone metastases in breast cancer by positron emission tomography. Radiol Clin North Am 2007;45(4):669–76, vi.
12. Blake G, Siddique M, Frost M, et al. Quantitative PET imaging using 18F sodium fluoride in the assessment of metabolic bone diseases and the monitoring of their response to therapy. PET Clin 2012;7(3):275–91.
13. Piert M, Zittel TT, Becker GA, et al. Assessment of porcine bone metabolism by dynamic. J Nucl Med 2001;42(7):1091–100.
14. Messa C, Goodman WG, Hoh CK, et al. Bone metabolic activity measured with positron emission tomography and [18F]fluoride ion in renal osteodystrophy: correlation with bone histomorphometry. J Clin Endocrinol Metab 1993;77(4):949–55.
15. Uchida K, Nakajima H, Miyazaki T, et al. Effects of alendronate on bone metabolism in glucocorticoid-induced osteoporosis measured by 18F-fluoride PET: a prospective study. J Nucl Med 2009;50(11):1808–14.
16. Haim S, Zakavi R, Saboury B, et al. Predictive value of 18F-NaF PET/CT in the assessment of osteoporosis: comparison with Dual-energy X-Ray Absorptiometry (DXA). Eur J Nucl Med Mol Imaging 2017;44(Suppl 2):S119.
17. Song IH, Carrasco-Fernandez J, Rudwaleit M, et al. The diagnostic value of scintigraphy in assessing sacroiliitis in ankylosing spondylitis: a systematic literature research. Ann Rheum Dis 2008;67(11):1535–40.
18. Blum U, Buitrago-Tellez C, Mundinger A, et al. Magnetic resonance imaging (MRI) for detection of active sacroiliitis–a prospective study comparing conventional radiography, scintigraphy, and contrast enhanced MRI. J Rheumatol 1996;23(12):2107–15.
19. Strobel K, Fischer DR, Tamborrini G, et al. 18F-fluoride PET/CT for detection of sacroiliitis in ankylosing spondylitis. Eur J Nucl Med Mol Imaging 2010;37(9):1760–5.
20. Li Y, Schiepers C, Lake R, et al. Clinical utility of (18)F-fluoride PET/CT in benign and malignant bone diseases. Bone 2012;50(1):128–39.
21. Weber U, Pfirrmann CW, Kissling RO, et al. Whole body MR imaging in ankylosing spondylitis: a descriptive pilot study in patients with suspected early and active confirmed ankylosing spondylitis. BMC Musculoskelet Disord 2007;8:20.
22. Fischer DR, Pfirrmann CW, Zubler V, et al. High bone turnover assessed by 18F-fluoride PET/CT in the spine and sacroiliac joints of patients with ankylosing spondylitis: comparison with inflammatory lesions detected by whole body MRI. EJNMMI Res 2012;2(1):38.
23. Bruijnen STG, Verweij NJF, van Duivenvoorden LM, et al. Bone formation in ankylosing spondylitis during anti-tumour necrosis factor therapy imaged by 18F-fluoride positron emission tomography. Rheumatology (Oxford) 2018;57(4):770.
24. Drubach LA, Johnston PR, Newton AW, et al. Skeletal trauma in child abuse: detection with 18F-NaF PET. Radiology 2010;255(1):173–81.
25. Grant FD. (1)(8)F-fluoride PET and PET/CT in children and young adults. PET Clin 2014;9(3):287–97.
26. Rauscher I, Beer AJ, Schaeffeler C, et al. Evaluation of 18F-fluoride PET/MR and PET/CT in patients with

foot pain of unclear cause. J Nucl Med 2015;56(3):
430–5.

27. Cronlein M, Rauscher I, Beer AJ, et al. Visualization of stress fractures of the foot using PET-MRI: a feasibility study. Eur J Med Res 2015;20:99.

28. Dua SG, Purandare NC, Shah S, et al. F-18 fluoride PET/CT in the detection of radiation-induced pelvic insufficiency fractures. Clin Nucl Med 2011;36(10): e146–9.

29. Strobel K, Vali R. (18)F NaF PET/CT versus conventional bone scanning in the assessment of benign bone disease. PET Clin 2012;7(3):249–61.

30. Hsu WK, Feeley BT, Krenek L, et al. The use of 18F-fluoride and 18F-FDG PET scans to assess fracture healing in a rat femur model. Eur J Nucl Med Mol Imaging 2007;34(8):1291–301.

31. Beheshti M, Mottaghy FM, Payche F, et al. (18)F-NaF PET/CT: EANM procedure guidelines for bone imaging. Eur J Nucl Med Mol Imaging 2015; 42(11):1767–77.

32. Hirschmann MT, Davda K, Rasch H, et al. Clinical value of combined single photon emission computerized tomography and conventional computer tomography (SPECT/CT) in sports medicine. Sports Med Arthrosc Rev 2011;19(2):174–81.

33. Love C, Tomas MB, Marwin SE, et al. Role of nuclear medicine in diagnosis of the infected joint replacement. Radiographics 2001;21(5):1229–38.

34. Kobayashi N, Inaba Y, Choe H, et al. Use of F-18 fluoride PET to differentiate septic from aseptic loosening in total hip arthroplasty patients. Clin Nucl Med 2011;36(11):e156–61.

35. Choe H, Inaba Y, Kobayashi N, et al. Use of 18F-fluoride PET to determine the appropriate tissue sampling region for improved sensitivity of tissue examinations in cases of suspected periprosthetic infection after total hip arthroplasty. Acta Orthop 2011;82(4):427–32.

36. Sterner T, Pink R, Freudenberg L, et al. The role of [18F]fluoride positron emission tomography in the early detection of aseptic loosening of total knee arthroplasty. Int J Surg 2007;5(2):99–104.

37. Rajender K, Rakesh K, Suhas S, et al. Role of 18F-fluoride PET/CT and 18-F FDG PET/CT for differentiating septic from aseptic loosening in patients with painful hip prosthesis. J Nucl Med 2011; 52(Supplement 1):458.

38. Zoccali C, Teori G, Salducca N. The role of FDG-PET in distinguishing between septic and aseptic loosening in hip prosthesis: a review of literature. Int Orthop 2009;33(1):1–5.

39. Farid K, El-Deeb G, Caillat Vigneron N. SPECT-CT improves scintigraphic accuracy of osteoid osteoma diagnosis. Clin Nucl Med 2010;35(3):170–1.

40. Lim R, Fahey FH, Drubach LA, et al. Early experience with fluorine-18 sodium fluoride bone PET in young patients with back pain. J Pediatr Orthop 2007;27(3):277–82.

41. Ovadia D, Metser U, Lievshitz G, et al. Back pain in adolescents: assessment with integrated 18F-fluoride positron-emission tomography-computed tomography. J Pediatr Orthop 2007;27(1):90–3.

42. Hakim SG, Bruecker CW, Jacobsen H, et al. The value of FDG-PET and bone scintigraphy with SPECT in the primary diagnosis and follow-up of patients with chronic osteomyelitis of the mandible. Int J Oral Maxillofac Surg 2006;35(9):809–16.

43. Berding G, Schliephake H, van den Hoff J, et al. Assessment of the incorporation of revascularized fibula grafts used for mandibular reconstruction with F-18-PET. Nuklearmedizin 2001;40(2):51–8.

44. Piert M, Winter E, Becker GA, et al. Allogenic bone graft viability after hip revision arthroplasty assessed by dynamic [18F]fluoride ion positron emission tomography. Eur J Nucl Med 1999;26(6):615–24.

45. Fischer DR, Maquieira GJ, Espinosa N, et al. Therapeutic impact of [(18)F]fluoride positron-emission tomography/computed tomography on patients with unclear foot pain. Skeletal Radiol 2010;39(10):987–97.

46. Laverick S, Bounds G, Wong WL. [18F]-fluoride positron emission tomography for imaging condylar hyperplasia. Br J Oral Maxillofac Surg 2009;47(3): 196–9.

47. Czernin J, et al. 18F-Fluoride PET/CT versus 99mTc-MDP scanning for detecting bone metastases: a randomized, multi-center trial to compare two bone imaging technique. In: American College of Radiology - Image Metrix World Molecular Imaging Society; 2012. Aviailable at: https://clinicaltrials.gov/ct2/show/NCT00882609. Accessed July 1, 2018.

48. Mosci C, Iagaru A. (18)F NaF PET/CT in the assessment of malignant bone disease. PET Clin 2012;7(3): 263–74.

49. NOPR. National Oncologic PET Registry. 2012. Available at: http://www.cancerpetregistry.org/what.htm. Accessed February 13, 2012.

50. Even Sapir E. Imaging of malignant bone involvement by morphologic, scintigraphic, and hybrid modalities. J Nucl Med 2005;46(8):1356–67.

51. Even Sapir E, Metser U, Mishani E, et al. The detection of bone metastases in patients with high-risk prostate cancer: 99mTc-MDP Planar bone scintigraphy, single- and multi-field-of-view SPECT, 18F-fluoride PET, and 18F-fluoride PET/CT. J Nucl Med 2006;47(2):287–97.

52. Krger S, Buck A, Mottaghy F, et al. Detection of bone metastases in patients with lung cancer: 99mTc-MDP planar bone scintigraphy, 18F-fluoride PET or 18F-FDG PET/CT. Eur J Nucl Med Mol Imaging 2009;36(11):1807–12.

53. Iagaru A, Mittra E, Dick D, et al. Prospective evaluation of (99m)Tc MDP Scintigraphy, (18)F NaF PET/CT, and (18)F FDG PET/CT for detection of skeletal metastases. Mol Imaging Biol 2011. https://doi.org/10.1007/s11307-011-0486-2.

54. Langsteger W, Rezaee A, Pirich C, et al. (18)F-NaF-PET/CT and (99m)Tc-MDP bone scintigraphy in the detection of bone metastases in prostate cancer. Semin Nucl Med 2016;46(6):491–501.

55. Beheshti M, Langsteger W. (18)F NaF PET/CT in the assessment of metastatic bone disease: comparison with specific PET tracers. PET Clin 2012;7(3):303–14.

56. Beheshti M. Clinical utility of 18NaF PET/CT in benign and malignant disorders, vol. 7. Elsevier; 2012.

57. Jemal A, Siegel R, Xu J, et al. Cancer statistics, 2010. CA Cancer J Clin 2010;60(5):277–300.

58. Siegel R, Naishadham D, Jemal A. Cancer statistics, 2012. CA Cancer J Clin 2012;62(1):10–29.

59. Im HJ, Kim TS, Park SY, et al. Prediction of tumour necrosis fractions using metabolic and volumetric 18F-FDG PET/CT indices, after one course and at the completion of neoadjuvant chemotherapy, in children and young adults with osteosarcoma. Eur J Nucl Med Mol Imaging 2012;39(1):39–49.

60. D'Adamo D. Appraising the current role of chemotherapy for the treatment of sarcoma. Semin Oncol 2011;38(Suppl 3):S19–29.

61. Hoh CK, Hawkins RA, Dahlbom M, et al. Whole body skeletal imaging with [18F]fluoride ion and PET. J Comput Assist Tomogr 1993;17(1):34–41.

62. Tse N, Hoh C, Hawkins R, et al. Positron emission tomography diagnosis of pulmonary metastases in osteogenic sarcoma. Am J Clin Oncol 1994;17(1): 22–5.

63. Franzius C, Daldrup Link HE, Sciuk J, et al. FDG-PET for detection of pulmonary metastases from malignant primary bone tumors: comparison with spiral CT. Ann Oncol 2001;12(4):479–86.

64. Kaira K, Okumura T, Ohde Y, et al. Correlation between 18F-FDG uptake on PET and molecular biology in metastatic pulmonary tumors. J Nucl Med 2011;52(5):705–11.

65. Iagaru A, Chawla S, Menendez L, et al. 18F-FDG PET and PET/CT for detection of pulmonary metastases from musculoskeletal sarcomas. Nucl Med Commun 2006;27(10):795–802.

66. Bernstein M, Kovar H, Paulussen M, et al. Ewing's sarcoma family of tumors: current management. Oncologist 2006;11(5):503–19.

67. Winterbottom AP, Shaw AS. Imaging patients with myeloma. Clin Radiol 2009;64(1):1–11.

68. Ludwig H, Kumpan W, Sinzinger H. Radiography and bone scintigraphy in multiple myeloma: a comparative analysis. Br J Radiol 1982;55(651): 173–81.

69. Kurdziel K, Lindenberg L, Mena E, et al. Temporal characterization of F-18 NaF PET/CT uptake. J Nucl Med Meeting Abstracts 2011;52(1_MeetingAbstracts):459.

70. Sachpekidis C, Goldschmidt H, Hose D, et al. PET/CT studies of multiple myeloma using (18) F-FDG and (18) F-NaF: comparison of distribution patterns and tracers' pharmacokinetics. Eur J Nucl Med Mol Imaging 2014;41(7):1343–53.

71. Nishiyama Y, Tateishi U, Shizukuishi K, et al. Role of 18F-fluoride PET/CT in the assessment of multiple myeloma: initial experience. Ann Nucl Med 2013; 27(1):78–83.

72. Dyrberg E, Hendel HW, Al-Farra G, et al. A prospective study comparing whole-body skeletal X-ray survey with 18F-FDG-PET/CT, 18F-NaF-PET/CT and whole-body MRI in the detection of bone lesions in multiple myeloma patients. Acta Radiol Open 2017;6(10). 2058460117738809.

73. Moreau P, Attal M, Caillot D, et al. Prospective evaluation of magnetic resonance imaging and [(18)F] Fluorodeoxyglucose positron emission tomography-computed tomography at diagnosis and before maintenance therapy in symptomatic patients with multiple myeloma included in the IFM/DFCI 2009 trial: results of the IMAJEM study. J Clin Oncol 2017;35(25):2911–8.

74. Even-Sapir E, Metser U, Flusser G, et al. Assessment of malignant skeletal disease: initial experience with 18F-fluoride PET/CT and comparison between 18F-fluoride PET and 18F-fluoride PET/CT. J Nucl Med 2004;45(2):272–8.

75. Picchio M, Messa C, Landoni C, et al. Value of [11C]choline-positron emission tomography for restaging prostate cancer: a comparison with [18F] fluorodeoxyglucose-positron emission tomography. J Urol 2003;169(4):1337–40.

76. Beheshti M, Haim S, Zakavi R, et al. Impact of 18F-choline PET/CT in prostate cancer patients with biochemical recurrence: influence of androgen deprivation therapy and correlation with PSA kinetics. J Nucl Med 2013;54(6):833–40.

77. Beheshti M, Imamovic L, Broinger G, et al. 18F choline PET/CT in the preoperative staging of prostate cancer in patients with intermediate or high risk of extracapsular disease: a prospective study of 130 patients. Radiology 2010;254(3): 925–33.

78. Jadvar H, Desai B, Conti P, et al. Preliminary evaluation of 18F-NaF and 18F-FDG PET/CT in detection of metastatic disease in men with PSA relapse after treatment for localized primary prostate cancer. J Nucl Med Meeting Abstracts 2011;52(1_MeetingAbstracts):1916.

79. Picchio M, Giovannini E, Messa C. The role of PET/computed tomography scan in the management of prostate cancer. Curr Opin Urol 2011; 21(3):230–6.

80. Langsteger W, Balogova S, Huchet V, et al. Fluorocholine (18F) and sodium fluoride (18F) PET/CT in the detection of prostate cancer: prospective comparison of diagnostic performance determined by masked reading. Q J Nucl Med Mol Imaging 2011; 55(4):448–57.

81. Beheshti M, Vali R, Waldenberger P, et al. Detection of bone metastases in patients with prostate cancer by 18F fluorocholine and 18F fluoride PET-CT: a comparative study. Eur J Nucl Med Mol Imaging 2008;35(10):1766–74.

82. Cook G, Parker C, Chua S, et al. 18F-fluoride PET: changes in uptake as a method to assess response in bone metastases from castrate-resistant prostate cancer patients treated with 223Ra-chloride (Alpharadin). EJNMMI Res 2011;1(1):4.

83. Coleman RE, Seaman JJ. The role of zoledronic acid in cancer: clinical studies in the treatment and prevention of bone metastases. Semin Oncol 2001; 28(2 Suppl 6):11–6.

84. Yamashita K, Koyama H, Inaji H. Prognostic significance of bone metastasis from breast cancer. Clin Orthop Relat Res 1995;(312):89–94.

85. Doot RK, Muzi M, Peterson LM, et al. Kinetic analysis of 18F-fluoride PET images of breast cancer bone metastases. J Nucl Med 2010;51(4):521–7.

86. Tritz DB, Doll DC, Ringenberg QS, et al. Bone marrow involvement in small cell lung cancer. Clinical significance and correlation with routine laboratory variables. Cancer 1989;63(4):763–6.

87. Bezwoda WR, Lewis D, Livini N. Bone marrow involvement in anaplastic small cell lung cancer. Diagnosis, hematologic features, and prognostic implications. Cancer 1986;58(8):1762–5.

88. Trillet V, Revel D, Combaret V, et al. Bone marrow metastases in small cell lung cancer: detection with magnetic resonance imaging and monoclonal antibodies. Br J Cancer 1989;60(1):83–8.

89. Schirrmeister H, Glatting G, Hetzel J, et al. Prospective evaluation of the clinical value of planar bone scans, SPECT, and 18F-labeled NaF PET in newly diagnosed lung cancer. J Nucl Med 2001;42(12): 1800–4.

90. Hetzel M, Arslandemir C, Knig H-H, et al. F-18 NaF PET for detection of bone metastases in lung cancer: accuracy, cost-effectiveness, and impact on patient management. J Bone Miner Res 2003; 18(12):2206–14.

91. Iagaru A, Mittra E, Yaghoubi SS, et al. Novel strategy for a cocktail 18F-fluoride and 18F-FDG PET/CT scan for evaluation of malignancy: results of the pilot-phase study. J Nucl Med 2009;50(4): 501–5.

92. Lin F, Rao J, Mittra E, et al. Prospective comparison of combined (18)F-FDG and (18)F-NaF PET/CT vs. (18)F-FDG PET/CT imaging for detection of malignancy. Eur J Nucl Med Mol Imaging 2012;39(2): 262–70.

93. Iagaru A, Mittra E, Sathekge M, et al. Combined 18F NaF and 18F FDG PET/CT: initial results of a multicenter trial. J Nucl Med Meeting Abstracts 2011; 52(1_MeetingAbstracts):34.

Radionuclide Therapy for Bone Metastases
Utility of Scintigraphy and PET Imaging for Treatment Planning

Hojjat Ahmadzadehfar, MD, MSc[a],*, Markus Essler, MD[a],
Kambiz Rahbar, MD[b], Ali Afshar-Oromieh, MD[c,d]

KEYWORDS

- Breast cancer • Prostate cancer • Lung cancer • Bone metastases • Radionuclide therapy
- Radium-223 • PET

KEY POINTS

- A Pain relief response is seen in approximately one-half of patients treated with radionuclides for painful osseous metastases.
- FDG PET plays an important role in the detection of bony metastases with higher detection rate compared with bone scintigraphy in a majority of tumor types and consistent with clinical status of the patients as it reflects tumor activity.
- Skeletal tumor burden measured by fluoride PET correlates with OS inpatients who underwent bone targeted therapies using radionuclides.

TREATMENT OF BONE METASTASES WITH RADIONUCLIDES

The skeleton is a common site for metastases of various malignant tumors. Bone metastases are the result of complex interactions between tumor cells, bone cells, and the microenvironment.[1] Some tumor types, such as prostate cancer and breast cancer, are more frequently associated with bone metastases compared with others.[2] For inducing bone metastases, the tumor cells must detach from the primary tumor, enter the systemic circulation, evade detection by the immune system, and finally adhere to capillaries in the bone marrow, leading to extravasation into the bone marrow space.[1,3–5] Bone metastases are a major cause of morbidity and mortality and are associated with pain, pathologic fractures, spinal cord compression, and decreased survival.[6] The pain from small metastases seems to be caused by irritation of nerve endings in the endosteum by a variety of chemical mediators. Larger bone metastases produce stretching of the periosteum, which leads to pain.[7]

Bone pain palliation with radionuclides has a long history of using various β-emitters, like phosphorus-32 (^{32}P),[8] strontium-89 (^{89}Sr),[8] rhenium-186 hydroxyethylidene diphosphonate (^{186}Re-HEDP),[9] samarium-153 ethylenediamine tetramethylene phosphonate (^{153}Sm-EDTMP),[9] and, recently, lutetium-177 EDTMP (^{177}Lu-EDTMP)[10] and (4-{[(bis(phosphonomethyl))

[a] Department of Nuclear Medicine, University Hospital Bonn, Sigmund-Freud-Str. 25, Bonn 53127, Germany;
[b] Department of Nuclear Medicine, University Hospital Muenster, Albert-Schweitzer-Campus 1, Muenster 48149, Germany; [c] Department of Nuclear Medicine, Heidelberg University Hospital, Im Neuenheimer Feld 400, Heidelberg 69120, Germany; [d] Clinical Cooperation Unit Nuclear Medicine, German Cancer Research Centre, Im Neuenheimer Feld 280, Heidelberg 69120, Germany
* Corresponding author. Department of Nuclear Medicine, University Hospital Bonn, Sigmund-Freud-Str. 25, Bonn 53127, Germany.
E-mail address: Hojjat.ahmadzadehfar@ukbonn.de

PET Clin 13 (2018) 491–503
https://doi.org/10.1016/j.cpet.2018.05.005
1556-8598/18/© 2018 Elsevier Inc. All rights reserved.

carbamoyl]methyl}-7,10-bis(carboxymethyl)-1,4,7, 10-tetraazacyclododec-1-yl)acetic acid ^{177}Lu-BPAMD.[11] The only approved α-emitter is radium-223 ([223]Ra).[12]

Bone-seeking radionuclides are classified into 2 groups: calcium analogs, like ^{89}Sr and [223]Ra, and radionuclides attached to phosphate, like [153]Sm-EDTMP and rhenium-186 hydroxyethylidene diphosphonate ([188]Re-HEDP). The various radionuclides have different physical characteristics, which are shown in **Table 1**.[13] In this article, apart from introduction of different bone-specific radionuclide therapies, the value of PET imaging for the treatment planning and also its predictive value are discussed. Radionuclides that can be used for the treatment of all types of metastases (soft tissue, lymph nodes, and bone), such as ^{131}I for metastatic thyroid cancer,[14] ^{131}I-MIBG for neuroblastoma,[15] ^{177}Lu–prostate-specific membrane antigen (PSMA) for prostate cancer,[16] or ^{177}Lu-DOTATATE for neuroendocrine tumors.[17] These substances, however, are not addressed in this article.

BONE-TARGETED THERAPY WITH BONE SPECIFIC β-EMITTERS
Phosphorus-32 and strontium-89

Typical response times to different β-emitters are shown in **Box 1** and **Table 2**. Pain reduction after the injection of ^{32}P and ^{89}Sr occurs after 5 days to 14 days and 14 days to 28 days postinjection, respectively. During treatment with ^{32}P, pain relief was reported by 50% to 87% of prostate cancer patients treated with 200 MBq to 800 MBq of ^{32}P administered in daily fractions of 20 weeks to 80 MBq after androgen priming. The main disadvantage of ^{32}P therapy is a dose-limiting reversible pancytopenia due to myelosuppression with a maximum at 5 weeks to 6 weeks after administration.[18]

The first studies using ^{89}Sr have demonstrated an efficacy for pain reduction as high as 80%.[19–24] A majority of treated patients in these studies suffered from prostate or breast cancer. [89]Sr was the first radiopharmaceutical to be approved for systemic radionuclide therapy in the palliation of painful bone metastases. In the largest study using ^{89}Sr, 622 patients were included. Of these, 15% showed complete pain relief and a partial response was documented in 81%.[25,26] In only 4% of the patients, no response was observed. In a randomized, controlled phase III trial, James and colleagues[27,28] compared the efficacy of zoledronic acid (ZA) with ^{89}Sr regarding clinical progression-free survival (CPFS) as the primary outcome and the skeletal-related event–free interval (SREFI), total skeletal-related events (SREs), overall survival (OS), and quality of life (QOL) as secondary outcomes. Each of the compounds (ZA and ^{89}Sr) was combined with docetaxel for the treatment of bone metastases of castration-resistant prostate cancer (CRPC) patients. In this trial, 757 patients were randomized to receive 6 cycles of docetaxel combined with prednisolone, with ZA, with a single ^{89}Sr dose after the sixth cycle of docetaxel, or with both ZA and a single ^{89}Sr dose. A Cox regression analysis adjusted for stratification variables and showed a CPFS benefit for [89]Sr (hazard ratio [HR] = 0.845, P = .036) and confirmed no effect of ZA (P = .46). ZA showed a significant SREFI effect (HR = 0.76; P = .008), however. Neither agent affected OS (^{89}Sr, P = .74; ZA, P = .91). QOL was well maintained in all treatment arms, with differing patterns of care resulting from the effects of ^{89}Sr on the time to progression and ZA on SREFI and total SREs. The investigators concluded that ^{89}Sr combined with docetaxel improved CPFS but did not improve OS, SREFI, or total SREs. Furthermore, ZA did not improve CPFS or OS

Table 1
Summary of main physical properties of different radionuclides clinically used for pain palliation

	Emission Type	Half-Life (d)	Maximum Energy (MeV)	Maximum Tissue Penetration Range (mm)
[32]P	ß-emitter	14.3	1.7	8.5
[89]Sr	ß-emitter	50.5	1.46	7
Samarium-153	ß and γ-emitter	1.9	0.81	4
[186]Re	ß and γ-emitter	3.7	1.07	5
[188]Re	ß and γ-emitter	0.7	2.1	10
[177]Lu	ß and γ-emitter	6.7	0.498	1.8
[223]Ra	α-Emitter and γ-emitter	11.4	27.78	0.1

Adapted from Ahmadzadehfar H. Targeted therapy for metastatic prostate cancer with radionuclides. In: Mohan R, editor. Prostate cancer - leading-edge diagnostic procedures and treatments. Croatia: InTech; 2016.

but significantly improved the median SREFI and reduced the total SREs by approximately one-third, suggesting a role in postchemotherapy maintenance therapy.

Several patient characteristics could predict a favorable response to [89]Sr. A normal serum hemoglobin (Hb) level prior to treatment is associated with a higher pain response rate.[29] Predictors of a poor pain response include a low performance status, a higher serum prostate-specific antigen (PSA), more extensive osseous metastases, and a poor PSA response.[30–33] The toxicity of ^{89}Sr is limited, with the common development of thrombocytopenia, with a nadir between the fourth week and sixth week. Recovery of thrombocytopenia is typically slow over the next 6 weeks and is dictated by the skeletal tumor extent and bone marrow reserve.[34]

Rhenium-186 hydroxyethylidene diphosphonate and Rhenium-188 hydroxyethylidene diphosphonate

Pain reduction after the injection of [186]Re-HEDP occurs 2 days to 7 days after application, and this effect lasts approximately 8 weeks to 10 weeks. Previous studies have shown a pain relief response rate of 60% to 86%.[31,35–37] Toxicity has been limited to temporary myelosuppression, with platelet and neutrophil nadirs at 4 weeks after therapy. Recovery occurs within 8 weeks and is usually complete.[38] Pain reduction after the injection of [188]Re-HEDP occurs 2 days to 7 days after application and this effect lasts approximately 8 weeks.[13] The overall response rate is 69% to 77%.[39–41] [188]Re is of special interest in clinical applications because of its excellent availability and cost-effectiveness, because it is the product of a [188]W ([188]W/[188]Re) generator.[41] The short physical half-life (0.7 days) and high dose rate are predicted to lead to a rapid symptom response. Fractionated therapy has been shown to prolong the response duration and progression-free survival (PFS).[42]

Table 2
Bone-seeking radionuclides

Radiopharmaceutical	Activity	Typical Response Time	Typical Response Duration	Retreatment Interval
[32]P	444 MBq (fractionated)	14 d	10 wk	>3 mo
[89]Sr-chloride	150–200 MBq	14–28 d	12–26 wk	>3 mo
[153]Sm -EDTMP	37 MBq/Kg	2–7 d	8 wk	>2 mo
[186]Re-HEDP	1.3 GBq	2–7 d	8–10 wk	>2 mo
[188]Re-HEDP	1.3–4.4 GBq	2–7 d	8 wk	2 mo
[223]Ra	55 KBq/Kg body weight	1–8 wk	6 wk	6 injections every 4 wk

Data from Refs.[34,104,105]

Palmedo and colleagues[43] showed that 2 injections of [188]Re-HEDP with an 8-week interval were more effective for pain palliation compared with only one injection, with response rate and time of response of 92% and 5.7 months, respectively ($P = .006$ and $P = .001$, respectively). Biersack and colleagues[42] also reported a positive effect of repeated therapy using [188]Re-HEDP on OS. They retrospectively analyzed 60 CRPC patients who had been assigned to 3 different groups according to the number of therapies. The mean survival after the initial therapy improved from 4.5 months in patients with only 1 therapy to 9.98 months in patients with 2 therapies, and 15.7 months in patients with 3 or more cycles of therapy.[42] A randomized phase II study of repeated [188]Re-HEDP cycles combined with docetaxel/prednisolone versus docetaxel and prednisone alone in CRPC patients has shown that the combined treatment with [188]Re-HEDP and docetaxel did not prolong PFS. The median OS was significantly longer in the [188]Re-HEDP group (33.8 months), than in the control group (docetaxel/prednisolone: 21.0 months; $P = .012$).[44] This OS prolongation warrants further studies in the combined treatment of chemotherapy and radiopharmaceuticals. Moderate thrombopenia and leukopenia have been reported in different studies.[41,43–45]

Samarium-153 ethylenediamine tetramethylene phosphonate

[153]Sm-EDTMP is one of the most widely used radionuclides for bone palliation. Since the clinical introduction of [223]Ra, however, it has been underestimated and not used as often as it could be. Pain reduction after the injection of [153]Sm-EDTMP occurs 2 days to 10 days after the application. Previous studies have shown a pain relief response rate of 59% to 86%.[46–50] Larger studies with more than 100 patients have demonstrated a median therapeutic efficacy of 80%. In a randomized, double-blind, placebo trial (n = 152), pain relief occurred in 65% of patients after [153]Sm-EDTMP treatment compared with 45% in the placebo group.[48] A significant decrease in pain between the [153]Sm-EDTMP and placebo groups was reported after 1 week and the analgesic intake was significantly reduced after 3 weeks and 4 weeks. [153]Sm-EDTMP can be administered prior to chemotherapy with docetaxel in CRPC patients. It neither reduces the antitumor efficacy of docetaxel nor causes additional toxicities.[51] Various studies with different protocols have shown the feasibility of a combination therapy of [153]Sm-EDTMP with the chemotherapeutic agent docetaxel in CRPC patients.[52–54] These studies have

concluded that [153]Sm-EDTMP can be safely combined with docetaxel in patients with CRPC. The authors, however, do not currently recommend this approach because of a new generation of antiandrogenic therapeutics, such as enzalutamide or abiraterone, which may be combined with β-emitters with a lower probability of hematotoxicities.[55]

Lutetium-177 ethylenediamine tetramethylene phosphonate

There is increasing evidence for the utility of ^{177}Lu labeled with different compounds for the treatment of various tumors, like neuroendocrine tumors and prostate cancer.[56–58] This is mainly due to the favorable physical characteristic of ^{177}Lu, including a short tissue penetration range, which reduces the probability of bone marrow suppression while simultaneously delivering an appropriate dose to the target due to its long half-life of 6.73 days.[59]

Alavi and colleagues[60] reported that, in 30 patients treated with ^{177}Lu-EDTMP, the pain relief began 2.53 ± 2.08 weeks after the injection, and the response lasted for 4.38 ± 3.34 weeks. Among these patients, 16 (53%) showed a complete palliative pain response, 9 (30%) revealed a partial response, and 5 (17%) showed no response to treatment. Thus, a total treatment response was achieved in 25 patients (83%).

In a phase II study, Yuan and colleagues[10] treated 16 breast cancer and prostate cancer patients with ^{177}Lu-EDTMP. The patients were divided into 2 groups according to the administered activity (group 1 with 1295 MBq vs group 2 with 2590 MBq). The rate of complete responses in bone pain palliation was 55% in group 1% and 80% in group 2 at 6 weeks after treatment. In group 1, 1 patient experienced a grade III toxicity in both the Hb and platelet counts; however, no grade IV toxicities were observed. In group 2, there were no grade III or IV toxicities in Hb, platelet, or leukocyte counts. Moreover, no clinically significant adverse effects were observed, and no significant differences in either efficacy or safety were detected between the 2 dose levels.[10] Another phase II study by Agarwal and colleagues[61] included 44 patients with CRPC and breast cancer treated with ^{177}Lu-EDTMP at a dose of 1295 MBq (group 1) and 2590 MBq (group 2). The overall response rate (in all 44 patients) was 86%, in group 1 the response rate was 77%, and it was 95% in group 2 ($P = .188$). Complete, partial, and minimal responses were seen in 6 patients (13%), 21 patients (48%), and 11 patients (25%), respectively. A favorable response was seen in 27 patients

(84%) with prostate cancer and in 11 patients (92%) with breast cancer. There was no statistically significant difference in response rates between the prostate and breast cancer patients ($P = .9$). No serious hematological toxicity (grade I/II) was observed in 15 patients (34%), whereas a serious toxicity (grade III/IV) occurred in 10 patients (23%). There was no statistically significant difference in hematological toxicity between the groups.

COMPARING THE PAIN RESPONSE BETWEEN DIFFERENT β-EMITTERS

Dickie and Macfarlane[62] compared ^{89}Sr with [153]Sm in 57 prostate cancer patients. They found no difference in the pain response rate and toxicity. Baczyk and colleagues[63] did a similar comparison between these radionuclides in 100 prostate and breast cancer patients. They reported that the analgesic effects of ^{89}Sr and [153]Sm-EDTMP were similar in both prostate and breast carcinoma patients.

van der Poel and colleagues[24] compared [186]Re-HEDP with ^{89}Sr and reported no differences in the response rate or toxicity. A nonrandomized comparison of [188]Re-HEDP and [153]Sm-EDTMP in patients with painful metastases from prostate and breast cancer by Liepe and colleagues[64] showed a comparable response and toxicity with both agents. Liepe and Kotzerke[9] also performed a comparative study of [188]Re-HEDP, [186]Re-HEDP, [153]Sm-EDTMP, and ^{89}Sr in the treatment of painful bone metastases. They reported that all radiopharmaceuticals were effective in pain palliation, without the induction of severe side effects or significant differences in therapeutic efficacy or toxicity. In a prospective study, Sharma and colleagues[65] compared the therapeutic efficacy of [153]Sm-EDTMP and ^{177}Lu-EDTMP in 30 patients suffering from breast and prostate cancer. Both [153]Sm-EDTMP and ^{177}Lu-EDTMP delivered similar absorbed doses to the metastatic sites. The mean absorbed doses to various other organs were comparable and within the safe limits. A complete response for each radionuclide was evaluated as 80.0%. No significant alteration in blood parameters and no untoward reactions were observed. In another study, Thapa and colleagues[66] showed a similar response efficacy between [153]Sm-EDTMP and ^{177}Lu-EDTMP.

BONE-TARGETED THERAPY WITH THE BONE-SPECIFIC α-EMITTER RADIUM-223 DICHLORIDE

The first, and currently the only, Food and Drug Administration–approved radiopharmaceutical for the treatment of symptomatic bone metastases of CRPC patients with a positive impact on OS is [223]Ra-dichloride.[67] It has a half-life of 11.4 days, with a total emitted energy of approximately 28 MeV. Radium-223 ([223]Ra) has a very high linear energy transfer and a very short penetration range in tissue (<100 μm). Therefore, despite the high energy, because of the short penetration range, bone marrow damage is minimal.[68] Double-strand breaks are induced even in quiescent cells and at low oxygen levels.[69] Thus, the α-particle is considerably more destructive to tumor cells than the β-particle.

In the randomized phase III Alpharadin in Symptomatic Prostate Cancer (ALSYMPCA) trial, 921 patients with progressive and symptomatic bone metastases with at least 2 or more metastases on bone scintigraphy and no known visceral metastases were recruited. Randomization was 2:1 in a double-blind fashion to receive 6 cycles of intravenous [223]Ra every 4 weeks with the best standard of care, or 6 infusions of placebo with the best standard of care. After treatment, there was a significant prolongation of OS (14.9 vs 11.3 months; $P<.001$), the frequency of SREs was reduced in the [223]Ra group, and the median time to a SRE increased (15.6 vs 9.8 months; $P<.001$). [223]Ra patients started subsequent chemotherapy later than placebo patients, and the chemotherapy duration was similar between the groups. In the [223]Ra and placebo patients receiving subsequent chemotherapy, the median hematological values (Hb, neutrophils, and platelets) remained nearly constant for up to 18 months after the start of chemotherapy, regardless of prior docetaxel treatment.[70] [223]Ra was well tolerated with low rates of grade 3/4 neutropenia (1.8% vs 0.8%) and thrombocytopenia (4% vs 2%).[12] An improvement of OS with [223]Ra was accompanied by significant QOL benefits, including a higher percentage of patients with a meaningful QOL improvement and a slower decline in QOL over time in patients with CRPC.[71]

In an open-label, phase IIIb trial,[55] 839 patients with CRPC were enrolled and, of these, 696 received at least 1 dose of [223]Ra, and 403 (58%) of these patients received the targeted 6 injections. The median follow-up period was 7.5 months. The investigators reported a median OS of 16 months. The median OS was longer in patients: with baseline alkaline phosphatase (ALP) concentration less than the upper limit of normal than for patients with ALP concentration equal to or greater than the upper limit of normal (median not reached vs 12 months); patients with baseline Hb levels of greater than or equal to 10 g/dL than for patients with Hb levels less than 10 g/dL (median 17 months vs 10 months); patients with a baseline Eastern

Cooperative Oncology Group (ECOG) performance status (PS) of 0 (median: not reached) than for patients with an ECOG PS of 1 (median: 13 months) or an ECOG PS of 2 or more (median: 7 months); and for patients with no reported baseline pain (median: not reached) than for those with mild pain (median: 14 months) or moderate to severe pain (median: 11 months, range: 9–13). The median OS was longer in patients who received ^{223}Ra plus abiraterone or enzalutamide, or both (median not reached), compared with those who did not receive these therapies (median: 13 months). The median OS was also longer in patients who received ^{223}Ra plus denosumab (median: not reached) compared with patients who received ^{223}Ra without denosumab (median: 13 months). Furthermore, the efficacy of ^{223}Ra in patients who were asymptomatic at baseline was well demonstrated by the investigators. The most common grade 3 or worse treatment-related adverse events were anemia in 5%, thrombocytopenia in 2%, neutropenia in 1%, and leukopenia in 1% of the patients. Any grade of serious adverse events was reported in 35% of the patients. The most common side effects, some of which were dose related, were diarrhea, fatigue, nausea, vomiting, and bone pain.[72–74] These side effects are easily manageable with symptomatic and supportive treatments.[75] Sartor and colleagues[76] have shown the feasibility of retreatment with ^{223}Ra in 44 patients who had undergone 6 initial ^{223}Ra injections. In this study, 66% of the patients received all 6 retreatment injections. No grade 4/5 hematologic treatment emergent adverse events occurred. The median OS and time to the first skeletal event were not reached.

Etchebehere and colleagues[77] retrospectively reviewed 110 patients with metastatic prostate cancer treated with ^{223}Ra. The end points of the study were OS, bone event–free survival (BeFS), PFS, and bone marrow failure. They evaluated the following parameters prior to the first therapy cycle: Hb, PSA, ALP, ECOG status, pain score, prior chemotherapy, and external beam radiation therapy (EBRT). Furthermore, during or after ^{223}Ra, the PSA doubling time (PSADT), the total number of radium cycles (RaTot), the use of chemotherapy, EBRT, enzalutamide, and abiraterone were evaluated. A significant reduction of ALP and pain scores occurred throughout the ^{223}Ra cycles. The risk of progression was associated with a declining ECOG status and a decrease in PSADT. RaTot, the initial ECOG status, ALP, the initial pain score, and the use of abiraterone were associated with OS ($P \leq .008$), PFS ($P \leq .003$), and BeFS ($P \leq .020$). RaTot, the initial ECOG status, ALP, and the initial pain score were significantly associated with

bone marrow failure ($P \leq .001$), as well as Hb (<.001) and EBRT ($P = .009$). In the multivariate analyses, only RaTot and abiraterone remained significantly associated with OS ($P<.001$ and $P = .033$, respectively), PFS ($P <.001$ and $P = .041$, respectively), and BeFS ($P<.001$ and $P = .019$, respectively). Additionally, RaTot ($P = .027$) and EBRT ($P = .013$) remained significantly associated with bone marrow failure. They concluded that the concomitant use of abiraterone and ^{223}Ra seems to have a beneficial effect, while the EBRT may increase the risk of bone marrow failure.

THE PROGNOSTIC UTILITY OF RADIONUCLIDE IMAGING FOR BONE-TARGETED THERAPY

As discussed previously, osteoblastic metastases show a better response to the bone-targeted therapies compared with osteolytic metastases. Different studies have demonstrated the prognostic value of quantitative assessments of bone scintigraphy and ^{18}F-PET for prognostication of clinical outcomes and hematological toxicity in patients treated with bone-specific radionuclides.

Prognostic Value of Bone Scintigraphy

Quantification of skeletal tumor burden on bone scintigraphy can be done by using the EXINI bone software (EXINI Diagnostics, Lund, Sweden), which calculates the percentage of total skeletal mass affected by metastases as the bone scan index (BSI). Fosbol and colleagues[78] reported the utility of the BSI as a prognostic biomarker of OS and hematological toxicity as well as a tool for the response assessment in 88 patients with CRPC treated with ^{223}Ra. BSI was significantly associated with OS in multivariate analysis. The median OS for patients with a BSI greater than 5 was 8.2 months versus 15 months for patients with a BSI less than or equal to 5 ($P = .001$). The baseline BSI was prognostic for the occurrence of hematological toxicity, and patients with a BSI greater than 5 had an odds ratio of 3.02 ($P = .02$) for toxicity. The BSI declined during therapy in 44% of patients who completed 3 cycles of ^{223}Ra ($n = 52$), and in 84% of patients after the end of therapy (n = 32). There was no significant association between BSI changes during therapy and OS. They concluded that the BSI is a promising biomarker for late-stage metastatic CRPC patients receiving ^{223}Ra for prognostication of OS and hematological toxicity.

Prognostic Value of PET

A quantification of a fluoride PET is easier than bone scintigraphy. Rohren and colleagues[79] described a quantification method to assess the skeletal tumor burden with fluoride PET scans. They used the volume of interest (VOI) on whole-body scans and adjusted the maximum standardized uptake value (SUV_{max}) at 10 (according to the established threshold of normal bone uptake), which excludes 99% of all normal bone uptake. They determined the skeletal tumor burden by calculating the fluoride tumor volume within the VOI (FTV_{10}) and the total lesion fluoride uptake as a product of the mean $SUV_{max} \times$ VOI (TLF_{10}).[79] The investigators evaluated the role of the skeletal tumor burden on baseline fluoride PET in predicting OS in patients who had undergone therapy with ^{223}Ra.[80] In this study, Etchebehere and colleagues[80] defined TLF_{10} and FTV_{10} in 42 CRPC patients. TLF_{10} and FTV_{10} at baseline were highly correlated and significant independent predictors of OS ($P = .0212$; HR = 5.990). A TLF_{10} cutoff value of 8000 discriminated the survivors from nonsurvivors after ^{223}Ra (with TLF_{10} values < 8,000, the median OS was not reached, whereas with TLF_{10} > 8,000, the median OS was 6.67 months).

^{18}F-fludeoxyglucose (FDG) PET/CT recognizes bone and bone marrow metastases with a high sensitivity in a majority of cancers compared with other modalities.[81–85]

It has been reported that lytic lesions have a higher SUV and are better detected by FDG PET than sclerotic lesions in patients with progressive disease.[86] Most lytic bone lesions heal with sclerosis, and FDG activity is expected to decrease or resolve after effective treatment.[84,87] At the same time these osteosclerotic lesions could be positive on bone scan suggesting that bone remodeling may continue for an extended period. Therefore, FDG PET may be a better indicator of active bony metastases.[84]

Compared with FDG PET/CT, FDG PET/MR imaging may offer a higher reader confidence without a significant difference in overall detection rate of bony metastases.[88]

In a meta-analysis of 17 article, including 2940 patients suffered from lung cancer, Qu and colleagues[85] reported that both ^{18}FDG PET/CT and ^{18}FDG PET were better imaging methods for diagnosing bone metastasis from lung cancer than MR imaging and bone scintigraphy. ^{18}FDG PET/CT has higher diagnostic value (sensitivity, specificity, and diagnostic odds ratios) for diagnosing bone metastasis from lung cancer than any other imaging methods.

The pooled sensitivity for the detection of bone metastasis in lung cancer using ^{18}FDG PET/CT, ^{18}FDG PET, MR imaging, and bone scintigraphy were 92%, 87%, 77% and 86%, respectively. The pooled specificity using ^{18}FDG PET/CT,

^{18}FDG PET, MR imaging, and bone scintigraphy were 98%, 94%, 92% and 88%, respectively.

In breast cancer, different meta-analysis showed the superiority of FDG PET/CT compared with bone scintigraphy in detection of bone and bone marrow metastases, with a sensitivity of 81% to 90% and specificity of more than 90%.[89–91] Regarding treatment response assessment of bone metastases in breast cancer, it has been reported that FDG PET/CT compared with bone scintigraphy is a powerful tool and consistent with clinical status of the patients because it reflects tumor activity. The investigators showed that bone scintigraphy is insufficient for response assessment of bone metastases because it reflects osteoblastic reaction of the bone against metastatic disease, which increases as the disease responds to treatment.[92]

In prostate cancer, most skeletal metastases have a low glycolytic rate, especially in the hormone-sensitive status of the disease. This could be one of the reasons for controversial reports of different studies regarding the detection rate of FDG PET in prostate cancer bony metastases. Morris and colleagues[93] reported that FDG PET can discriminate active osseous disease from scintigraphically quiescent lesions in patients with progressive metastatic prostate cancer. They showed that post-treatment changes in the SUV tend to correlate with changes in PSA.

Two other studies, however, reported lower sensitivity of FDG PET compared with bone scintigraphy in the detection of bony metastases[94,95]

PET/CT using ^{68}Ga-labelled ligands targeting the PSMA is a sensitive and specific diagnostic modality in prostate cancer diagnostic imaging.[96–98] Bräuer and colleagues[99] reported that ^{68}Ga-PSMA PET/CT revealed, in 15% of patients evaluated for a therapy with ^{223}Ra, previously unknown visceral metastases. In addition, ^{68}Ga-PSMA PET/CT revealed more extended tumor involvement in the bone compared with bone scintigraphy in 9 patients (33%). One other study[100] has demonstrated the utility of ^{68}Ga-PSMA PET as a gatekeeper for the treatment planning of metastatic prostate cancer with ^{223}Ra. The investigators showed that ^{68}Ga-PSMA PET can better select eligible patients for a bone-targeted therapy compared with a bone scan 63 patients who had undergone a total of 307 cycles of therapy with ^{223}Ra were analyzed. In 31 patients, bone scans and radiological imaging were performed for pretherapeutic imaging (group 1). In 32 patients, bone scans and ^{68}Ga-PSMA PET were performed before therapy (group 2). Patients with small lymph node metastases as well as local recurrence were not excluded from treatment, consistent with current guidelines. PSA and ALP

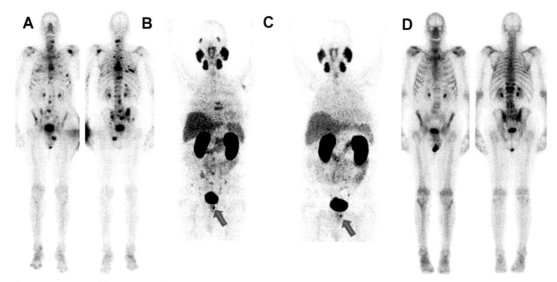

Fig. 1. A 74-year-old patient with CRPC and an increasing PSA level during a running abiraterone and leuprolide acetate therapy. He had a history of radiation therapy for prostate. The bone scintigraphy with ^{99m}Tc-MDP (*A*) showed multiple osteoblastic bone metastases; however, in the same time, the ^{68}Ga-PSMA PET scan showed only a few bone metastases (*B*), which were significantly less in number compared with bone scintigraphy and no lymph node metastases but a small local recurrence (*red arrow*). The PSA and ALP levels prior to the first cycle of ^{223}Ra therapy were 17 ng/mL and 463 U/L, respectively. The patient received 6 cycles of ^{223}Ra and the PSA level decreased continuously during cycles from 17 ng/mL to 1.05 ng/mL (4 weeks after the last cycle). The ALP showed also a decreasing value from 463 to 107 U/L (4 weeks after the last cycle). The PSMA PET (*C*) and bone scintigraphy (*D*) 4 weeks after the last cycle showed a significant response with regression of osteoblastic activity and the PSMA expression.

were measured prior to each treatment cycle and again 4 weeks after the final cycle. In group 1, 4 patients (12.9%) showed a PSA decline, with 1 patient who had a PSA decline greater than 50%. In contrast, in group 2, 14 patients (43.8%) showed a PSA decline, 8 of whom showed a decline greater than 50% ($P = .007$). Overall, 37 patients had a high ALP level (19 from group 1 and 18 from group 2). Twelve (63.2%) and 16 (88.9%) patients from groups 1 and 2, respectively, showed an ALP decline. This difference was not statistically significant; however, 7 (36%) and 13 (72.2%) patients in groups 1 and 2, respectively, showed an ALP decline greater than 30% ($P = .04$). The investigators concluded that using ^{68}Ga-PSMA PET as a gatekeeper, radionuclide therapy with ^{223}Ra may be more effective and successful (**Fig. 1**). The determination of a therapy response with a bone scan may take 4 months to 6 months, meaning that patients may stay on potentially ineffective and toxic treatments for longer than necessary.[101] It seems that metabolic imaging, such as ^{68}Ga-PSMA PET, may be a better option compared with a bone scan for the purpose of follow-up.[102,103] This, however, demands prospective studies be performed.

SUMMARY

A pain relief response is seen in approximately one-half of patients treated with radionuclides for painful osseous metastases. The ALSYMPCA study has shown an OS benefit for patients treated with the α-emitter ^{223}Ra. Other radiopharmaceuticals (exclusively β-emitters) discussed in this review have not yet been tested in prospective multicenter trials with large numbers of patients. They have also shown an OS benefit, however, in various studies.

A combination of hormone therapy with bone-targeted therapy may be more effective compared with a single therapy approach. Radionuclide imaging can improve the planning of bone-targeted therapies and, therefore, potentially lead to improvements in OS, PFS, and toxicity. Radionuclide imaging, especially using PET and PET/CT, is one of the most important modalities for the treatment planning and follow-ups.

FDG PET plays an important role in the detection of bony metastases with higher detection rate compared with bone scintigraphy in a majority of tumor types and consistent with clinical status of the patients as it reflects tumor activity. In prostate cancer, PSMA PET together with bone scintigraphy can be used as a gatekeeper for selection of eligible patients for a radionuclide therapy for bony metastases. Skeletal tumor burden measured by fluoride PET correlates with OS in patients who underwent bone targeted therapies using radionuclides.

REFERENCES

1. Chiang AC, Massague J. Molecular basis of metastasis. N Engl J Med 2008;359:2814–23.
2. Coleman RE. Clinical features of metastatic bone disease and risk of skeletal morbidity. Clin Cancer Res 2006;12:6243s–9s.
3. Yin JJ, Pollock CB, Kelly K. Mechanisms of cancer metastasis to the bone. Cell Res 2005;15: 57–62.
4. Waning DL, Guise TA. Molecular mechanisms of bone metastasis and associated muscle weakness. Clin Cancer Res 2014;20:3071–7.
5. Guise TA, Mohammad KS, Clines G, et al. Basic mechanisms responsible for osteolytic and osteoblastic bone metastases. Clin Cancer Res 2006; 12:6213s–6s.
6. Costa L, Badia X, Chow E, et al. Impact of skeletal complications on patients' quality of life, mobility, and functional independence. Support Care Cancer 2008;16:879–89.
7. Crawford ED, Kozlowski JM, Debruyne FM, et al. The use of strontium 89 for palliation of pain from bone metastases associated with hormone-refractory prostate cancer. Urology 1994;44:481–5.
8. Nair N. Relative efficacy of 32P and 89Sr in palliation in skeletal metastases. J Nucl Med 1999;40: 256–61.
9. Liepe K, Kotzerke J. A comparative study of 188Re-HEDP, 186Re-HEDP, 153Sm-EDTMP and 89Sr in the treatment of painful skeletal metastases. Nucl Med Commun 2007;28:623–30.
10. Yuan J, Liu C, Liu X, et al. Efficacy and safety of 177Lu-EDTMP in bone metastatic pain palliation in breast cancer and hormone refractory prostate cancer: a phase II study. Clin Nucl Med 2013;38: 88–92.
11. Meckel M, Nauth A, Timpe J, et al. Development of a [177Lu]BPAMD labeling kit and an automated synthesis module for routine bone targeted endoradiotherapy. Cancer Biother Radiopharm 2015; 30:94–9.
12. Parker C, Nilsson S, Heinrich D, et al. Alpha emitter radium-223 and survival in metastatic prostate cancer. N Engl J Med 2013;369:213–23.
13. Ahmadzadehfar H. Targeted therapy for metastatic prostate cancer with radionuclides. In: Mohan R, editor. Prostate cancer - leading-edge diagnostic procedures and treatments. Croatia: InTech; 2016.
14. Dietlein M, Eschner W, Grunwald F, et al. Procedure guidelines for radioiodine therapy of differentiated thyroid cancer. Version 4. Nuklearmedizin 2016; 55:77–89 [in German].
15. Franzius C, Schmidt M, Hero B, et al. [Procedure guidelines for MIBG-scintigraphy in children]. Nuklearmedizin 2008;47:132–8.
16. Fendler WP, Kratochwil C, Ahmadzadehfar H, et al. 177Lu-PSMA-617 therapy, dosimetry and follow-up in patients with metastatic castration-resistant prostate cancer. Nuklearmedizin 2016;55:123–8 [in German].
17. Bodei L, Cremonesi M, Grana CM, et al. Peptide receptor radionuclide therapy with (1)(7)(7)Lu-DOTA-TATE: the IEO phase I-II study. Eur J Nucl Med Mol Imaging 2011;38:2125–35.
18. Silberstein EB, Elgazzar AH, Kapilivsky A. Phosphorus-32 radiopharmaceuticals for the treatment of painful osseous metastases. Semin Nucl Med 1992;22:17–27.
19. Lewington VJ, McEwan AJ, Ackery DM, et al. A prospective, randomised double-blind crossover study to examine the efficacy of strontium-89 in pain palliation in patients with advanced prostate cancer metastatic to bone. Eur J Cancer 1991;27: 954–8.
20. Laing AH, Ackery DM, Bayly RJ, et al. Strontium-89 chloride for pain palliation in prostatic skeletal malignancy. Br J Radiol 1991;64:816–22.
21. Mertens WC, Stitt L, Porter AT. Strontium 89 therapy and relief of pain in patients with prostatic carcinoma metastatic to bone: a dose response relationship? Am J Clin Oncol 1993;16:238–42.
22. Mertens WC, Porter AT, Reid RH, et al. Strontium-89 and low-dose infusion cisplatin for patients with hormone refractory prostate carcinoma metastatic to bone: a preliminary report. J Nucl Med 1992; 33:1437–43.
23. Buchali K, Correns HJ, Schuerer M, et al. Results of a double blind study of 89-strontium therapy of skeletal metastases of prostatic carcinoma. Eur J Nucl Med 1988;14:349–51.
24. van der Poel HG, Antonini N, Hoefnagel CA, et al. Serum hemoglobin levels predict response to strontium-89 and rhenium-186-HEDP radionuclide treatment for painful osseous metastases in prostate cancer. Urol Int 2006;77:50–6.
25. Robinson RG, Blake GM, Preston DF, et al. Strontium-89: treatment results and kinetics in patients with painful metastatic prostate and breast cancer in bone. Radiographics 1989;9:271–81.
26. Robinson RG, Preston DF, Schiefelbein M, et al. Strontium 89 therapy for the palliation of pain due to osseous metastases. JAMA 1995;274: 420–4.
27. James ND, Pirrie SJ, Pope AM, et al. Clinical outcomes and survival following treatment of

metastatic castrate-refractory prostate cancer with docetaxel alone or with Strontium-89, Zoledronic Acid, or both: the TRAPEZE randomized clinical trial. JAMA Oncol 2016;2:493–9.

28. James N, Pirrie S, Pope A, et al. TRAPEZE: a randomised controlled trial of the clinical effectiveness and cost-effectiveness of chemotherapy with zoledronic acid, strontium-89, or both, in men with bony metastatic castration-refractory prostate cancer. Health Technol Assess 2016;20:1–288.

29. Windsor PM. Predictors of response to strontium-89 (Metastron) in skeletal metastases from prostate cancer: report of a single centre's 10-year experience. Clin Oncol (R Coll Radiol) 2001;13: 219–27.

30. Oosterhof GO, Roberts JT, de Reijke TM, et al. Strontium(89) chloride versus palliative local field radiotherapy in patients with hormonal escaped prostate cancer: a phase III study of the European Organisation for Research and Treatment of Cancer, Genitourinary Group. Eur Urol 2003;44:519–26.

31. Dafermou A, Colamussi P, Giganti M, et al. A multicentre observational study of radionuclide therapy in patients with painful bone metastases of prostate cancer. Eur J Nucl Med 2001;28: 788–98.

32. Porter AT, McEwan AJ, Powe JE, et al. Results of a randomized phase-III trial to evaluate the efficacy of strontium-89 adjuvant to local field external beam irradiation in the management of endocrine resistant metastatic prostate cancer. Int J Radiat Oncol Biol Phys 1993;25:805–13.

33. Zyskowski A, Lamb D, Morum P, et al. Strontium-89 treatment for prostate cancer bone metastases: does a prostate-specific antigen response predict for improved survival? Australas Radiol 2001;45: 39–42.

34. Lewington VJ. Bone-seeking radionuclides for therapy. J Nucl Med 2005;46(Suppl 1):38S–47S.

35. Maxon HR 3rd, Schroder LE, Hertzberg VS, et al. Rhenium-186(Sn)HEDP for treatment of painful osseous metastases: results of a double-blind crossover comparison with placebo. J Nucl Med 1991;32:1877–81.

36. Liepe K, Franke WG, Kropp J, et al. Comparison of rhenium-188, rhenium-186-HEDP and strontium-89 in palliation of painful bone metastases. Nuklearmedizin 2000;39:146–51 [in German].

37. Sciuto R, Tofani A, Festa A, et al. Short- and long-term effects of 186Re-1,1-hydroxyethylidene diphosphonate in the treatment of painful bone metastases. J Nucl Med 2000;41:647–54.

38. O'Sullivan JM, McCready VR, Flux G, et al. High activity Rhenium-186 HEDP with autologous peripheral blood stem cell rescue: a phase I study in progressive hormone refractory prostate cancer metastatic to bone. Br J Cancer 2002;86:1715–20.

39. Lange R, Overbeek F, de Klerk JM, et al. Treatment of painful bone metastases in prostate and breast cancer patients with the therapeutic radiopharmaceutical rhenium-188-HEDP. Clinical benefit in a real-world study. Nuklearmedizin 2016;55:188–95.

40. Liepe K, Hliscs R, Kropp J, et al. Rhenium-188-HEDP in the palliative treatment of bone metastases. Cancer Biother Radiopharm 2000;15:261–5.

41. Palmedo H, Manka-Waluch A, Albers P, et al. Repeated bone-targeted therapy for hormone-refractory prostate carcinoma: tandomized phase II trial with the new, high-energy radiopharmaceutical rhenium-188 hydroxyethylidenediphosphonate. J Clin Oncol 2003;21:2869–75.

42. Biersack HJ, Palmedo H, Andris A, et al. Palliation and survival after repeated (188)Re-HEDP therapy of hormone-refractory bone metastases of prostate cancer: a retrospective analysis. J Nucl Med 2011; 52:1721–6.

43. Palmedo H, Guhlke S, Bender H, et al. Dose escalation study with rhenium-188 hydroxyethylidene diphosphonate in prostate cancer patients with osseous metastases. Eur J Nucl Med 2000;27: 123–30.

44. van Dodewaard-de Jong JM, de Klerk JMH, Bloemendal HJ, et al. A randomised, phase II study of repeated rhenium-188-HEDP combined with docetaxel and prednisone versus docetaxel and prednisone alone in castration-resistant prostate cancer (CRPC) metastatic to bone; the Taxium II trial. Eur J Nucl Med Mol Imaging 2017;44: 1319–27.

45. Liepe K, Kropp J, Runge R, et al. Therapeutic efficiency of rhenium-188-HEDP in human prostate cancer skeletal metastases. Br J Cancer 2003;89: 625–9.

46. Kolesnikov-Gauthier H, Lemoine N, Tresch-Bruneel E, et al. Efficacy and safety of 153Sm-EDTMP as treatment of painful bone metastasis: a large single-center study. Support Care Cancer 2018;26(3):751–8.

47. Tian JH, Zhang JM, Hou QT, et al. Multicentre trial on the efficacy and toxicity of single-dose samarium-153-ethylene diamine tetramethylene phosphonate as a palliative treatment for painful skeletal metastases in China. Eur J Nucl Med 1999;26:2–7.

48. Sartor O, Reid RH, Hoskin PJ, et al. Samarium-153-Lexidronam complex for treatment of painful bone metastases in hormone-refractory prostate cancer. Urology 2004;63:940–5.

49. Ayati N, Aryana K, Jalilian A, et al. Treatment efficacy of (153)Sm-EDTMP for painful bone metastasis. Asia Ocean J Nucl Med Biol 2013; 1:27–31.

50. Enrique O, Zhongyun P, Parma EP, et al. Efficacy and toxicity of Sm-153 EDTMP in the palliative

treatment of painful bone metastases. World J Nucl Med 2002;1(1):21–7.

51. Borso E, Boni G, Pastina I, et al. Safety and antitumor efficacy of (153)Sm-EDTMP and docetaxel administered sequentially to patients with metastatic castration-resistant prostate cancer. Nucl Med Commun 2014;35:88–94.

52. Autio KA, Pandit-Taskar N, Carrasquillo JA, et al. Repetitively dosed docetaxel and (1)(5)(3) samarium-EDTMP as an antitumor strategy for metastatic castration-resistant prostate cancer. Cancer 2013;119:3186–94.

53. Fizazi K, Beuzeboc P, Lumbroso J, et al. Phase II trial of consolidation docetaxel and samarium-153 in patients with bone metastases from castration-resistant prostate cancer. J Clin Oncol 2009;27: 2429–35.

54. Lin J, Sinibaldi VJ, Carducci MA, et al. Phase I trial with a combination of docetaxel and (1)(5)(3)Sm-lexidronam in patients with castration-resistant metastatic prostate cancer. Urol Oncol 2011;29: 670–5.

55. Saad F, Carles J, Gillessen S, et al. Radium-223 and concomitant therapies in patients with metastatic castration-resistant prostate cancer: an international, early access, open-label, single-arm phase 3b trial. Lancet Oncol 2016;17:1306–16.

56. Yordanova A, Mayer K, Brossart P, et al. Safety of multiple repeated cycles of 177Lu-octreotate in patients with recurrent neuroendocrine tumour. Eur J Nucl Med Mol Imaging 2017;44:1207–14.

57. Ahmadzadehfar H, Eppard E, Kurpig S, et al. Therapeutic response and side effects of repeated radioligand therapy with 177Lu-PSMA-DKFZ-617 of castrate-resistant metastatic prostate cancer. Oncotarget 2016;7:12477–88.

58. Afshar-Oromieh A, Hetzheim H, Kratochwil C, et al. The theranostic PSMA ligand PSMA-617 in the diagnosis of prostate cancer by PET/CT: biodistribution in humans, radiation dosimetry, and first evaluation of tumor lesions. J Nucl Med 2015; 56:1697–705.

59. Fakhari A, Jalilian AR, Yousefnia H, et al. Radiolabeling and evaluation of two 177Lu-labeled bisphosphonates. Iran J Nucl Med 2015;23:108–15.

60. Alavi M, Omidvari S, Mehdizadeh A, et al. Metastatic bone pain palliation using (177)Lu-ethylenediaminetetramethylene phosphonic acid. World J Nucl Med 2015;14:109–15.

61. Agarwal KK, Singla S, Arora G, et al. (177)Lu-EDTMP for palliation of pain from bone metastases in patients with prostate and breast cancer: a phase II study. Eur J Nucl Med Mol Imaging 2015;42:79–88.

62. Dickie GJ, Macfarlane D. Strontium and samarium therapy for bone metastases from prostate carcinoma. Australas Radiol 1999;43:476–9.

63. Baczyk M, Czepczynski R, Milecki P, et al. 89Sr versus 153Sm-EDTMP: comparison of treatment efficacy of painful bone metastases in prostate and breast carcinoma. Nucl Med Commun 2007;28: 245–50.

64. Liepe K, Runge R, Kotzerke J. The benefit of bone-seeking radiopharmaceuticals in the treatment of metastatic bone pain. J Cancer Res Clin Oncol 2005;131:60–6.

65. Sharma S, Singh B, Koul A, et al. Comparative therapeutic efficacy of 153Sm-EDTMP and 177Lu-EDTMP for bone pain palliation in patients with skeletal metastases: patients' pain score analysis and personalized dosimetry. Front Med (Lausanne) 2017;4:46.

66. Thapa P, Nikam D, Das T, et al. Clinical efficacy and safety comparison of 177Lu-EDTMP with 153Sm-EDTMP on an equidose basis in patients with painful skeletal metastases. J Nucl Med 2015;56:1513–9.

67. Parker C, Sartor O. Radium-223 in prostate cancer. N Engl J Med 2013;369:1659–60.

68. Hafeez S, Parker C. Radium-223 for the treatment of prostate cancer. Expert Opin Investig Drugs 2013;22:379–87.

69. Anderson RM, Stevens DL, Sumption ND, et al. Effect of linear energy transfer (LET) on the complexity of alpha-particle-induced chromosome aberrations in human CD34+ cells. Radiat Res 2007;167:541–50.

70. Sartor O, Hoskin P, Coleman RE, et al. Chemotherapy following radium-223 dichloride treatment in ALSYMPCA. Prostate 2016;76:905–16.

71. Nilsson S, Cislo P, Sartor O, et al. Patient-reported quality-of-life analysis of radium-223 dichloride from the phase III ALSYMPCA study. Ann Oncol 2016;27:868–74.

72. Nilsson S, Larsen RH, Fossa SD, et al. First clinical experience with alpha-emitting radium-223 in the treatment of skeletal metastases. Clin Cancer Res 2005;11:4451–9.

73. Nilsson S, Franzen L, Parker C, et al. Bone-targeted radium-223 in symptomatic, hormone-refractory prostate cancer: a randomised, multicentre, placebo-controlled phase II study. Lancet Oncol 2007;8:587–94.

74. Parker CC, Pascoe S, Chodacki A, et al. A randomized, double-blind, dose-finding, multicenter, phase 2 study of radium chloride (Ra 223) in patients with bone metastases and castration-resistant prostate cancer. Eur Urol 2013;63:189–97.

75. Pacilio M, Ventroni G, De Vincentis G, et al. Dosimetry of bone metastases in targeted radionuclide therapy with alpha-emitting (223)Ra-dichloride. Eur J Nucl Med Mol Imaging 2016;43: 21–33.

76. Sartor O, Heinrich D, Mariados N, et al. Re-treat-ment with radium-223: first experience from an international, open-label, phase I/II study in pa-tients with castration-resistant prostate cancer and bone metastases. Ann Oncol 2017;28: 2464–71.

77. Etchebehere EC, Milton DR, Araujo JC, et al. Fac-tors affecting (223)Ra therapy: clinical experience after 532 cycles from a single institution. Eur J Nucl Med Mol Imaging 2016;43:8–20.

78. Fosbol MO, Petersen PM, Kjaer A, et al. Radium-223 therapy of advanced metastatic castration-resistant prostate cancer: quantitative assessment of skeletal tumor burden for prognostication of clin-ical outcome and hematological toxicity. J Nucl Med 2018;59(4):596–602.

79. Rohren EM, Etchebehere EC, Araujo JC, et al. Determination of skeletal tumor burden on 18F-Fluoride PET/CT. J Nucl Med 2015;56: 1507–12.

80. Etchebehere EC, Araujo JC, Fox PS, et al. Prog-nostic factors in patients treated with 223Ra: the role of skeletal tumor burden on baseline 18F-Fluo-ride PET/CT in predicting overall survival. J Nucl Med 2015;56:1177–84.

81. Liu FY, Yen TC, Chen MY, et al. Detection of hema-togenous bone metastasis in cervical cancer: 18F-fluorodeoxyglucose-positron emission tomog-raphy versus computed tomography and magnetic resonance imaging. Cancer 2009;115:5470–80.

82. Mahner S, Schirrmacher S, Brenner W, et al. Comparison between positron emission tomogra-phy using 2-[fluorine-18]fluoro-2-deoxy-D-glucose, conventional imaging and computed tomography for staging of breast cancer. Ann Oncol 2008;19: 1249–54.

83. Kim MR, Roh JL, Kim JS, et al. 18F-fluorodeoxyglu-cose-positron emission tomography and bone scintigraphy for detecting bone metastases in pa-tients with malignancies of the upper aerodigestive tract. Oral Oncol 2008;44:148–52.

84. Costelloe CM, Chuang HH, Madewell JE. FDG PET for the detection of bone metastases: sensitivity, specificity and comparison with other imaging mo-dalities. PET Clin 2010;5:281–95.

85. Qu X, Huang X, Yan W, et al. A meta-analysis of (1)(8)FDG-PET-CT, (1)(8)FDG-PET, MRI and bone scintigraphy for diagnosis of bone metastases in patients with lung cancer. Eur J Radiol 2012;81: 1007–15.

86. Cook GJ, Houston S, Rubens R, et al. Detection of bone metastases in breast cancer by 18FDG PET: differing metabolic activity in osteoblastic and os-teolytic lesions. J Clin Oncol 1998;16:3375–9.

87. Israel O, Goldberg A, Nachtigal A, et al. FDG-PET and CT patterns of bone metastases and their rela-tionship to previously administered anti-cancer therapy. Eur J Nucl Med Mol Imaging 2006;33: 1280–4.

88. Samarin A, Hullner M, Queiroz MA, et al. 18F-FDG-PET/MR increases diagnostic confidence in detection of bone metastases compared with 18F-FDG-PET/CT. Nucl Med Commun 2015;36:1165–73.

89. Isasi CR, Moadel RM, Blaufox MD. A meta-analysis of FDG-PET for the evaluation of breast cancer recurrence and metastases. Breast Cancer Res Treat 2005;90:105–12.

90. Shie P, Cardarelli R, Brandon D, et al. Meta-anal-ysis: comparison of F-18 Fluorodeoxyglucose-positron emission tomography and bone scintigraphy in the detection of bone metastases in patients with breast cancer. Clin Nucl Med 2008;33:97–101.

91. Rong J, Wang S, Ding Q, et al. Comparison of 18 FDG PET-CT and bone scintigraphy for detection of bone metastases in breast cancer patients. A meta-analysis. Surg Oncol 2013;22:86–91.

92. Al-Muqbel KM, Yaghan RJ. Effectiveness of 18F-FDG-PET/CT vs bone scintigraphy in treatment response assessment of bone metastases in breast cancer. Medicine (Baltimore) 2016;95: e3753.

93. Morris MJ, Akhurst T, Osman I, et al. Fluorinated deoxyglucose positron emission tomography im-aging in progressive metastatic prostate cancer. Urology 2002;59:913–8.

94. Shreve PD, Grossman HB, Gross MD, et al. Metastatic prostate cancer: initial findings of PET with 2-deoxy-2-[F-18]fluoro-D-glucose. Radiology 1996;199:751–6.

95. Yeh SD, Imbriaco M, Larson SM, et al. Detection of bony metastases of androgen-independent pros-tate cancer by PET-FDG. Nucl Med Biol 1996;23: 693–7.

96. Afshar-Oromieh A, Avtzi E, Giesel FL, et al. The diagnostic value of PET/CT imaging with the (68) Ga-labelled PSMA ligand HBED-CC in the diag-nosis of recurrent prostate cancer. Eur J Nucl Med Mol Imaging 2015;42:197–209.

97. Afshar-Oromieh A, Haberkorn U, Eder M, et al. [68Ga]Gallium-labelled PSMA ligand as superior PET tracer for the diagnosis of prostate cancer: comparison with 18F-FECH. Eur J Nucl Med Mol Imaging 2012;39:1085–6.

98. Afshar-Oromieh A, Holland-Letz T, Giesel FL, et al. Diagnostic performance of 68Ga-PSMA-11 (HBED-CC) PET/CT in patients with recurrent prostate can-cer: evaluation in 1007 patients. Eur J Nucl Med Mol Imaging 2017;44:1258–68.

99. Bräuer A, Rahbar K, Konnert J, et al. Diagnostic value of additional 68Ga-PSMA-PET before 223Ra-dichloride therapy in patients with metasta-tic prostate carcinoma. Nuklearmedizin 2017;56: 14–22.

100. Ahmadzadehfar H, Azgomi K, Hauser S, et al. 68Ga-PSMA-11 PET as a gatekeeper for the treatment of metastatic prostate cancer with 223Ra: proof of concept. J Nucl Med 2017;58: 438–44.

101. Azad GK, Taylor B, Rubello D, et al. Molecular and functional imaging of bone metastases in breast and prostate cancers: an overview. Clin Nucl Med 2016;41:e44–50.

102. Ahmadzadehfar H, Schlenkhoff CD, Rogenhofer S, et al. 68Ga-PSMA-11 PET represents the tumoricidal effect of 223Ra in a patient with castrate-resistant metastatic prostate cancer. Clin Nucl Med 2016;41:695–6.

103. Hama Y. Antitumor effect of 89Sr for multiple bone metastases of breast cancer: diagnosis by 18F-FDG PET/CT. Clin Nucl Med 2014;39:e290–1.

104. Pandit-Taskar N, Larson SM, Carrasquillo JA. Bone-seeking radiopharmaceuticals for treatment of osseous metastases, Part 1: alpha therapy with 223Ra-dichloride. J Nucl Med 2014;55:268–74.

105. Falkmer U, Jarhult J, Wersall P, et al. A systematic overview of radiation therapy effects in skeletal metastases. Acta Oncol 2003;42:620–33.

Whole-Body MR Imaging
The Novel, "Intrinsically Hybrid," Approach to Metastases, Myeloma, Lymphoma, in Bones and Beyond

Frederic E. Lecouvet, MD, PhD[a,*],
Sandy Van Nieuwenhove, MD[a], François Jamar, MD, PhD[b],
Renaud Lhommel, MD[b], Ali Guermazi, MD, PhD[c],
Vassiliki P. Pasoglou, MD, PhD[a]

KEYWORDS

- WB-MR imaging • DWI • Bone metastases • Rheumatology • PET

KEY POINTS

- Using anatomic and functional sequences, whole-body MR imaging (WB-MR imaging) offers a "hybrid" approach to global cancer staging, maximizing early detection of different lesion types for all-organ screening and assessment of therapeutic response.
- WB-MR imaging is now a commonly applied and recommended modality for bone screening for "osteophilic" metastases in the case of solid cancers, lymphoma, and multiple myeloma and expands screening to visceral and nodal involvement.
- Efforts have been made for the optimization of the technique, minimization of acquisition times, and harmonization in sequence acquisition, reading, reporting, and evaluation of lesion response to treatment.

INTRODUCTION

Since its advent almost 20 years ago, whole-body MR imaging (WB-MR imaging), using bone and visceral organ-targeting anatomic T1 and short-tau inversion recovery (STIR) sequences, has become a powerful, global tool for detecting skeletal involvement by metastases and to match or exceed available imaging standards, that is, bone scintigraphy and computed tomography (CT).[1,2] The efficacy of WB-MR imaging has increased because of the development of the diffusion-weighted imaging (DWI) sequences, refinements in sequence combinations, and extension of anatomic imaging targets from the skeleton to all organs.[3] Through its combination of anatomic and functional sequences, WB-MR imaging has become a unique, intrinsically hybrid technique, now available for use in oncology.[4]

Its diagnostic accuracy for multiorgan screening is comparable to PET for many indications, without the need to combine nuclear and radiological

Disclosures: F.E. Lecouvet, S. Van Nieuwenhove, and V.P. Pasoglou's works have been supported by grants from the Belgian nonprofit organizations Fonds de la Recherche Scientifique (FRS-FNRS), Fondation Contre le Cancer, Fondation Saint Luc, and Fonds de Recherche Clinique (Cliniques Universitaires Saint-Luc).
[a] Department of Radiology, Centre du Cancer and Institut de Recherche Expérimentale et Clinique (IREC–IMAG), Cliniques Universitaires Saint-Luc, Université Catholique de Louvain (UCL), Avenue Hippocrate 10/2942, Brussels B-1200, Belgium; [b] Department of Nuclear Medicine, Centre du Cancer and Institut de Recherche Expérimentale et Clinique (IREC–IMAG), Cliniques Universitaires Saint-Luc, Université Catholique de Louvain (UCL), Avenue Hippocrate 10/2942, Brussels B-1200, Belgium; [c] Department of Radiology, Boston University School of Medicine, 820 Harrison Avenue, FGH Building, 3rd floor, Boston, MA 02118, USA
* Corresponding author.
E-mail address: frederic.lecouvet@uclouvain.be

PET Clin 13 (2018) 505–522
https://doi.org/10.1016/j.cpet.2018.05.006
1556-8598/18/© 2018 Elsevier Inc. All rights reserved.

imaging methods or use radioactive tracers. Extensive knowledge of pathologic processes is required for WB-MR imaging reading, because of the quantity of information provided on all organs within the body.[5]

The usefulness of WB-MR imaging has recently been expanded to rheumatology, probing axial and extra-axial involvement in disorders such as spondyloarthropathies, detecting and mapping bone, muscle, tendon, fascia, vessels or nerves.[5]

This article illustrates the general principles of WB-MR imaging, explains how the technique combines anatomic and metabolic information, describes novel state-of-the-art sequences, and provides an overview of established oncologic indications and developing applications. The comparison to alternative imaging modalities is also provided.

GENERAL PRINCIPLES AND IMAGING PLANES

To generate WB-MR images, reconstructive software fuses consecutive stacks of high-spatial-resolution images covering consecutive 20- to 50-cm fields of view from either "head to toe" or "eyes to thighs."[6] The feasibility of all anatomic and functional pulse sequences has been demonstrated with both 1.5- and 3-T magnets.[7–10]

Anatomic images are most often acquired in the coronal or axial planes, offering extensive coverage of body.[11] Sagittal sequences on the spine are necessary for evaluating the neurologic and skeletal consequences of complicated tumors.[12–16] This choice of imaging planes may become superfluous shortly with the increasing use of 3-dimensional anatomic sequences with thin slices and isotropic voxel size, allowing multiplanar reformatting and extensive body coverage.[17]

Gadolinium injection is used only for WB-MR imaging if screening for meningeal carcinomatosis or epiduritis, or liver or brain metastases, is required, depending on the primary cancer.[16,18] Gadolinium-enhanced MR imaging can be used in disease staging in multiple myeloma (MM) and lymphoma, but the use of WB-DWI often renders this injection unnecessary.[19]

DWI sequences are usually acquired in the axial plane and read on workstations as multiplanar reformatted (MPR) or maximal intensity projection (MIP) views, often as inverted-grayscale images, linked to corresponding anatomic sequences for optimal correlations and lesion interpretation (**Figs. 1** and **2**).

ANATOMIC SEQUENCES

MR imaging sequences include anatomic pulse sequences, which delineate organs and show physicochemical tissue content, and metabolic pulse sequences, that is, DWI, which probe tissue cellularity, viability, and vascularity. For anatomic pulse sequences, the T1-weighted sequence is most useful for evaluating the bone marrow composition in oncologic conditions.[20] The extension of cancer screening to organs beyond bones may require dedicated, "fluid-sensitive" pulse sequences depending on clinical indication,[9] including T2-, fat-suppressed T2-, or STIR-weighted images.[21]

Regardless of the skeletal region, bone marrow replacement by neoplastic cells has consistent characteristics on T1-weighted images. Tumor cells are indicated by focal or diffuse low signal intensity with a lower intensity signal in the marrow than skeletal muscles and intervertebral disks.[20,22] In MM with diffuse low-grade infiltration, the bone marrow may present an additional "salt and pepper" appearance due to the presence of multiple tiny abnormalities, or may even appear normal.[20,23] The signal of bone lesions on T2-, fat-suppressed T2-weighted, and STIR images is variable, depending on the water content and lesion phenotype, that is, its more or less hydrated or sclerotic composition.[21,24] Previous research highlighted that STIR is particularly sensitive in detecting bone involvement by breast cancer metastases and lymphoma, whereas more recent research suggests that it could be abandoned from most oncologic protocols.[24] T2 images are mainly used for visceral organs and lymph node evaluations.

FUNCTIONAL SEQUENCES: DIFFUSION-WEIGHTED IMAGING

DWI has been introduced to WB-MR imaging studies for oncologic lesion screening and whole-body examination as a functional pulse sequence.[25,26] Fat-suppressed single-shot spin-echo echo-planar DWI sequences use high-diffusion sensitizing gradients combining several b values, which allow the concurrent acquisition of diagnostic images and calculation of apparent diffusion coefficients (ADC). These quantitative parameters enable tissue probing and quantification of tissue diffusion characteristics throughout treatment.[25,27] Its high contrast makes DWI particularly useful for detecting bone lesions in areas difficult to study with anatomic pulse sequences (ribs, thoracic girdle) and for detecting visceral lesions, especially lymphadenopathies and peritoneal nodules (see **Figs. 1** and **2**).[14]

DWI effectively detects tumor involvement through its sensitivity to the impediment on water molecule diffusion, which differs in tumors

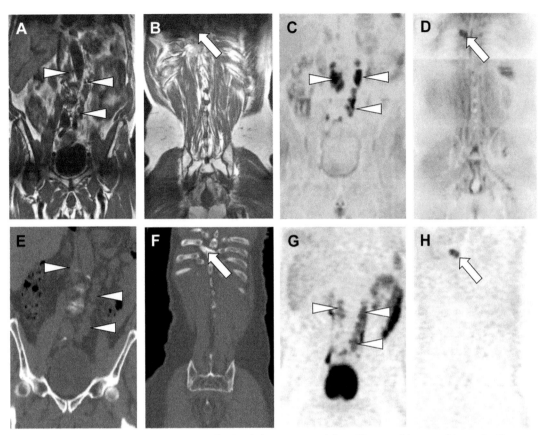

Fig. 1. WB-MR imaging and PSMA PET/CT obtained the same week in a 68-year-old man with newly diagnosed prostate cancer evaluated for N and M staging. (A–D) WB-MR imaging consisting of (A, B) anatomic T1 and (C, D) functional DWI sequences show multiple abnormal lymph nodes in the lumboaortic area (arrowheads in A and C) and bone metastasis in the right transverse process of a midthoracic vertebra (arrows in B and D). (E–H) PSMA PET/CT using corresponding (E, F) reformatted coronal CT images and (G, H) metabolic PET images show the same abnormal lymph nodes area (arrowheads in E and G) and sclerotic bone metastasis (arrow in F and H).

compared with normal tissue, depending on many cellular factors.[28] Impeded diffusion and decreased ADC values observed in tumors are often attributed to the accumulation of membrane interfaces and loss of extracellular spaces resulting from the high cell density in tumors.[8,29] In bones, the detection of tumoral foci relies on a higher lesion signal intensity on high b-value DWI images and increased ADC values in tumors compared with normal marrow, increased T1 and T2 relaxation times, increased water content, increased vascularity, and absence of fat.[30] Interestingly, DWI allows noninvasive evaluation of treatment response through follow-up over time of the global tumor volume as measured by ADC values from high b-value images and of individual lesion changes after treatment.[31,32]

Although high b-value DWI images offer outstanding sensitivity, allowing an "at a glance"

and global view of tumoral foci, they must be correlated to ADC maps and anatomic pulse sequences to avoid false positive observations, which can occur with benign conditions (ie, hemangiomas, benign fractures, degenerative joint disorders) that present as abnormal foci on high b-value images.[33–35] The "T2 shine-through" phenomenon makes tissues with a long T2 decay time, in particular necrotic tumors or edema, present a high signal intensity suggestive of a tumoral lesion on high b-value images.[36,37] This uncertainty is solved by correlating the DWI with anatomic pulse sequences and demonstrating high ADC values in "shine-through" areas and low ADC values in tumors.[38] Subtle diffuse bone marrow infiltration seen in early stages of MM and primarily or treatment-related sclerotic bone metastases may represent false negative of DWI, but are detected easily by study of anatomic sequences.[28,39]

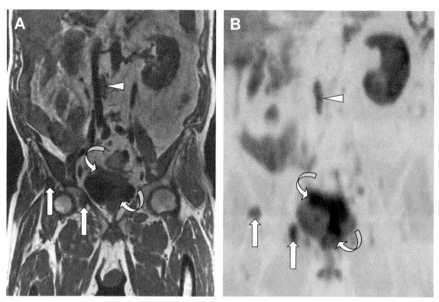

Fig. 2. WB-MR imaging for "all-in-one" TNM staging in a 65-year-old man with recurrent prostate cancer. (*A*) Anatomic T1 and (*B*) functional DWI MR images show, in one nonirradiating examination, the local (T) recurrence with infiltration of the prostate, bladder, and seminal vesicles (*curved arrows*), nodes in the lumboaortic area (N) (*arrowheads*), and 2 bone metastasis (M) within the right iliac bone (*arrows*).

METASTATIC CANCER

WB-MR imaging was first used in cancers that occur in bone (eg, MM, lymphoma) or commonly result in osseous metastases (eg, prostate, breast).[9,14,15,40,41] It allows earlier and more reliable detection of metastases than bone scintigraphy and CT, leading to earlier treatment initiation and reliable treatment response evaluation.[42–44] **Table 1** provides an overview of WB-MR imaging oncologic indications, and **Table 2** provides the multiparametric sequences used for metastatic cancers, lymphoma, and MM.

"Osteophilic" (Prostate and Breast) Cancers

In prostate cancer, WB-MR imaging's combined anatomic and functional sequences outperform bone scintigraphy in bone staging and thoracoadbominopelvic CT for a one-step node (N) and visceral (M) staging (see **Fig. 1**).[14] WB-MR imaging has also been proposed for concurrent local (T), N, and M staging in particular patients, either at diagnosis or by the time of biochemical recurrence in prostate cancer (see **Fig. 2**).[45,46]

A meta-analysis reported that MR imaging had a sensitivity of 95% and specificity of 96% for detecting bone metastases, with a significantly higher area under a receiver operating characteristic curve (AUC) of 0.987 than either choline PET (sensitivity: 87%, specificity: 97%, AUC: 0.951) or bone scintigraphy (sensitivity: 79%, specificity:

82%, AUC: 0.888).[59] Another meta-analysis of 10 studies including 1031 patients with prostate cancer found a sensitivity of 96% and a specificity of 98% and suggested the use of at least 2 imaging planes for optimal sensitivity.[60]

Another recent application of WB-MR imaging in prostate cancer is the reliable detection of oligometastatic disease, for which specific treatments with a curative intent have been developed. Conde-Moreno and colleagues[61] showed that choline-PET/CT with a higher sensitivity and WB-MR imaging with DWI may be complementary techniques in this setting. Larbi and colleagues[62] in another study demonstrated the interest of WB-MR imaging screening for oligometastatic disease as most metastases were located outside the usual anatomic targets of salvage surgery and radiotherapy performed in recurrent prostate cancer.

WB-MR imaging with DWI now rivals choline-PET/CT and should be compared in further studies with prostate-specific membrane antigen-PET (PSMA-PET) and other emerging nuclear medicine tracers in prostate cancer (see **Fig. 1**).[61] Preliminary results suggest that PSMA-PET/CT improves nodal staging in initial workup of prostate cancer compared with pelvic MR imaging.[63]

Concerning breast cancer metastases, WB-MR imaging is the favored technique for patients who exhibit bone predominant or exclusive metastatic diseases, for staging and assessment of treatment

Table 1
Current applications of whole-body-MR imaging in oncology

Cancer Categories	Indications
Prostate cancer	Newly diagnosed, high risk for metastases (upfront or after negative or nonconclusive bone scintigraphy)[4] Biochemical recurrence (as general staging aside from local staging with multiparametric MR imaging of the prostate and pelvis for salvage therapy planning)[45,46] Response assessment in advanced disease, castrate-resistant state when PSA and clinical symptoms are less valuable, and in primary aggressive variants (adenocarcinoma, small cell, neuroendocrine) or oligosecretory forms[5,47] All stages: oligometastatic disease (detection, treatment planning, and monitoring)
Breast cancer	High-risk patients; metastatic disease with preferential or exclusive bone tropism (upfront or after negative or nonconclusive bone scintigraphy)[48] Response assessment in predominant or exclusive bone metastatic disease[49] All stages: oligometastatic disease (detection, treatment planning, and monitoring)
Lung, melanoma, thyroid, neuroendocrine, renal, ovarian, testicular cancers; myxoid liposarcoma	First line or as alternative to other imaging modalities (see text)
MM	Asymptomatic and smoldering myeloma, solitary plasmocytoma (primary indication

(continued on next page)

Table 1
(continued)

Cancer Categories	Indications
	IMWG guidelines)[50] First-line imaging in suspected MM (NICE guidelines UK)[51] Non- or hyposecretory myeloma for initial assessment, follow-up, and response to treatment
Lymphoma	Lymphomas especially variable or poorly FDG avid forms[52] All lymphomas with potential bone involvement[53] Response assessment[54,55]
(Predisposition to) cancer with emphasis on absence of irradiation	Pediatric lymphoma or solid cancer (Ewing sarcoma, osteosarcoma, rhabdomyosarcoma)[56] Li-Fraumeni and other cancer-predisposing syndromes[57] Pregnancy[58] Multiple exostosis, neurofibromatosis

Abbreviations: IMWG, International Myeloma Working Group; PSA, prostate-specific antigen.

response. WB-MR imaging also outperforms fluorodeoxyglucose (FDG) PET/CT in detecting bone and liver lesions (**Fig. 3**).[9] Di Gioia and colleagues[18] found that a reproducible tumor marker increase followed by either WB-MR imaging or FDG-PET/CT scan is a highly effective follow-up care paradigm for detecting asymptomatic breast cancer recurrence.

In a study including both patients with breast and patients with prostate cancer, Jambor and colleagues[64] found sensitivity of 100% and specificity of 88% to 97% for WB-MR imaging with DWI sequences and sensitivity of 95% to 100% and specificity of 82% to 97% for fluoride PET/CT, significantly exceeding the diagnostic accuracy of bone scintigraphy and single-photon emission CT.

Other Cancers

In non–small-cell lung cancer, the diagnostic accuracy of WB-MR imaging with anatomic and DWI pulse sequences is higher than that of either sequence alone and of PET/CT.[34,65] In a study of 96 consecutive postoperative patients with non–

Table 2
Basic components of whole-body-MR imaging "multiparametric" protocols in metastatic cancer, myeloma and lymphoma

Sequence Types	Planes and Technique	Indications

Anatomic, WB coverage
  T1-weighted
  STIR
  T2-weighted
  Optional: contrast-enhanced
  T1-weighted
	Axial or coronal acquisition
	"Eyes to thighs"
	2D FSE or GE; 3D FSE or GE (Dixon technique)
	Adapted inversion time
	2D FSE without fat suppression
		Bones; nodes
		Increases sensitivity in bones; nodes and liver
		Nodes and liver
		Brain and liver (breast, lung)

Functional sequences, WB coverage DWI	Axial or coronal acquisition Fat suppressed, at least 2 b values (50–150 s/mm^2, 800–1000 s/mm^2) MPR or MIP reading, inverted gray scale	High b-value images for detection (bones, nodes, solid organs) Low b-value images as alternative to T2 images, nodes and liver ADC maps for characterization

Optional, anatomic spine coverage (superfluous if anatomic sequences use 3D option)
  T1-weighted
  STIR
	Sagittal	Vertebrae
		Vertebrae, canal compromise, neurologic compression

Abbreviations: FSE, fast spin echo; GE, gradient echo.

small-cell lung cancer, whole-body FDG-PET/MR imaging and WB-MR imaging with DWI were found to be more specific and accurate than FDG-PET/CT and routine radiological examinations for assessment of recurrence. However, MR imaging and MR imaging with DWI demonstrated slightly lower sensitivity than PET/CT.[66]

Current staging guidelines for both lung and colorectal cancers recommend sequential use of various imaging modalities, including CT and PET, for detection of metastases. To determine a staging alternative, the multicenter Streamline trials plan to assess whether WB-MR imaging improves identification of the metastases of non–small-cell lung and colorectal cancers, but no conclusions have been yet reported.[67]

In thyroid cancer, WB-MR imaging with DWI and PET/CT has significantly better accuracy compared with WB-MR imaging anatomic sequences alone, indicating that combinations of sequences or modalities improve the diagnostic performance.[68]

In malignant melanoma, preliminary research investigating WB-MR imaging has reached varied conclusions. Mosavi and colleagues[69] determined that WB-MR imaging is not yet a suitable substitute for CT in staging, but it is valuable for bone lesion detection if conventional sequences and DWI are combined. Petralia and colleagues[70] found that WB-MR imaging with DWI was promising for detecting extracranial metastases, but that contrast-enhanced MR imaging was necessary for evaluating the brain.

Comparisons have shown that both PET-CT and WB-MR imaging have high diagnostic accuracy with differing organ-specific detection rates: WB-MR imaging had higher performance in detecting hepatic, skeletal, and brain metastases, whereas PET-CT had a higher accuracy in N staging and in pulmonary and soft tissue metastases.[71] In the authors' experience, WB-MR imaging is an effective diagnostic modality, especially if DWI and Dixon-T1 with fat-suppressed (water) images are included, combining sensitivity to impeded diffusion and melanin content (**Fig. 4**).

In neuroendocrine tumors, CT is the current reference standard cross-sectional imaging modality for staging. Moryoussef and colleagues[72] retrospectively analyzed 22 abnormal WB-MR imaging with and without DWI to determine the efficacy of WB-MR imaging as a new staging paradigm for neuroendocrine tumor staging and observed that adding DWI sequences to standard MR imaging revealed additional metastases and significantly affected therapeutic decisions. A study by Schraml and colleagues[73] that compared WB-MR imaging to [^{68}GA]DOTATOC multiphase PET/CT determined that PET/CT and WB-MR imaging exhibited comparable overall lesion-based metastasis detection rates, but differed in organ-

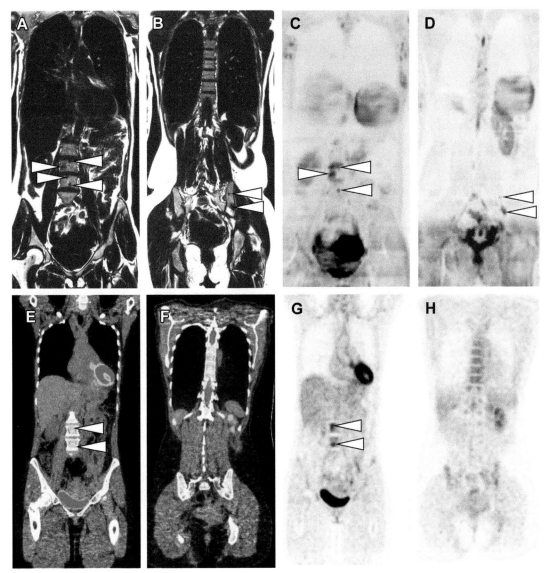

Fig. 3. Comparison of WB-MR imaging and [18]FDG PET findings in a 28-year-old woman with breast cancer. (A–D) WB-MR imaging combining (A, B) anatomic T1 and (C, D) functional DWI sequences show bone lesions with a low signal on T1 (*arrowheads* in A and B) and high signal on DWI (*arrowheads* in C and D) corresponding to metastases in the lumbar spine and posterior iliac crest. (E–H) [18]FDG PET/CT correlation (E, F) corresponding to reformatted fused PET/CT images and (G, H) metabolic PET images show the same abnormal lumbar metastases (*arrowheads* in E and G) but do not detect the posterior iliac lesions.

based detection rates; PET/CT was superior for lymph node and pulmonary lesions, and WB-MR imaging was superior for liver and bone metastases. Another study using hepatobiliary phase imaging (HBP), in addition to PET-CT and whole-body PET-MR imaging, confirmed these findings but demonstrated the superiority of HBP over all modalities to identify liver lesions.[74] WB-MR imaging has shown similar accuracy to OctreoScan PET in staging neuroendocrine tumors,[75] but using both PET/CT and WB-MR imaging has been recommended.[73]

In ovarian cancer, WB-MR imaging represents an auspicious alternative to current CT and PET/CT approaches, with WB-MR imaging being superior to PET/CT for M (peritoneal) staging, whereas both techniques have similar performances for T and N staging.[76] WB-MR imaging with DWI appears superior to CT for primary tumor characterization, staging, and prediction of operability.[77]

In testicular cancer, Mosavi and colleagues[78] demonstrated that of WB-MR imaging with DWI is a nonirradiating alternative to CT for the detection of residual active masses in this young patient

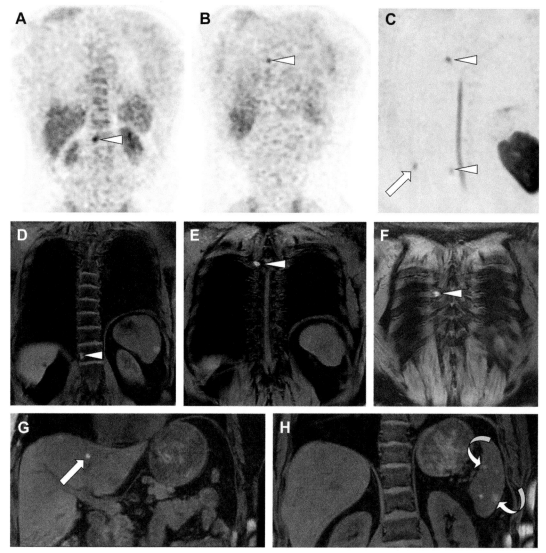

Fig. 4. Comparison of ¹⁸FDG PET and WB-MR imaging findings in a 62-year-old man with melanoma. (*A*, *B*) Coronal reformatted PET images show 2 costal and vertebral foci of ¹⁸FDG uptake, suspect for bone metastases (*arrowheads*). (*C*) Corresponding reformatted WB-MR imaging DWI shows the same vertebral foci (*arrowheads*), and one additional presumably hepatic lesion (*arrow*). (*D–H*) Coronal water images from T1 gradient echo Dixon sequence, sensitive to melanin content because of fat signal suppression show 3 bone lesions (*arrowheads*): one hepatic metastasis (*arrow* in *G*) and multiple spleen metastases (*curved arrows* in *H*).

population. WB-MR imaging is progressively adopted for the routine nonirradiating imaging tool for the prospective surveillance of this young patient population.

Myxoid liposarcoma is a soft tissue tumor that tends to metastasize to unusual sites. PET-FDG has been shown unreliable for the diagnosis and staging of this disease.[79] Conversely, WB-MR imaging has been demonstrated to be effective in metastasis identification and displays a larger quantity of metastatic disease sites than CT.[80] In a case series of 15 patients exhibiting metastatic disease, WB-MR imaging showed a sensitivity of 80%, a specificity of 97.0%, and a positive predictive value of 57.1% for soft tissue lesions.[79] For bone lesions, WB-MR imaging scored 84.6%, 98.9%, and 68.8%, respectively.[79]

Evaluation of the Response to Treatment

Assessing the response to treatment of metastatic disease is a cardinal step in oncologic imaging. Bone lesions have been excluded from response assessment because of the poor reliability of bone scintigraphy and CT.[81] WB-MR imaging effectively allows an evaluation of treatment response based on the demonstration of morphologic and size changes on both anatomic and functional sequences, on the evaluation of the global tumor load on DWI images, and on the observation of changes in ADC values in individual lesions.[28,31,82,83] WB-MR imaging refines response assessment, as underlined in a study showing that CT and WB-MR imaging differed in 28.0% of cases for the assessment of response to systemic anti–cancer therapy. Within this study, the most common discrepancy was a classification of progressive disease from WB-MR imaging instead of a stable disease classification from CT.[84]

MULTIPLE MYELOMA

In MM, aggressive treatment is often necessary, triggered by the detection of bone involvement. WB-MR imaging has been established as the imaging modality of choice for the detection of this bone marrow involvement. The 2015 consensus from the International Myeloma Working Group positions WB-MR imaging as the reference standard imaging for detecting MM bone marrow involvement and recommends systematic WB-MR imaging in patients with smoldering and asymptomatic disease.[50] More recently, the National Institute for Health and Care Excellence (NICE) guidelines in the United Kingdom placed WB-MR imaging at the forefront of everyday practice, indicating that WB-MR imaging should be the first-line imaging modality in MM, replacing the radiographic survey and outperforming WB-CT and PET-CT.[51]

WB-MR imaging surveys of the axial skeleton have showed superiority over radiological skeletal surveys,[20,85,86] which should be used only for imaging the skull and ribs, where the sensitivity of WB-MR imaging might still be lower.[31,87–89] WB-MR imaging exhibits a high sensitivity for the visualization of focal lesions, which are significant prognostic factors for asymptomatic MM patients (**Fig. 5**).[90] The use of high b-value DWI images for MM allows easy detection of diffuse or focal bone marrow involvement; ADC map calculations show correlation between high ADC values and high vessel density/bone marrow cellularity.[91] MR imaging also detects vertebral compression fractures, which often complicate the disease.[92]

WB-MR imaging has demonstrated a better accuracy in the identification of bone involvement in MM than WB multiple detector CT.[40] In an early comparison, WB-MR imaging had higher sensitivity (68%) and specificity (83%) than FDG-PET/CT (59% and 75%, respectively).[93] Pawlyn and colleagues[94] have also shown the advantage

WB-MR imaging with DWI has over FDG PET/CT for detecting the presence of diffuse and multifocal marrow infiltration.

In treated MM patients, WB-MR imaging with DWI allows quantification of tumor load, and visual scoring of WB-MR imaging with DWI and quantitative analysis of segmented ADC values appears able to differentiate between treatment responders and nonresponders with 100% specificity and 90% sensitivity.[31] In patients treated with bone marrow transplantation, the severity of pretreatment alterations and the presence of residual bone marrow disease detected on MR imaging studies correlate with a poorer outcome and earlier relapse.[95,96]

LYMPHOMA

In lymphoma, given that the sensitivity and specificity of WB-MR imaging are similar or superior to those of FDG PET/CT, and with its lack of ionizing radiation, WB-MR imaging is a promising imaging method. When compared with contrast-enhanced CT (CE-CT), WB-MR imaging/DWI was found to be superior in the visualization of both nodal and extranodal localization (CE-CT sensitivity: 89% and 52%, respectively; MR imaging sensitivity: 91% and 97%, respectively).[97]

The detection of bone involvement indicates advanced Ann Arbor stage 4 disease and influences treatment and prognosis. WB-MR imaging has been compared with FDG-PET/CT for detecting this skeletal involvement in lymphoma and has been shown to have similar diagnostic accuracy.[53,98] Regarding bone marrow involvement, Albano and colleagues[99] discovered that WB-MR imaging and FDG-PET/CT showed excellent agreement (Cohen's Kappa = 0.935), and WB-MR imaging correlated better with bone marrow biopsy. However, the combination of PET and MR imaging leads to a higher diagnostic accuracy than WB-MR imaging alone.[100]

Despite the high sensitivity, comparable to that of PET/CT, of WB-MR imaging/DWI for detecting bone marrow involvement in aggressive lymphomas, the lower sensitivity of WB-MR imaging/DWI for indolent lymphomas indicates that bone marrow biopsy should not be replaced as the reference standard.[101] Mayerhoefer and colleagues[52] confirmed that WB-MR imaging/DWI was comparable to PET/CT for detecting bone marrow involvement in patients with FDG-avid lymphomas; WB-MR imaging was superior to PET/CT in patients with variable or poorly FDG-avid lymphomas, with sensitivity of 94.4% and specificity of 100% compared with 60.9% and 99.8% for PET/CT.

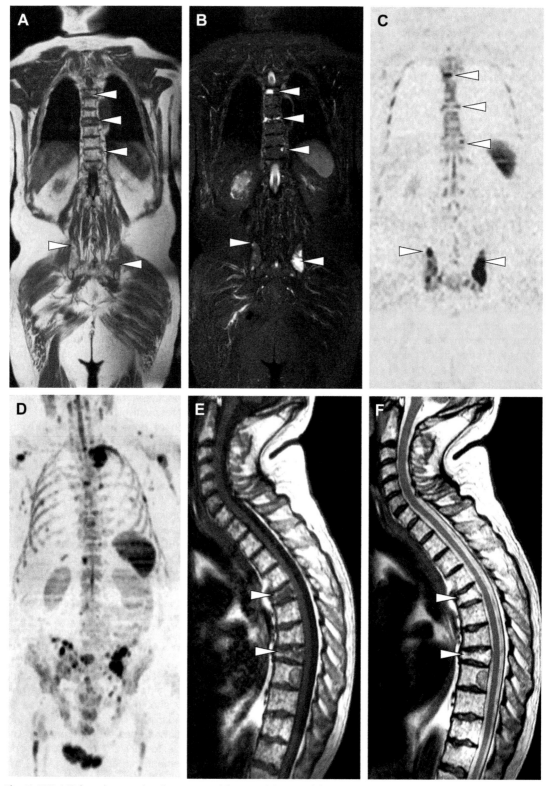

Fig. 5. WB-MR imaging staging in 55-year-old man with MM. (*A*) Coronal anatomic T1, (*B*) STIR, and (*C*) functional DWI (inverted grayscale, b = 1000 s/mm²) MR images show multiple vertebral and iliac bone lesions (*arrowheads*). (*D*) MIP of the DWI sequence shows "at a glance" the multiple foci of bone marrow involvement, located in the spine and pelvis, but also ribs and proximal femurs and humerus. (*E*) Sagittal T1- and (*F*) T2-weighted MR images show the bone marrow lesions and better demonstrate vertebral compression fractures (*arrowheads*).

The effectiveness of WB-MR imaging for a con-current detection of bone and visceral involvement by the time of lymphoma staging has been demonstrated in multiple studies[102–105] and matches that of PET/CT (**Fig. 6**).[106] The combination of WB-MR imaging, including DWI to PET in PET/MR imaging examinations, has been shown to provide similar or better results than PET/CT, thanks to the

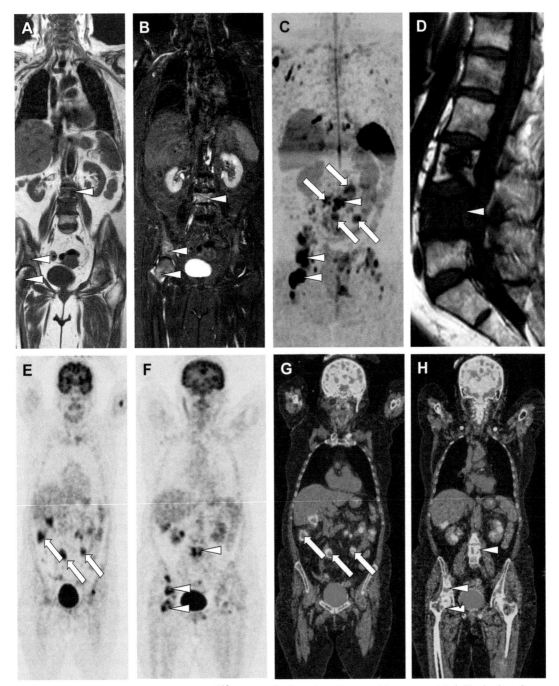

Fig. 6. Comparison of WB-MR imaging and [18]FDG PET findings in a 65-year-old woman with follicular lymphoma. (*A*) Coronal anatomic T1 and (*B*) STIR show bone involvement of a lumbar vertebral body and right iliac acetabular region and proximal femur (*arrowheads*). (*C*) Functional DWI (MIP view, inverted grayscale, b value = 1000 s/mm²) MR images show the same bone lesions (*arrowheads*) and reveals multiple abdominal lymph nodes (*arrows*). (*D*) Sagittal image of the lumbar spine additionally shows L3 and L4 vertebral lesions and anterior epidural extension in L4 (*arrowhead*). (*E, F*) Coronal reformatted [18]FDG PET image and (*G, H*) fused PET/CT images show the same bony (*arrowheads* in *F* and *H*) and nodal (*arrows* in *E* and *G*) lesions.

combination of the sensitivity of FDG PET to that of DWI, the latter being higher in mucosa-associated lymphoid tissue lymphomas.[107,108]

Concerning the response assessment in lymphomas, Mayerhoefer and colleagues[54] found that WB-MR imaging/DWI and PET/CT exhibited agreement for 97% of lymphoma cases, across different types. Littooij and colleagues[55] confirmed the diagnostic accuracy of WB-MR imaging/DWI to detect residual disease after treatment, especially with the addition of ADC measurements, providing information on tissue viability, which increased the specificity of findings.

NICHE INDICATIONS IN SPECIFIC PATIENT POPULATIONS

The diagnostic accuracy of WB-MR imaging has been shown to match or exceed that of FDG-PET and bone scintigraphy for detecting and staging of bone metastases and lymphoma in pediatric oncology. Its lack of ionizing radiation makes it particularly attractive in this population.[56,104] This lack of radiation exposure also promotes WB-MR imaging as the imaging technique of choice for one-step staging of malignancies that appear during pregnancy.[64,109,110]

For the same reason, WB-MR imaging is preferable for patients with conditions predisposing to cancer. WB-MR imaging demonstrated 100% sensitivity and 94% specificity for revealing malignancies in a study of 24 children with genetic predispositions to cancer.[111]

In a study of 578 patients with Li-Fraumeni syndrome, WB-MR imaging was able to detect 42 cancers in 39 individuals with a 7% detection rate.[57] WB-MR imaging was also able to detect cancer earlier in baseline screenings in which non-MR imaging techniques were ineffective.[112] Other studies corroborated the high sensitivity and specificity of WB-MR imaging for Li-Fraumeni and several other cancer-predisposing syndromes, including rhabdoid tumor syndrome and hereditary paraganglioma-pheochromocytoma syndrome; despite a low positive predictive value (25%), screenings using WB-MR imaging have been recommended to allow earlier treatment without introducing risks associated with ionizing radiation.[111]

The same screening for malignant transformation underlies the use of WB-MR imaging to track multiple exostoses and enchondromas in multifocal forms at risk for pejorative evolution.[113] Multiparametric WB-MR imaging also provides information on the growth configuration, dynamics, and coverage of nerve sheath tumors, making it the reference standard for identifying neurofibromatosis-associated nerve sheath tumors.[114] In neurofibromatosis, using both anatomic and functional sequences allows identification and characterization of neoplasms, disease tracking, and detection of malignant transformation.[115]

PRESENT AND FUTURE IN THE ONCOLOGIC IMAGING LANDSCAPE

WB-MR imaging acquisition, reading, reporting, and response evaluation criteria are currently being harmonized across clinical applications.[5,47] Its diagnostic accuracy and reproducibility have been evaluated for an ever-broadening range of indications. Analytical efforts have been made to reduce costs and minimize scan times, to optimize the diagnostic value, and to harmonize acquisitions and readings. The simplification of anatomic sequences by introduction of 3DT1 TSE imaging has allowed faster examinations by reducing the number of sequences and avoiding redundant acquisition of sagittal sequences on the spine.[4] In addition, 3DT1 Dixon sequences offer promising innovations in that they provide different contrasts, are faster than 3DT1 TSE, and have diagnostic value in metastatic disease and MM.[116] This reduction in imaging times offers the perspective of an all organ screening in cancer in as few as 20 minutes, with no need of contrast material in most cases, which will improve the acceptance from both patients and radiologists.[4]

Because of the many similarities in the indications and images for PET/CT and WB-MR imaging, it is essential that their comparative efficacies be evaluated. Like PET and its cancer-specific tracers, WB-MR imaging, including anatomic and DWI sequences, allows a multiorgan screening capability and offers a "one-step" imaging paradigm for the detection of skeletal and visceral involvement in many cancers (see Fig. 2).[14,64] The main strength of WB-MR imaging is its "one size fits all" approach for identifying bone marrow infiltration by metastases from most solid tumors, lymphoma, and MM, because bone marrow replacement has consistent appearance on morphologic images, and water diffusion is impeded on DWI, regardless of the origin and phenotype of neoplastic cells. This strength is an advantage, at least in those cancers where specific PET tracers are not available locally or simply do not exist. The availability of PET-MR imaging should be considered a wonderful research tool that will allow for optimal comparisons of the performances of PET and MR imaging to detect the same lesions in the same patients at the same time, and comparisons between anatomic and functional MR imaging sequences.[117]

The comparison should assess the diagnostic effectiveness, financial feasibility, and ability to evaluate response to treatment. The diagnostic method to use in the future may vary according to the primary cancer, the target organ, the availability of cancer-specific PET tracers, and the underlying medical questions, like disease staging at diagnosis, detection of recurrences, and response assessment.

These research goals, as well as the need for optimization of diagnostic approaches and patient care, offer perspectives for collaboration between radiologists and nuclear medicine physicians. This collaboration will also likely result in the emergence of a new "crossover" medical subspecialty, that is, "oncoimaging," as hybrid anatomic and functional approaches provided by PET/CT, PET MR imaging, and WB-MR imaging show extreme similarity in appearances and require the same knowledge of pathologies and complex cancer-specific staging systems.

SUMMARY

WB-MR imaging has been advanced into clinical practice for the study of a growing number of oncologic disorders, providing advances in the workup and management of diseases. The technique allows for early diagnosis, staging, assessment of therapeutic response, with a superior diagnostic performance compared with historical imaging tools. Other advantages are the absence of ionizing radiation, the lack of contrast material injection necessity for many indications, and the convenience for the patient, because it allows a global skeletal and multiorgan disease workup in one step.

WB-MR imaging, including anatomic and functional (DWI) sequences, offers a "hybrid" approach to maximize detection of different lesion types and to probe all organs. WB-MR imaging outperforms bone scintigraphy and CT for metastatic screening in solid cancers, emerges as first-line modality for skeletal lesion detection in MM, and challenges PET/CT in lymphoma. It was recently recommended by national and international authorities. WB-MR imaging is progressively integrated in the diagnostic strategy in oncology practice, and comparisons are ongoing with PET and its cutting-edge cancer-specific tracers. PET imaging keeps the advantage of cell specificity, provided adequate and multiple tracers are developed, such as PSMA or somatostatin analogues nowadays. Hence, a combination of tissue-specific PET tracers and WB-MR imaging seems to be the Holy Grail for this endeavor. To what extent PET/MR imaging will apply to limited or larger groups of patients in the concept of *Oncoimaging* remains to be established.

REFERENCES

1. Eustace S, Tello R, DeCarvalho V, et al. A comparison of whole-body turboSTIR MR imaging and planar 99mTc-methylene diphosphonate scintigraphy in the examination of patients with suspected skeletal metastases. AJR Am J Roentgenol 1997;169(6):1655–61.
2. Horvath LJ, Burtness BA, McCarthy S, et al. Total-body echo-planar MR imaging in the staging of breast cancer: comparison with conventional methods–early experience. Radiology 1999;211(1):119–28.
3. Berzaczy D, Giraudo C, Haug AR, et al. Whole-Body 68Ga-DOTANOC PET/MRI versus 68Ga-DOTANOC PET/CT in Patients with neuroendocrine tumors: a prospective study in 28 patients. Clin Nucl Med 2017;42(9):669–74.
4. Lecouvet FE. Whole-body MR imaging: musculoskeletal applications. Radiology 2016;279(2): 345–65.
5. Lecouvet FE, Michoux N, Nzeusseu Toukap A, et al. The increasing spectrum of indications of whole-body MRI beyond oncology: imaging answers to clinical needs. Semin Musculoskelet Radiol 2015;19(4):348–62.
6. Lauenstein TC, Freudenberg LS, Goehde SC, et al. Whole-body MRI using a rolling table platform for the detection of bone metastases. Eur Radiol 2002;12(8):2091–9.
7. Koh DM, Lee JM, Bittencourt LK, et al. Body diffusion-weighted mr imaging in oncology: imaging at 3 T. Magn Reson Imaging Clin N Am 2016; 24(1):31–44.
8. Schick F. Whole-body MRI at high field: technical limits and clinical potential. Eur Radiol 2005;15(5):946–59.
9. Schmidt GP, Baur-Melnyk A, Haug A, et al. Comprehensive imaging of tumor recurrence in breast cancer patients using whole-body MRI at 1.5 and 3 T compared to FDG-PET-CT. Eur J Radiol 2008;65(1):47–58.
10. Azzedine B, Kahina MB, Dimitri P, et al. Whole-body diffusion-weighted MRI for staging lymphoma at 3.0T: comparative study with MR imaging at 1.5T. Clin Imaging 2015;39(1):104–9.
11. Schmidt GP, Baur-Melnyk A, Herzog P, et al. High-resolution whole-body magnetic resonance image tumor staging with the use of parallel imaging versus dual-modality positron emission tomography-computed tomography: experience on a 32-channel system. Invest Radiol 2005;40(12):743–53.
12. Dutoit JC, Vanderkerken MA, Verstraete KL. Value of whole body MRI and dynamic contrast enhanced MRI in the diagnosis, follow-up and evaluation of disease activity and extent in multiple myeloma. Eur J Radiol 2013;82(9):1444–52.
13. Nakanishi K, Kobayashi M, Nakaguchi K, et al. Whole-body MRI for detecting metastatic bone

tumor: diagnostic value of diffusion-weighted images. Magn Reson Med Sci 2007;6(3):147–55.

14. Lecouvet FE, El Mouedden J, Collette L, et al. Can whole-body magnetic resonance imaging with diffusion-weighted imaging replace Tc 99m bone scanning and computed tomography for single-step detection of metastases in patients with high-risk prostate cancer? Eur Urol 2012;62(1):68–75.

15. Lecouvet FE, Simon M, Tombal B, et al. Whole-body MRI (WB-MRI) versus axial skeleton MRI (AS-MRI) to detect and measure bone metastases in prostate cancer (PCa). Eur Radiol 2010;20(12):2973–82.

16. Mosher TJ. Diagnostic effectiveness of gadolinium-enhanced MR imaging in evaluation of abnormal bone marrow signal. Radiology 2002;224(2):320–2.

17. Pasoglou V, Michoux N, Peeters F, et al. Whole-body 3D T1-weighted MR imaging in patients with prostate cancer: feasibility and evaluation in screening for metastatic disease. Radiology 2015;275(1):155–66.

18. Di Gioia D, Stieber P, Schmidt GP, et al. Early detection of metastatic disease in asymptomatic breast cancer patients with whole-body imaging and defined tumour marker increase. Br J Cancer 2015;112(5):809–18.

19. Squillaci E, Bolacchi F, Altobelli S, et al. Pre-treatment staging of multiple myeloma patients: comparison of whole-body diffusion weighted imaging with whole-body T1-weighted contrast-enhanced imaging. Acta Radiol 2015;56(6):733–8.

20. Lecouvet FE, Vande Berg BC, Michaux L, et al. Stage III multiple myeloma: clinical and prognostic value of spinal bone marrow MR imaging. Radiology 1998;209(3):653–60.

21. Mirowitz SA, Apicella P, Reinus WR, et al. MR imaging of bone marrow lesions: relative conspicuousness on T1-weighted, fat-suppressed T2-weighted, and STIR images. AJR Am J Roentgenol 1994;162(1):215–21.

22. Vogler JB 3rd, Murphy WA. Bone marrow imaging. Radiology 1988;168(3):679–93.

23. Angtuaco EJ, Fassas AB, Walker R, et al. Multiple myeloma: clinical review and diagnostic imaging. Radiology 2004;231(1):11–23.

24. Pearce T, Philip S, Brown J, et al. Bone metastases from prostate, breast and multiple myeloma: differences in lesion conspicuity at short-tau inversion recovery and diffusion-weighted MRI. Br J Radiol 2012;85(1016):1102–6.

25. Takahara T, Imai Y, Yamashita T, et al. Diffusion weighted whole body imaging with background body signal suppression (DWIBS): technical improvement using free breathing, STIR and high resolution 3D display. Radiat Med 2004;22(4):275–82.

26. Padhani AR, Koh DM, Collins DJ. Whole-body diffusion-weighted MR imaging in cancer: current status and research directions. Radiology 2011;261(3):700–18.

27. Kwee TC, Takahara T, Ochiai R, et al. Diffusion-weighted whole-body imaging with background body signal suppression (DWIBS): features and potential applications in oncology. Eur Radiol 2008;18(9):1937–52.

28. Blackledge MD, Collins DJ, Tunariu N, et al. Assessment of treatment response by total tumor volume and global apparent diffusion coefficient using diffusion-weighted MRI in patients with metastatic bone disease: a feasibility study. PLoS One 2014;9(4):e91779.

29. Padhani AR, Liu G, Koh DM, et al. Diffusion-weighted magnetic resonance imaging as a cancer biomarker: consensus and recommendations. Neoplasia 2009;11(2):102–25.

30. Padhani AR, van Ree K, Collins DJ, et al. Assessing the relation between bone marrow signal intensity and apparent diffusion coefficient in diffusion-weighted MRI. AJR Am J Roentgenol 2013;200(1):163–70.

31. Giles SL, Messiou C, Collins DJ, et al. Whole-body diffusion-weighted MR imaging for assessment of treatment response in myeloma. Radiology 2014;271(3):785–94.

32. Padhani AR, Makris A, Gall P, et al. Therapy monitoring of skeletal metastases with whole-body diffusion MRI. J Magn Reson Imaging 2014;39(5):1049–78.

33. Koh DM, Blackledge M, Padhani AR, et al. Whole-body diffusion-weighted MRI: tips, tricks, and pitfalls. AJR Am J Roentgenol 2012;199(2):252–62.

34. Ohno Y, Koyama H, Onishi Y, et al. Non-small cell lung cancer: whole-body MR examination for M-stage assessment–utility for whole-body diffusion-weighted imaging compared with integrated FDG PET/CT. Radiology 2008;248(2):643–54.

35. Lecouvet FE, Vande Berg BC, Malghem J, et al. Diffusion-weighted MR imaging: adjunct or alternative to T1-weighted MR imaging for prostate carcinoma bone metastases? Radiology 2009;252(2):624.

36. Burdette JH, Elster AD, Ricci PE. Acute cerebral infarction: quantification of spin-density and T2 shine-through phenomena on diffusion-weighted MR images. Radiology 1999;212(2):333–9.

37. Le Bihan D, Breton E, Lallemand D, et al. MR imaging of intravoxel incoherent motions: application to diffusion and perfusion in neurologic disorders. Radiology 1986;161(2):401–7.

38. Koh DM, Collins DJ. Diffusion-weighted MRI in the body: applications and challenges in oncology. AJR Am J Roentgenol 2007;188(6):1622–35.

39. Messiou C, Collins DJ, Morgan VA, et al. Use of apparent diffusion coefficient as a response

biomarker in bone: effect of developing sclerosis on quantified values. Skeletal Radiol 2014;43(2):205–8.

40. Baur-Melnyk A, Buhmann S, Becker C, et al. Whole-body MRI versus whole-body MDCT for staging of multiple myeloma. AJR Am J Roentgenol 2008;190(4):1097–104.

41. Kwee TC, Fijnheer R, Ludwig I, et al. Whole-body magnetic resonance imaging, including diffusion-weighted imaging, for diagnosing bone marrow involvement in malignant lymphoma. Br J Haematol 2010;149(4):628–30.

42. Cascini GL, Falcone C, Console D, et al. Whole-body MRI and PET/CT in multiple myeloma patients during staging and after treatment: personal experience in a longitudinal study. Radiol Med 2013;118(6):930–48.

43. Falcone C, Cipullo S, Sannino P, et al. Whole Body Magnetic Resonance and CT/PET in patients affected by multiple myeloma during staging before treatment. Recenti Prog Med 2012;103(11):444–9 [in Italian].

44. Ohlmann-Knafo S, Kirschbaum M, Fenzl G, et al. Diagnostic value of whole-body MRI and bone scintigraphy in the detection of osseous metastases in patients with breast cancer–a prospective double-blinded study at two hospital centers. Rofo 2009;181(3):255–63 [in German].

45. Pasoglou V, Larbi A, Collette L, et al. One-step TNM staging of high-risk prostate cancer using magnetic resonance imaging (MRI): toward an upfront simplified "all-in-one" imaging approach? Prostate 2014;74(5):469–77.

46. Robertson NL, Sala E, Benz M, et al. Combined whole body and multiparametric prostate magnetic resonance imaging as a 1-step approach to the simultaneous assessment of local recurrence and metastatic disease after radical prostatectomy. J Urol 2017;198(1):65–70.

47. Padhani AR, Lecouvet FE, Tunariu N, et al. METastasis reporting and data system for prostate cancer: practical guidelines for acquisition, interpretation, and reporting of whole-body magnetic resonance imaging-based evaluations of multiorgan involvement in advanced prostate cancer. Eur Urol 2017;71(1):81–92.

48. Liu T, Cheng T, Xu W, et al. A meta-analysis of 18FDG-PET, MRI and bone scintigraphy for diagnosis of bone metastases in patients with breast cancer. Skeletal Radiol 2011;40(5):523–31.

49. Woolf DK, Padhani AR, Makris A. Assessing response to treatment of bone metastases from breast cancer: what should be the standard of care? Ann Oncol 2015;26(6):1048–57.

50. Dimopoulos MA, Hillengass J, Usmani S, et al. Role of magnetic resonance imaging in the management of patients with multiple myeloma: a consensus statement. J Clin Oncol 2015;33(6):657–64.

51. Pratt G, Morris TC. Review of the NICE guidelines for multiple myeloma. Int J Lab Hematol 2017;39(1):3–13.

52. Mayerhoefer ME, Karanikas G, Kletter K, et al. Evaluation of diffusion-weighted MRI for pretherapeutic assessment and staging of lymphoma: results of a prospective study in 140 patients. Clin Cancer Res 2014;20(11):2984–93.

53. Ribrag V, Vanel D, Leboulleux S, et al. Prospective study of bone marrow infiltration in aggressive lymphoma by three independent methods: whole-body MRI, PET/CT and bone marrow biopsy. Eur J Radiol 2008;66(2):325–31.

54. Mayerhoefer ME, Karanikas G, Kletter K, et al. Evaluation of diffusion-weighted magnetic resonance imaging for follow-up and treatment response assessment of lymphoma: results of an 18F-FDG-PET/CT-controlled prospective study in 64 patients. Clin Cancer Res 2015;21(11):2506–13.

55. Littooij AS, Kwee TC, de Keizer B, et al. Whole-body MRI-DWI for assessment of residual disease after completion of therapy in lymphoma: a prospective multicenter study. J Magn Reson Imaging 2015;42(6):1646–55.

56. Daldrup-Link HE, Franzius C, Link TM, et al. Whole-body MR imaging for detection of bone metastases in children and young adults: comparison with skeletal scintigraphy and FDG PET. AJR Am J Roentgenol 2001;177(1):229–36.

57. Ballinger ML, Best A, Mai PL, et al. Baseline surveillance in li-fraumeni syndrome using whole-body magnetic resonance imaging: a meta-analysis. JAMA Oncol 2017;3(12):1634–9.

58. Eustace SJ, Nelson E. Whole body magnetic resonance imaging. BMJ 2004;328(7453):1387–8.

59. Shen G, Deng H, Hu S, et al. Comparison of choline-PET/CT, MRI, SPECT, and bone scintigraphy in the diagnosis of bone metastases in patients with prostate cancer: a meta-analysis. Skeletal Radiol 2014;43(11):1503–13.

60. Woo S, Suh CH, Kim SY, et al. Diagnostic performance of magnetic resonance imaging for the detection of bone metastasis in prostate cancer: a systematic review and meta-analysis. Eur Urol 2018;73(1):81–91.

61. Conde-Moreno AJ, Herrando-Parreno G, Muelas-Soria R, et al. Whole-body diffusion-weighted magnetic resonance imaging (WB-DW-MRI) vs choline-positron emission tomography-computed tomography (choline-PET/CT) for selecting treatments in recurrent prostate cancer. Clin Transl Oncol 2017;19(5):553–61.

62. Larbi A, Dallaudiere B, Pasoglou V, et al. Whole body MRI (WB-MRI) assessment of metastatic spread in prostate cancer: therapeutic perspectives

on targeted management of oligometastatic disease. Prostate 2016;76(11):1024–33.

63. Gupta M, Choudhury PS, Hazarika D, et al. A comparative study of 68gallium-prostate specific membrane antigen positron emission tomography-computed tomography and magnetic resonance imaging for lymph node staging in high risk prostate cancer patients: an initial experience. World J Nucl Med 2017;16(3):186–91.

64. Jambor I, Kuisma A, Ramadan S, et al. Prospective evaluation of planar bone scintigraphy, SPECT, SPECT/CT, F-NaF PET/CT and whole body 1.5T MRI, including DWI, for the detection of bone metastases in high risk breast and prostate cancer patients: SKELETA clinical trial. Acta Oncol 2016; 55(1):59–67.

65. Takenaka D, Ohno Y, Matsumoto K, et al. Detection of bone metastases in non-small cell lung cancer patients: comparison of whole-body diffusion-weighted imaging (DWI), whole-body MR imaging without and with DWI, whole-body FDG-PET/CT, and bone scintigraphy. J Magn Reson Imaging 2009;30(2):298–308.

66. Ohno Y, Yoshikawa T, Kishida Y, et al. Diagnostic performance of different imaging modalities in the assessment of distant metastasis and local recurrence of tumor in patients with non-small cell lung cancer. J Magn Reson Imaging 2017;46(6):1707–17.

67. Taylor SA, Mallett S, Miles A, et al. Streamlining staging of lung and colorectal cancer with whole body MRI; study protocols for two multicentre, non-randomised, single-arm, prospective diagnostic accuracy studies (Streamline C and Streamline L). BMC Cancer 2017;17(1):299.

68. Sakurai Y, Kawai H, Iwano S, et al. Supplemental value of diffusion-weighted whole-body imaging with background body signal suppression (DWIBS) technique to whole-body magnetic resonance imaging in detection of bone metastases from thyroid cancer. J Med Imaging Radiat Oncol 2013;57(3): 297–305.

69. Mosavi F, Ullenhag G, Ahlstrom H. Whole-body MRI including diffusion-weighted imaging compared to CT for staging of malignant melanoma. Ups J Med Sci 2013;118(2):91–7.

70. Petralia G, Padhani A, Summers P, et al. Whole-body diffusion-weighted imaging: is it all we need for detecting metastases in melanoma patients? Eur Radiol 2013;23(12):3466–76.

71. Pfannenberg C, Schwenzer N. Whole-body staging of malignant melanoma: advantages, limitations and current importance of PET-CT, whole-body MRI and PET-MRI. Radiologe 2015;55(2):120–6 [in German].

72. Moryoussef F, de Mestier L, Belkebir M, et al. Impact of liver and whole-body diffusion-weighted mri for neuroendocrine tumors on patient management: a pilot study. Neuroendocrinology 2017; 104(3):264–72.

73. Schraml C, Schwenzer NF, Sperling O, et al. Staging of neuroendocrine tumours: comparison of [(6)(8)Ga]DOTATOC multiphase PET/CT and whole-body MRI. Cancer Imaging 2013;13:63–72.

74. Ferdinandy P, Hausenloy DJ, Heusch G, et al. Interaction of risk factors, comorbidities, and comedications with ischemia/reperfusion injury and cardioprotection by preconditioning, postconditioning, and remote conditioning. Pharmacol Rev 2014;66(4):1142–74.

75. Bezerra R, Gumz BP, Etchebehere E, et al. Whole-body diffusion-weighted MRI (DWMR) compared with [68Ga] DOTATOC-PET/CT (68Ga) and Octreo-Scan (OCT) for staging neuroendocrine tumors (NET). J Clin Oncol 2014;32(15_suppl):e15167.

76. Michielsen K, Vergote I, Op de Beeck K, et al. Whole-body MRI with diffusion-weighted sequence for staging of patients with suspected ovarian cancer: a clinical feasibility study in comparison to CT and FDG-PET/CT. Eur Radiol 2014;24(4):889–901.

77. Michielsen K, Dresen R, Vanslembrouck R, et al. Diagnostic value of whole body diffusion-weighted MRI compared to computed tomography for pre-operative assessment of patients suspected for ovarian cancer. Eur J Cancer 2017;83: 88–98.

78. Mosavi F, Laurell A, Ahlstrom H. Whole body MRI, including diffusion-weighted imaging in follow-up of patients with testicular cancer. Acta Oncol 2015;54(10):1763–9.

79. Seo SW, Kwon JW, Jang SW, et al. Feasibility of whole-body MRI for detecting metastatic myxoid liposarcoma: a case series. Orthopedics 2011; 34(11):e748–54.

80. Stevenson JD, Watson JJ, Cool P, et al. Whole-body magnetic resonance imaging in myxoid liposarcoma: a useful adjunct for the detection of extra-pulmonary metastatic disease. Eur J Surg Oncol 2016;42(4):574–80.

81. Therasse P, Arbuck SG, Eisenhauer EA, et al. New guidelines to evaluate the response to treatment in solid tumors. European Organization for Research and Treatment of Cancer, National Cancer Institute of The United States, National Cancer Institute of Canada. J Natl Cancer Inst 2000;92(3):205–16.

82. Padhani AR, Gogbashian A. Bony metastases: assessing response to therapy with whole-body diffusion MRI. Cancer Imaging 2011;11(Spec No A): S129–45.

83. Lecouvet FE, Larbi A, Pasoglou V, et al. MRI for response assessment in metastatic bone disease. Eur Radiol 2013;23(7):1986–97.

84. Kosmin M, Makris A, Joshi PV, et al. The addition of whole-body magnetic resonance imaging to body

computerised tomography alters treatment decisions in patients with metastatic breast cancer. Eur J Cancer 2017;77:109–16.

85. Lecouvet FE, Malghem J, Michaux L, et al. Skeletal survey in advanced multiple myeloma: radiographic versus MR imaging survey. Br J Haematol 1999;106(1):35–9.

86. Walker R, Barlogie B, Haessler J, et al. Magnetic resonance imaging in multiple myeloma: diagnostic and clinical implications. J Clin Oncol 2007;25(9):1121–8.

87. Bauerle T, Hillengass J, Fechtner K, et al. Multiple myeloma and monoclonal gammopathy of undetermined significance: importance of whole-body versus spinal MR imaging. Radiology 2009; 252(2):477–85.

88. Ghanem N, Altehoefer C, Kelly T, et al. Whole-body MRI in comparison to skeletal scintigraphy in detection of skeletal metastases in patients with solid tumors. In Vivo 2006;20(1):173–82.

89. Giles SL, deSouza NM, Collins DJ, et al. Assessing myeloma bone disease with whole-body diffusion-weighted imaging: comparison with x-ray skeletal survey by region and relationship with laboratory estimates of disease burden. Clin Radiol 2015; 70(6):614–21.

90. Zamagni E, Nanni C, Patriarca F, et al. A prospective comparison of 18F-fluorodeoxyglucose positron emission tomography-computed tomography, magnetic resonance imaging and whole-body planar radiographs in the assessment of bone disease in newly diagnosed multiple myeloma. Haematologica 2007;92(1):50–5.

91. Hillengass J, Bauerle T, Bartl R, et al. Diffusion-weighted imaging for non-invasive and quantitative monitoring of bone marrow infiltration in patients with monoclonal plasma cell disease: a comparative study with histology. Br J Haematol 2011; 153(6):721–8.

92. Lecouvet FE, Vande Berg BC, Michaux L, et al. Development of vertebral fractures in patients with multiple myeloma: does MRI enable recognition of vertebrae that will collapse? J Comput Assist Tomogr 1998;22(3):430–6.

93. Shortt CP, Gleeson TG, Breen KA, et al. Whole-Body MRI versus PET in assessment of multiple myeloma disease activity. AJR Am J Roentgenol 2009;192(4):980–6.

94. Pawlyn C, Fowkes L, Otero S, et al. Whole-body diffusion-weighted MRI: a new gold standard for assessing disease burden in patients with multiple myeloma? Leukemia 2016;30(6):1446–8.

95. Lecouvet FE, Dechambre S, Malghem J, et al. Bone marrow transplantation in patients with multiple myeloma: prognostic significance of MR imaging. AJR Am J Roentgenol 2001; 176(1):91–6.

96. Mai EK, Hielscher T, Kloth JK, et al. A magnetic resonance imaging-based prognostic scoring system to predict outcome in transplant-eligible patients with multiple myeloma. Haematologica 2015;100(6):818–25.

97. Balbo-Mussetto A, Cirillo S, Bruna R, et al. Whole-body MRI with diffusion-weighted imaging: a valuable alternative to contrast-enhanced CT for initial staging of aggressive lymphoma. Clin Radiol 2016;71(3):271–9.

98. Littooij AS, Kwee TC, Barber I, et al. Whole-body MRI for initial staging of paediatric lymphoma: prospective comparison to an FDG-PET/CT-based reference standard. Eur Radiol 2014;24(5):1153–65.

99. Albano D, Patti C, Lagalla R, et al. FDG-PET/CT, and bone marrow biopsy, for the assessment of bone marrow involvement in patients with newly diagnosed lymphoma. J Magn Reson Imaging 2017;45(4):1082–9.

100. Kirchner J, Deuschl C, Schweiger B, et al. Imaging children suffering from lymphoma: an evaluation of different 18F-FDG PET/MRI protocols compared to whole-body DW-MRI. Eur J Nucl Med Mol Imaging 2017;44(10):1742–50.

101. Adams HJ, Kwee TC, Vermoolen MA, et al. Whole-body MRI for the detection of bone marrow involvement in lymphoma: prospective study in 116 patients and comparison with FDG-PET. Eur Radiol 2013;23(8):2271–8.

102. Toledano-Massiah S, Luciani A, Itti E, et al. Whole-body diffusion-weighted imaging in hodgkin lymphoma and diffuse large B-cell lymphoma. Radiographics 2015;35(3):747–64.

103. Punwani S, Taylor SA, Bainbridge A, et al. Pediatric and adolescent lymphoma: comparison of whole-body STIR half-Fourier RARE MR imaging with an enhanced PET/CT reference for initial staging. Radiology 2010;255(1):182–90.

104. Klenk C, Gawande R, Uslu L, et al. Ionising radiation-free whole-body MRI versus (18)F-fluorodeoxyglucose PET/CT scans for children and young adults with cancer: a prospective, non-randomised, single-centre study. Lancet Oncol 2014;15(3):275–85.

105. Kwee TC. Can whole-body MRI replace (18)F-fluorodeoxyglucose PET/CT? Lancet Oncol 2014; 15(3):243–4.

106. Regacini R, Puchnick A, Shigueoka DC, et al. Whole-body diffusion-weighted magnetic resonance imaging versus FDG-PET/CT for initial lymphoma staging: systematic review on diagnostic test accuracy studies. Sao Paulo Med J 2015; 133(2):141–50.

107. Heacock L, Weissbrot J, Raad R, et al. PET/MRI for the evaluation of patients with lymphoma: initial observations. AJR Am J Roentgenol 2015;204(4): 842–8.

108. Giraudo C, Raderer M, Karanikas G, et al. 18F-Fluorodeoxyglucose positron emission tomography/magnetic resonance in lymphoma: comparison with 18F-Fluorodeoxyglucose positron emission tomography/computed tomography and with the addition of magnetic resonance diffusion-weighted imaging. Invest Radiol 2016; 51(3):163–9.

109. Antoch G, Vogt FM, Freudenberg LS, et al. Whole-body dual-modality PET/CT and whole-body MRI for tumor staging in oncology. JAMA 2003; 290(24):3199–206.

110. Lecouvet FE, Talbot JN, Messiou C, et al. Monitoring the response of bone metastases to treatment with magnetic resonance imaging and nuclear medicine techniques: a review and position statement by the European organisation for research and treatment of cancer imaging group. Eur J Cancer 2014;50(15):2519–31.

111. Anupindi SA, Bedoya MA, Lindell RB, et al. Diagnostic performance of whole-body MRI as a tool for cancer screening in children with genetic cancer-predisposing conditions. AJR Am J Roentgenol 2015;205(2):400–8.

112. Mai PL, Khincha PP, Loud JT, et al. Prevalence of cancer at baseline screening in the national cancer institute li-fraumeni syndrome cohort. JAMA Oncol 2017;3(12):1640–5.

113. Schmidt GP, Reiser MF, Baur-Melnyk A. Whole-body imaging of bone marrow. Semin Musculoskelet Radiol 2009;13(2):120–33.

114. Salamon J, Mautner VF, Adam G, et al. Multimodal imaging in neurofibromatosis type 1-associated nerve sheath tumors. Rofo 2015;187(12):1084–92.

115. Cai W, Kassarjian A, Bredella MA, et al. Tumor burden in patients with neurofibromatosis types 1 and 2 and schwannomatosis: determination on whole-body MR images. Radiology 2009;250(3): 665–73.

116. Bray TJP, Singh S, Latifoltojar A, et al. Diagnostic utility of whole body Dixon MRI in multiple myeloma: a multi-reader study. PLoS One 2017; 12(7):e0180562.

117. Eiber M, Takei T, Souvatzoglou M, et al. Performance of whole-body integrated 18F-FDG PET/MR in comparison to PET/CT for evaluation of malignant bone lesions. J Nucl Med 2014;55(2): 191–7.

MR Imaging of Joint Infection and Inflammation with Emphasis on Dynamic Contrast-Enhanced MR Imaging

Mikael Boesen, MD, PhD[a,b,*], Olga Kubassova, MSc, PhD[c],
Iwona Sudoł-Szopińska, MD, PhD[d,e],
Mario Maas, MD, PhD[f,g], Philip Hansen, MD, PhD[a],
Janus Damm Nybing, MSc[a], Edwin H. Oei, MD, PhD[h,i],
Robert Hemke, MD, PhD[f,g], Ali Guermazi, MD, PhD[j]

KEYWORDS

- Musculoskeletal radiology • MR imaging • Dynamic contrast-enhanced MR imaging • Infection
- Inflammation • Arthritis • Synovitis • Osteitis

KEY POINTS

- Dynamic contrast-enhanced MR imaging (DCE-MR imaging) can provide robust and sensitive quantitative information on perfusion in the joint tissues for diagnosis and monitoring of infectious and most inflammatory joint diseases.
- There is increasing evidence of clinical and research utility of DCE-MR imaging in inflammatory and degenerative joint diseases, and to a lesser degree in septic arthritis and spondyloarthropathies.
- High sensitivity and reproducibility of quantitative perfusion markers can be obtained from DCE-MR imaging in healthy individuals and patients when appropriate postprocessing imaging software is used.
- Quantitative DCE-MR imaging perfusion markers correlate highly with synovial vascularity and inflammatory cell infiltrates and allows differentiation of patients with distinct inflammatory joint diseases.
- DCE-MR imaging–based outcome measures show high sensitivity to treatment response following steroid injection and biologic treatments and correlate closely with clinical scores of pain and function in patients with inflammatory and degenerative joint diseases.

Disclosure Statement: M. Boesen is chairman of the clinical and scientific advisory board and shareholder of Image Analysis Group. O. Kubassova is CEO and shareholder of Image Analysis Group; E.H. Oei receives research support from GE Healthcare. A. Guermazi is the President of Boston Imaging Core Laboratory, LLC, and is a consultant to MerckSerono, TissueGene, OrthoTrophix, GE Healthcare, AstraZeneca, Pfizer, and Sanofi. I. Sudoł-Szopińska, P. Hansen, J. Damm Nybing, M. Maas, and R. Hemke: No conflict of interest.

[a] Department of Radiology, Bispebjerg and Frederiksberg Hospital, Bispebjerg Bakke 23, 2400, Copenhagen Nv, Denmark; [b] Parker Institute, Bispebjerg and Frederiksberg Hospital, Nordrefasanvej 57, 2000 Copenhagen F, Denmark; [c] Image Analysis Group (IAG), AQBC Minster House, 272-274 Vauxhall Bridge Road, SW1V 1BA, London, UK; [d] Department of Radiology, National Institute of Geriatrics, Rheumatology and Rehabilitation, Warsaw, Poland; [e] Department of Diagnostic Imaging, Warsaw Medical University, Warsaw, Poland; [f] Department of Radiology, Faculty of Medicine, Academic Medical Center (AMC) Amsterdam, University of Amsterdam, Amsterdam, The Netherlands; [g] Department of Nuclear Medicine, Faculty of Medicine, Academic Medical Center (AMC) Amsterdam, University of Amsterdam, Amsterdam, The Netherlands; [h] Department of Radiology, Erasmus MC, University Medical Center Rotterdam, Rotterdam, The Netherlands; [i] Department of Nuclear Medicine, Erasmus MC, University Medical Center Rotterdam, Rotterdam, The Netherlands; [j] Department of Radiology, Boston University School of Medicine, Boston, MA, USA
* Corresponding author. Department of Radiology, Bispebjerg and Frederiksberg Hospital, Bispebjerg Bakke 23, 2400 Copenhagen NV, Denmark.
E-mail address: mikael.ploug.boesen@regionh.dk

PET Clin 13 (2018) 523–550
https://doi.org/10.1016/j.cpet.2018.05.007

INTRODUCTION

Inflammation is the hallmark and main driver of both inflammatory and infectious joint diseases[1,2] that will lead to rapid destruction of the joint structures if appropriate diagnosis and treatments are delayed.[3] Radiography is currently the first-line imaging modality for most musculoskeletal diseases, including malignancies, fractures, and inflammatory or infectious diseases. In the early stages of inflammatory and infectious joint diseases, radiographs may show juxta articular nonspecific thickening and increased density of periarticular soft tissues, osteoporosis, periosteal reactions, and radiographic signs of growth disorders in children may be present. In late disease stages, the development of bone cysts, erosions, joint space narrowing, and reactive juxta articular sclerosis, osteoproliferative lesions, joint destructions, or ankylosis are helpful to make a more specific diagnosis.[1,2,4]

MR imaging with intravenous (IV) Gadolinium (Gd) is often recommended for early diagnosis and monitoring of infectious and inflammatory joint diseases, except for sacroiliitis in the course of spondyloarthritis (SpA).[1,2,5–8] IV Gd facilitates separation of enhancing soft and bony tissue from the fluid collections, infectious debris, and abscesses on postcontrast T1-weighted (T1w) images.[1,2,5,8] When IV Gd is used, a dynamic contrast-enhanced MR imaging (DCE-MR imaging) sequence can be applied on both high-field and low-field MR imaging scanners,[9–11] using a fast T1w sequence just before and for several minutes after the injection of the contrast. DCE-MR imaging is a widely used MR imaging method, especially in oncology, where it provides information about the blood flow and capillary permeability. DCE-MR imaging has in this context been used to visualize neovascularity and assess disease (tumor) grade.[9] For similar reasons, the use of DCE-MR imaging within the field of infectious and inflammatory musculoskeletal diseases is increasing, because it allows for comprehensive investigation of perfusion of the joint tissue.[9,10,12–16] With the use of appropriate postprocessing methods and software, DCE-MR imaging allows quantification of the degree of perfusion in the synovium, bone marrow, cartilage, muscle, and fat tissue, which can be used to complement the static imaging changes.[13,14,16]

This review describes principles of DCE-MR imaging for the assessment of infectious and inflammatory joint diseases.

TECHNICAL REQUIREMENTS FOR DYNAMIC CONTRAST-ENHANCED MR IMAGING

To perform a DCE-MR imaging sequence of a given anatomy, dedicated scanner hardware is required, such as appropriate scanner gradients, parallel imaging techniques, and preferably a send/receive phase array coil along with a power injector that can time the contrast injection and injection speed.

DCE-MR imaging sequences are based on sequential acquisition of rapid MR images of a specific anatomy of interest before and during the IV injection of a bolus infusion of Gd contrast.

Two distinctly different DCE-MR imaging acquisition methods using IV Gd contrast to assess perfusion have been used in the literature: susceptibility-weighted (ie, T2*-weighted) and T1-weighted (T1w) DCE-MR imaging. Susceptibility-weighted imaging is primarily used for brain studies, which is beyond the scope of this review to address. The method has been extensively described elsewhere[9,17–19] and to our knowledge it has never been applied in studies of joint diseases.

T1-WEIGHTED DYNAMIC CONTRAST-ENHANCED MR IMAGING

T1w DCE-MR imaging, which in the following will be referred to DCE-MR imaging, is usually built on a gradient echo (GRE) sequence with a short repetition time (TR) and echo time (TE). A low flip angle between 10° and 20° is to maintain good T1 contrast and a high temporal resolution of 1 to 10 seconds. Spin-echo techniques also can be used, but will generally suffer from longer acquisition times and thus a lower temporal resolution (>10 seconds).

BASIC CONCEPTS OF POSTPROCESSING T1-WEIGHTED DYNAMIC CONTRAST-ENHANCED MR IMAGING

DCE-MR images are obtained when a Gd contrast agent is injected into the bloodstream by acquiring a time series of T1w images of the same anatomy with intervals of a few seconds. Following the IV injection of the contrast agent, which is preferentially taken up at sites with high perfusion, a temporal variation of the MR imaging signal intensity occurs.[9,19,20] When the contrast distributes through the intravascular and extravascular spaces, the MR signal intensity in the image volume elements (voxels) of the target tissue changes over time, generating so-called signal intensity (SI) curves. These curves can be analyzed to derive parameters related to tissue perfusion.[18,19] In most cases in which single contrast dose is used, the SI increase over time corresponds to the underlying changes in tissue concentration of the contrast agent. In this way, generation of SI curves in regions of interest (ROIs) or in every image voxel can be used to separate areas with high perfusion, such as vessels and inflamed tissue from healthy tissue.[20,21] The most common approaches for analyzing the change in MR signal over time include (1) visual assessment (qualitative), (2) quantitative pharmacokinetic or heuristic parameters and (3) descriptive (semiquantitative) heuristic parameters.[17–19] **Table 1** highlights examples of the various T1w DCE-MR imaging protocols and studies published on infectious and inflammatory joint diseases over the past decade.

Qualitative (Visual) Analysis

The qualitative analysis method is based on the observer's visual evaluation of the DCE-MR imaging contrast enhancement within a tissue of interest.[17] The enhancement kinetics can be analyzed qualitatively on native, subtraction, or maximum intensity projection images by running a movie focusing on a visual grading of contrast kinetics, such as speed of wash-in (filling phase), peak intensity after wash-in, plateau, and washout time.[17] This approach can be performed on most imaging platforms and does not depend on the use of a particular technology or software, but it relies on the reader's experience and is vulnerable to the reader's bias as well as the image acquisition protocol.[19] As a consequence of this variability, the DCE-MR imaging sequence is often replaced by the acquisition of "only" a static postcontrast image sequence. This reduces the number of images the reader needs to scroll through and assess. Such systems are known as "criteria-based" systems, meaning that each joint will be scored by an observer using specific criteria; for example, a joint is scored for synovitis on scale

from 0 to 3, with 0 indicating no synovitis and 3 indicating "the worst imaginable." To aid the assessment, standardized case atlases for various diseases have been published and can be used as guidance. This method is widely used when scoring static MR images that within inflammatory and degenerative joint diseases include Rheumatoid Arthritis MRI Scoring (RAMRIS)[22] for rheumatoid arthritis (RA), Psoriatic MRI Scoring (PSAMRIS)[23] for psoriatic arthritis, MRI Osteoarthritis Knee Score (MOAKS)[24] for knee osteoarthritis (OA), and many others. However, such simplification hinders objective identification of the time point and speed of maximum contrast enhancement.

Quantitative (Computer-Aided) Analysis

Quantitative analysis of DCE-MR imaging can be performed using pharmacokinetics or heuristics approaches,[17–19] which both rely on the underlying principle of computer-aided assessment of SI curves.

Pharmacokinetic Analysis

A pharmacokinetics-based approach uses a predefined model to characterize difference in perfusion between the blood vessels and the tissues. The blood flow is modeled and several such models are in use. We describe and provide examples of the 2-compartment model introduced by Tofts and Kermode,[25] but further information can be found elsewhere.[17–19]

The model of Tofts and Kermode[25] describes the contrast agent distribution between 2 compartments: the plasma space (C_p) and the tissue space (C_t) and outputs the values of K^{trans}, the volume transfer constant between C_p and C_t, and

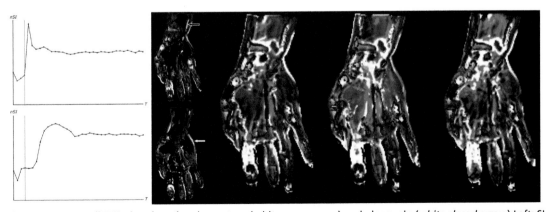

Fig. 1. From a small ROI placed on the ulnar artery (*white open arrow*) and ulnar vein (*white closed arrow*) Left: SI versus time curves from the artery (*top*) and the vein (*bottom*) needed to construct the AIF. The red vertical line indicates onset of Gadolinium contrast agent in the artery. Pharmacokinetic maps of a hand from a patient with active RA (*left to right*: Ktrans, Ve, IAU60) calculated using AIF values). Note both wrist joint synovitis and tenosynovitis in the second finger.

Table 1
Examples of studies using dynamic contrast-enhanced MR imaging published within the past 10 years within inflammatory and infectious joint diseases

Study	Joint	Disease	Field Strength	Temporal Resolution/ Duration	K^{trans}/SI Curve	Year	TR/TE/FA	Contrast Agent, Amount, Rate	Sequence	Analysis ROI/VBV
Lavini et al,[16] 2007	Ankle, knee, wrist	Arthritis, osteoblastoma, chondrosarcoma	1.5 T	20 s/7.2 min	SI curve	2007	8.1/3.4/30	Gd-DTPA, NA, 5 mL/s	T1-FSGRE	VBV
Kubassova et al,[13,14] 2007	MCP	RA	1.5 T	7 s/2.3 min	SI curve	2007	14/3.8/40	Gd-DTPA, NA	T1-SGRE	VBV
Zierhut et al,[54] 2007	MCP	RA, synovitis	1.5 T	10 s/5.7 min	K^{trans}	2007	35/4.2/70	Gd-DTPA, NA, 20 mL	T1-GRE	VBV
van der Leij et al,[29] 2009	Knee	Synovitis	1.5 T	22 s/7 min	SI curve	2009	8.1/3.5/30	Gd-DTPA, 0.1 mg/kg, 5 mL/s	T1-GRE	VBV
Malattia et al,[90] 2010	Wrist, hip	Juvenile idiopathic arthritis	1.5 T	5 s/3.3 min	SI curve	2010	6/1.7/40	Gd-DTPA, 0.1 mmol/kg, 2 mL/s	T1-FFE	VBV
van de Sande et al,[15] 2012	Knee	Early RA and non RA	1.5 T	20 s/7 min	SI curve	2012	8.1/3.5/30	Gd-DTPA, 0.1 mg/kg, 5 mL/s	T1-GRE	VBV
Kim et al,[127] 2012	Hip	Septic arthritis, synovitis	1.5 T	30 s/6 min	SI curve	2012	75–100/ 1.4–1.7/70	Gd-DTPA, 0.1 mmol/kg, NA	T1	VBV
Boesen et al,[56] 2012	Wrist	RA	0.2 T	10 s/5 min	SI curve	2012	60/6/75	Gd-BOPTA, 0.1 mmol/kg manual	T1-GRE	VBV
Axelsen et al,[60] 2012	Knee	RA	1.5 T	10 s/4.7 min	SI curve	2012	40/12/70	Gd-DTPA, 0.05 mmol/kg	FLASH	VBV
Cimmino et al,[65] 2012	Wrist	PsA, synovitis, BME	0.2 T	18 s/6 min	SI curve	2012	100/16/NA	Gd-DTPA, 0.2 mL/kg, manual	T1SE	VBV
Wojciechowski et al,[55] 2013	Wrist	RA, synovitis, BME	0.2 T	10 s/NA	SI curve	2012	NA/NA/NA	Gd-DTPA, 0.1 mL/kg, manual	T1-GRE	VBV
Poggenborg et al,[102] 2014	MCP, PIP, DIP	PsA	0.6 T	3.6 s/1.8 min	SI curve	2013	33/4.2/25	Gd-DOTA, 0.2 mL/kg, 2 mL/s	NA	VBV
Ballegaard et al,[106] 2014	Knee (IPFP)	OA	3.0 T	9 s/4.4 min	SI curve	2014	5.5/1.9/15	Gd-HP-DO3A, 0.1 mL/kg, 2 mL/s	VIBE	VBV
Teruel et al,[85] 2014	Wrist	RA, BME	3.0 T	12 s/6.4 min	SI curve	2014	6.4/2.1/12	Gd-DTPA, NA, NA	SPGR	VBV

Study	Joint	Application	Field strength	TR/TE	Analysis	Year	TR/TE/FA	Contrast	Sequence	Method
Vordenbäume et al,[61] 2014	MCP	RA, Synovitis	3.0 T	1.7 s/5.7 min	SI curve	2014	333/1.5/8	Gd-DTPA, 0.4 mL/kg, NA	FLASH	ROI
Wenham et al,[113] 2014	Knee	OA	3.0 T	10 s/5 min	SI curve	2014	4.3/2.5/30	Gd-DOTA, 0.1 mmol/kg, 4 mL/s	GRE	ROI
Müller-Lutz et al,[74] 2015	MCP	RA	3.0 T	1.7 s/5.7 min	SI curve	2014	333/1.5/8	Gd-DTPA, 0.4 mL/kg, NA	FLASH	ROI
Axelsen et al,[62] 2014	MCP, Wrist	RA, Synovitis, erosion, JSN, tenosynovitis	0.6 T	NA	SI curve	2015	33/4.2/25	Gd-DOTA, 0.2 mL/kg, NA	T1-GRE	VBV
Maijer et al,[64] 2016	Knee	RA, Synovitis	1.5 T	21 s/7 min	K^{trans}	2016	4.6/8.1/30	Gd-DTPA, 0.1 mmol/kg, 3-5 mL/s	FSGRE	VBV
Anwander et al,[104] 2016	Hip	THA	1.5 T	7.8/4 min	K^{trans}	2016	865/6.8/NA	Gd-DTPA, 0.1 mmol/kg, 2.5 mL/s	FSE (Bookend)	VBV
Conaghan et al,[73] 2016	Wrist, MCP	RA, BME, synovitis	1.5/3.0 T	NA	SI curve	2016	NA	NA, 0.1 mmol/Kg, NA	NA	VBV
Riis et al,[107] 2016; Riis et al,[114] 2017	Knee	OA	3.0 T	9 s/4.4 min	SI curve	2016	1.9/5.5/15	Gd-DOTA, 0.1 mL/kg, 2 mL/s	VIBE	VBV
Budzik et al,[122] 2017	Knee	OA	3.0 T	11 s/4.1 min	SI curve/K^{trans}	2017	4.8/2.1/20	Gd-DOTA, 0.1 mL/kg, NA	FSGRE	ROI
Nusman et al,[93,98] 2017	Knee	Juvenile idiopathic arthritis	1.0 T	15.7 s/4.1 min	SI curve	2017	8.1/6.9/NA	Gd-DO3A-butriol, 0.1 mmol/kg, 3 mL/s	FSGRE	VBV
Swaminathan et al,[115] 2017	Knee	OA, Synovitis	1.5 T	22 s/NA	K^{trans}	2017	NA/NA/NA	Gd-DOTA	NA	VBV

Abbreviations: BME, bone marrow edema; DIP, distal interphalangeal joint; FA, flip angle; FFE, Fast field echo; FLASH, fast low angle shot; FSE, fast spin echo; FSGRE, fat saturated gradient echo; GRE, Gradient echo; Gd-DOTA, Dotarem® Gadolinum contrat; IPFP, infrapatellar fat pad (Hoffa's fat pad); JSN, Joint space narrowing; MCP, metacarpophalangeal; NA, not available; OA, osteoarthritis; PIP, proximal interphalangeal joint; PsA, psoriatic arthritis; RA, rheumatoid arthritis; ROI, region of interest; SI-curve, signal intensity versus time curve; T1SE, T1 spin echo; TE, echo time; TR, repetition time; VBV, voxel by voxel; VIBE, volumetric interpolated breath-hold.

K_{ep}, the redistribution rate constant between C_t and C_p, as well as the plasma and tissue volume fractions, which are denoted as v_p and v_e.[19] These measurements may not precisely reflect the true physiologic processes in vivo; however, they seem to be reproducible when performed with identical acquisition techniques at a single center.[17] Generally for all quantitative data measurements, the SI changes over time must be converted to dynamic change in contrast agent concentration in the tissue, which usually requires acquisition of DCE-MR imaging with a very high temporal resolution (a few seconds between images) and obtaining a T1 map sequence of the tissue of interest,[19] before contrast infusion.

Methods to quantify the precontrast native T1 maps of the tissues of interest vary in accuracy and length of acquisition, and the resulting T1 map values will always suffer from inaccuracies related to magnetic field inhomogeneity and various artifacts, such as flow artifacts.[19] To simplify this, "tissue population averages" of T1 values can be used; however, these measurements are not accurately replicated across different patients and scanners.

Another key component of most types of pharmacokinetics modeling is to initially determine the changes in contrast concentration over time in a blood vessel feeding the tissue of interest: the so-called Arterial Input Function (AIF)[19] (see **Fig. 1**). Although current best practice is to draw a small ROI over an artery within the field of view and measuring the AIF values from the average ROI curve, this can be difficult because of flow artifacts, partial volume effects, and nonlinear saturation effects of high contrast agent concentrations.[19] Therefore, many investigators use either a mathematical approximation or population-based average function. Unfortunately, these approaches are also known to weaken the reproducibility of the results across patients.[19]

The tracer kinetic models applied to the data vary in the literature depending on the clinical problem, the unique tissue physiology, anatomy, and the temporal MR imaging data resolution required for accurate depiction of contrast agent uptake.[19] Despite this challenge, a large number of clinical trials primarily in oncology have used K^{trans} and other similar parameters as primary imaging endpoints, which is described in recent comprehensive reviews.[17–19,26] In most cases, efficacy was determined by observing a reduction in K^{trans}; however, there was little standardization in both how the K^{trans} values were determined and what constituted a significant reduction. In addition, the parameters of pharmacokinetic analysis did not only differ between clinical and research applications, but also between individual hospital institutions. The lack of method standardization has prevented multicenter comparison of raw K^{trans} values, limiting establishment of quantitative cutoff values for use as imaging biomarkers in the assessment of drug efficacy or monitoring of disease progression. Standardization of quantitative biomarkers such as K^{trans} has therefore become a priority for radiologists, illustrated by formation of the Quantitative Imaging Biomarkers Alliance (QIBA) initiative sponsored by the Radiological Society of North America. This group has aimed to, and published, basic standards for DCE-MR imaging measurements and quality controls that provide reliable DCE-MR imaging protocols for more reproducible K^{trans} value measurements across imaging platforms, clinical sites, and over time[27].

Descriptive (Semiquantitative) Heuristic Analysis

An alternative methodology is based on the direct measurement of changes in tissue perfusion as captured by the individual SI curves located within the tissue of interest called heuristic analysis. Here the pattern of contrast uptake is used to classify various SI curves during the acquisition. Many clinical research groups have used 4 different curve "shapes" that seem to reflect the underlying contrast behavior in vivo, described as (1) baseline (reflecting no contrast uptake), (2) baseline and uptake (persistent enhancement), (3) baseline uptake and a plateau, and (4) baseline, uptake, plateau, and a washout pattern. **Fig. 2** shows the 4 SI curves approximated by the 4 model types described by

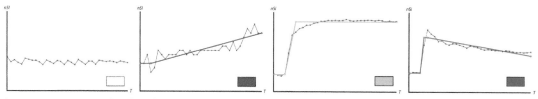

Fig. 2. SI curves normalized to the baseline (nSI) versus time (T). The curves are approximated by the linear segments showing different stages of tissue response to Gd contrast injection: baseline, wash-in, plateau, and washout. These linear segments are automatically fitted into the normalized SI curves. From left: type 0 (*transparent*), no enhancement; type 1 (*blue*), persistent enhancement; type 2 (*green*), plateau enhancement; type 3 (*red*), washout enhancement patterns.

Kubassova and colleagues.[13,14] Note that the x-axis reflects the time of acquisition and the y-axis reflects the normalized SI (nSI). The normalization of original SI curves is done to reduce variability between examinations on the same scanner in follow-up acquisitions. All SI values are divided by the mean of the first few precontrast values, so that nSI starts from approximately 1.[13,14]

The speed of distribution and the volume of absorption of Gd contrast by a particular tissue and the scan time will influence the type of model appropriate for a particular SI curve that for visual aid can be color-coded.

- Type 0: No enhancement. SI curve models as such will correspond to pixels located in the noisy background of the image, nonenhancing bone interior, or healthy tissue.
- Type 1: Persistent enhancement. Tissues exhibiting baseline and wash-in phases, but not reaching a plateau during the acquisition time; for example, showing a continuous slow rise-up. Often, such SI curves are located in skin, muscle, bone, and soft tissue boundaries or artifacts.
- Type 2: Plateau enhancement. Tissues are vascular to the extent that SI curves show baseline, wash-in, and plateau phase with *no* washout. They are normally located within inflamed synovium, muscle, and bone marrow edema (BME).
- Type 3: Washout enhancement. Tissue exhibits baseline, wash-in, plateau, and washout phases; they are often located in arteries, some veins and within highly perfused and/or severely inflamed tissue.

This DCE-MR imaging analysis approach was developed by Kubassova and colleagues[13,14,20,21,28] for musculoskeletal applications and has been validated in various inflammatory joint diseases. The strength of this heuristic approach is the fully automated decision on which model is used for which SI curve. The decision is based on the use of the noise level in the MR sequence and statistical principals of Kolmogorov-Smirnov test for noise distribution comparison. Such approach leads to a 100% reproducible observer-independent choice of model in the same image data.

Fig. 3 shows an example of Gd map build in every voxel in a fully automated manner from the sagittal DCE-MR imaging sequences acquired in a patient with inflammatory reactive knee arthritis scanned for 5 minutes. In the Gd map of the knee, each voxel is color-coded according to the pattern type of enhancement: blood vessels are clearly shown as tubular structures in the posterior knee in red (type 3), synovial tissue mostly in green (type 2), but in the posterior capsular area there is enhancement in red (type 3); tissues with no reaction to contrast agent are shown in native grayscale with no color (type 0).

Other groups like Lavini and colleagues[16] have used up to 7 different models, as shown in **Fig. 4.** Here, instead of linear segments, a continuous function is fitted into the SI curve based on the use of threshold to choose the model that in

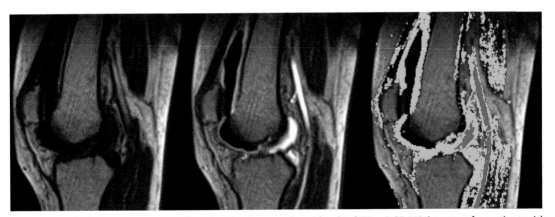

Fig. 3. From the left: precontrast and postcontrast grayscale midsagittal T1w DCE-MR images of a patient with reactive arthritis of the knee and a corresponding parametric map showing pattern of Gd uptake (Gd map). Images are mid-sagittal T1w DCE-MR imaging acquired at time 0 (*left*) and 5 minutes (*center*) after Gd injection. In the Gd map of the knee (*right*), each voxel is color-coded according to the pattern type of enhancement. The artery behind the knee joint is clearly shown as tubular structures in red (type 3), synovial tissue in the anterior and central part of the knee mostly in green (type 2), and the posterior capsular and synovial enhancement are shown in red (type 3) reflecting washout. Tissues with no color shown in native grayscale represent areas of no significant contrast in enhancement (type 0).

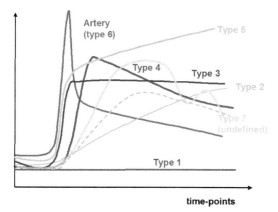

Fig. 4. Multiple models representing behaviors of SI curves. Type 1 (*gray*), no enhancement; type 2 (*green*), slow enhancement, maximum of the curve is reached after half scan; type 3 (*blue*), quick enhancement, followed by a signal plateau; type 4 (*magenta*), fast enhancement and quick washout; type 5 (*yellow*), quick enhancement, followed by a slow constant enhancement; type 6 (*red*), artery; type 7 (*white/light gray*), all others.

their article is referred to as time intensity curves. This approach has also shown relatively high reproducibility and has been applied in various inflammatory joint disease.[15,29]

To further understand the functional pattern of inflammatory changes and to differentiate tissues on the basis of their vascularity and enhancement following contrast injection, the height, slope, time of update, and washout can be calculated and parameterized. For each SI curve approximated by a model, parameters such as Maximum Enhancement (ME), Initial Rate of Enhancement (IRE), Initial rate of Washout (IRW), Time of Onset of Enhancement (Tonset), and Time of Washout (Twashout) can be extracted as shown in **Fig. 5**.

As shown in **Figs. 6** and **7**, the inflamed synovial membrane can show heterogeneous enhancement patterns within 1 joint. Therefore, it can be helpful to assess the SI curve shape of every pixel in the whole synovial volume; as such, a pixel-by-pixel analysis method allows direct visualization of heterogeneously distributed disease activity.[16,21]

DCE-MR imaging protocols for most musculoskeletal joint diseases have temporal resolution of less than 10 seconds. DCE-MR imaging is acquired at several anatomic locations usually in 2-dimensional (2D) imaging to cover the anatomy of interest, and by summing the slices, the data form the full volume of the joint. To extract quantitative measures from DCE-MR imaging, each temporal slice in the 2D image can automatically be processed using methodology published by Kubassova and colleagues[21] or Lavini and colleagues.[16] These pixel-by-pixel approaches help to visualize the differently shaped SI curves within a volume of interest, which helps to allocate zones with specific types of SI curves for computer-guided placement of an ROI around the anatomy of interest[13,14,16] in one or all slices. In adults, the

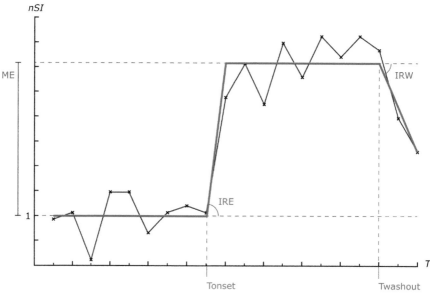

Fig. 5. SI curve (*in black*) approximated by linear segments (*in red*) to show the stages of Gd uptake by a tissue: baseline, uptake, plateau and washout phases. The quantitative modeled parameters of ME, IRE, Tonset, Twashout, and IRW are shown.

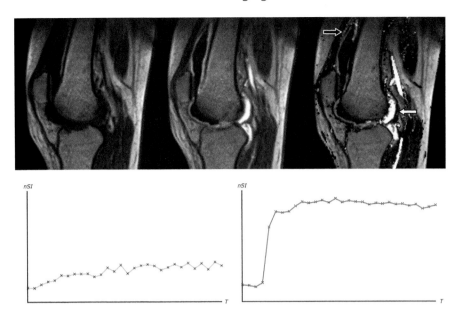

Fig. 6. Midsagittal precontrast and postcontrast images from DCE-MR imaging sequences acquired from the same patient as **Fig. 3** with inflammatory reactive knee arthritis and secondary osteoarthritis to illustrate the added value of DCE-MR imaging to separate low perfused and high perfused synovitis. Top row: the DCE-MR imaging sequence before Gd contrast (*left*) followed by the DCE-MR imaging image 5 minutes after IV Gd injection (*center*). The image on the right shows the map of IRE superimposed on the original grayscale MR image. The highest perfusion is shown in the capsular area (*solid white arrow*) in the posterior part of the knee with the corresponding SI curve in red (*lower right*) showing high IRE and ME. Note also the low perfusion depicted in the thick synovium of the suprapatellar pouch (*open arrow*) illustrated by the green SI curve in the lower left figure. Using static imaging scoring of synovitis will give the same score to both of these 2 areas, illustrating the strength of the parameterized maps to understand distribution of perfusion and inflammatory activity.

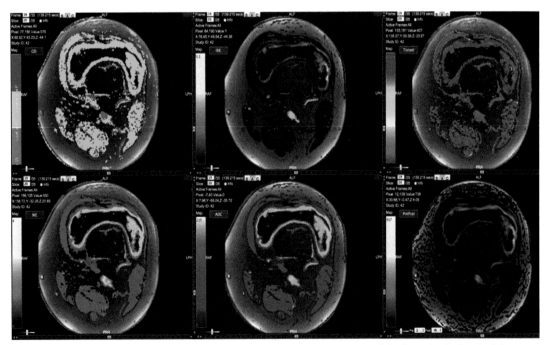

Fig. 7. Various multiparametric maps calculated from axial DCE-MR imaging of the knee in the level of the suprapatellar recess in a patient with knee OA. Top row from left maps of Gd, IRE, and time of onset. Bottom row from left maps of ME, AUC, and a subtraction map of the first and the last dynamic temporal series. Note the heterogeneous perfusion in the synovial membrane with the highest perfusion in the right side of the image in the proliferative synovial lining.

ROI is usually placed roughly around the enhancing area and only the enhancing voxels within the ROI are counted. In children, however, a more cautious delineation is important to exclude the hypervascular growth plate from the ROIs. An example of 3-slice coronal acquisition of a hand and the corresponding ROIs around the metacarpophalangeal (MCP) joints in a patient with RA is shown in **Figs. 8** and **9**. The figures show how the different SI curves can be extracted from different joints and have the same static scores on the postcontrast images.

Once the ROIs are placed, all voxels are counted in an automated manner. From the map of Gd uptake, the quantitative volume of inflammation can be extracted as a total number of enhancing pixels; the volume of inflammation is weighted by the degree of severity of inflammation, extracted from the map of ME and IRE. These 2 measures have been validated in several trials of inflammatory joint diseases and referred to as dynamic contrast-enhanced MR imaging quantification volume (DEMRIQ-Volume) and DEMRIQ-Inflammation, in which the use of parametric maps to guide ROI placement saves significant time and increases the reproducibility of the results to 95% and higher.[28,30]

When using heuristic SI curve analysis, it is also important to note that all DCE-MR imaging datasets ideally should be corrected for patient motion before the analysis, which both can increase the signal-to-noise ratio of the data up to 300% but also significantly affect the curve classification in each voxel[21,31] exemplified in **Figs. 10–12**.

Figs. 10 and **11** show DCE-MR imaging data from inflamed MCP joints in a patient with RA. Regardless of proper patient positioning and the use of a dedicated coil, the DCE-MR imaging data, acquired over a 5-minute interval, suffers from the introduced noise due to the patient's internal micro movement and shivering. Note that there is a significant misalignment between the first few and the last few images, as illustrated by the blue and red joint outlines in **Fig. 10**.

Use of patient motion correction will also impact the shape of the classified curves and therefore the outcome measures of the analysis, as shown in **Fig. 11**.

Fig. 12 illustrates in 2 cases the importance of the patient motion correction, showing the parametric maps of ME constructed for images without and with motion correction applied.

Advantages of nonparametric DCE-MR imaging analysis include that it is less time-consuming and complex acquisition requirements with no need of knowing the tissue T1 value, no need for conversion of MR imaging SI into contrast concentration,

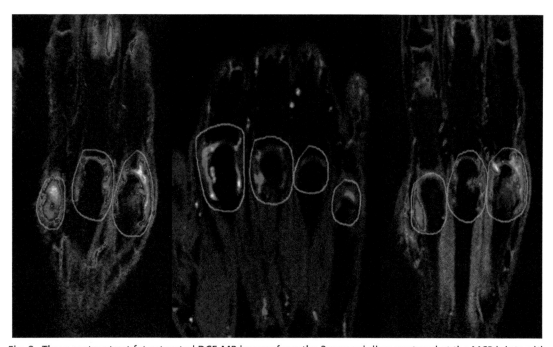

Fig. 8. Three postcontrast fat-saturated DCE-MR images from the 3 coronal slices centered at the MCP joints with maps of ME superimposed on the MR images. On the visual scale, the bright yellow-white colors in each map show the higher degree of perfusion and the darker red shows the lower. ROIs are places around the joints to capture the inflammatory activity within synovial tissue and BME of the joints.

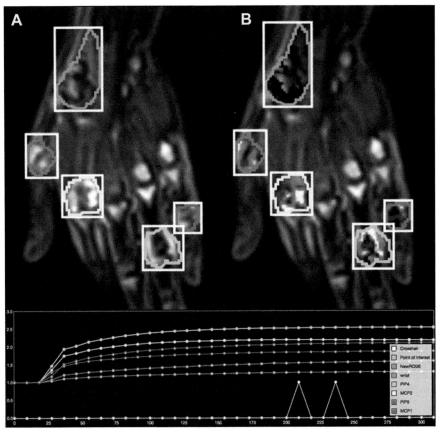

Fig. 9. Coronal DCE-MR images from a patient with active RA. Note the rough ROIs encircled around the various joints with similar volume of enhancing synovitis shown with different colors. Image at top row left (*A*) shows an example of the last grayscale postcontrast DCE-MR imaging series. Image to the right (*B*) is the same with overlay of IRE map. The corresponding SI curve according to the colors can be seen in the bottom of the figure: green, fourth proximal interphalangeal joint (PIP); yellow, second MCP joint; purple, fifth PIP; red, first MCP; orange, radial part of the wrist; white, background noise.

and no need for measurement AIF. However, because the analysis is based on MR imaging SI, the scan time, acquisition parameters, selected Gd contrast agent, MR imaging scanner field

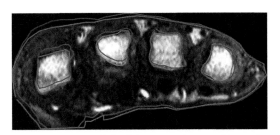

Fig. 10. Contour of the joints' envelope and bone interiors outlined in the original MR image (*blue*) and following motion correction (*red*) superimposed on the target image. The difference in the joint and bone interiors demonstrates the impact of patient movement during the acquisition of DCE-MR imaging sequence.

strength, and the used heuristic analysis methods will influence these semiquantitative measurements and limit comparison of results from different patients and especially between scanners.[11,17–19] By standardizing the DCE-MR imaging acquisition to 5 minutes, in which normal tissue should have reached enhancement equilibrium, and by using the same scanner, sequence, contrast media, speed of contrast injection, and analysis method, the variability between trials and patients can be diminished and observed differences in tissue enhancement properties between normal tissue and tissue with disease can better be distinguished.[21,32]

INFLAMMATORY JOINT DISEASES

According to 1983 American Rheumatism Association (ARA; currently American Colleague of Rheumatology [ACR]) classification, rheumatic diseases are divided into several groups.[33] The first involves

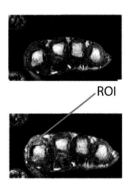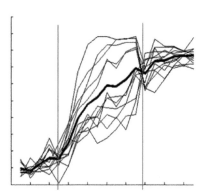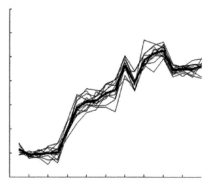

ROI

Fig. 11. Left: Precontrast (*upper*) and postcontrast images (*lower*) from an axial DCE-MR imaging sequence acquired over the MCP joints in a patient with RA and active synovitis of the MCP joints. A small ROI in red is placed inside the inflamed synovium (*lower left image*). The patient's hand has moved during the acquisition, thus creating misalignment between all images in the DCE-MR imaging sequences, in particular during the contrast uptake phase illustrated in the SI curves in the center. Center: SI curves from the red ROI without motion correction. The curves extracted from the ROI (*thin lines* are voxel-based nSI and the bold line is the mean of the pixel nSI). It is clearly visible that the motion affects the shape of the individual nSI curves. Right: nSI voxel-based and the mean curve (*in bold*) extracted from the same red ROI after the patient motion correction was applied to align the temporal images in the DCE-MR imaging sequence. This significantly changes the mean curve from type 2 (plateau) to type 3 (washout).

typical inflammatory rheumatic connective tissue diseases, such as RA, juvenile idiopathic arthritis (JIA), lupus erythematosus, scleroderma, dermatomyositis and polymyositis, Sjögren syndrome. The second group includes spondyloarthritis (SpA), such as ankylosing spondylitis (AS), reactive SpA, psoriatic SpA (PsA), SpA in the course of inflammatory bowel diseases, and undifferentiated forms. Osteoarthritis is the third group in the ARA classification[34] and numerous studies confirm the presence of low-grade inflammation along with mechanical, genetic, hormonal, metabolic, and immunologic factors in the pathogenesis.[35–41] For the most common inflammatory arthritis in adults and children, RA and JIA, inflammation affects subchondral bone, synovium, tenosynovium, intra-articular and extra-articular fat tissue, and leads to subsequent cartilage loss, formation of bony cysts and erosions, tendons tears, joint malalignment, and ankyloses, especially if left untreated.[42,43]

SpA may affect peripheral joints as well as sacroiliac joints (SIJs) and spine. In the peripheral joints, SpA features resembles RA with typical presence of soft tissue thickening, osteoporosis, cysts, and joint space narrowing, but without severe bony destruction. In the SIJs, sacroiliitis is typical for SpA, which first affects the subchondral bone of SIJ and is seen on MR imaging as BME. Additional active inflammatory lesions include SIJ synovitis, capsulitis, and enthesitis. In the later disease stages, subsequent structural lesions are seen, which include fatty metaplasia, sclerosis,

erosions, backfill, nonbridging bone buds, and ankylosis.[44]

In the spine, MR imaging findings include inflammatory corner lesions (BME in the corners of the spinal vertebrae), aseptic noninfectious discitis, endplate erosions, zygo-apophyseal joint inflammation, costovertebral joint inflammation, inflammation of the posterior spinal elements, and subsequent ankylosis in the end stage. One of the most diversified SpA subgroups is PsA, which usually involves the peripheral joints, spine, SIJs, and entheses. In the peripheral joints, the classic features of PsA include dactylitis, cysts, and classic erosions coexisting with proliferative lesions at the distal interphalangeal joint level, phalangeal tuft acroosteolysis, osteolyses, enthesopatic lesions, and bone ankylosis. In SIJs and spine, typical asymmetric sacroiliitis and thick, fluffy asymmetric syndesmophytes, called parasyndesmophytes in the spine may be seen.[45]

OA affects synovial joints of both the axial and peripheral skeleton, and shows a low degree synovitis with synovial hypertrophy and mild postcontrast enhancement on T1w MR imaging in addition to bony osteophytes, focal or diffuse cartilage destruction, bony cysts, bone marrow lesions, and meniscal and ligamentous damage. Finally, crystal deposition diseases, the fifth group of rheumatic diseases according to the ARA, is characterized by inflammation in the soft tissues and/or bone induced by crystal deposition, with subsequent soft tissue lesions, tendon delamination, and/or tears, cartilage damage, subchondral

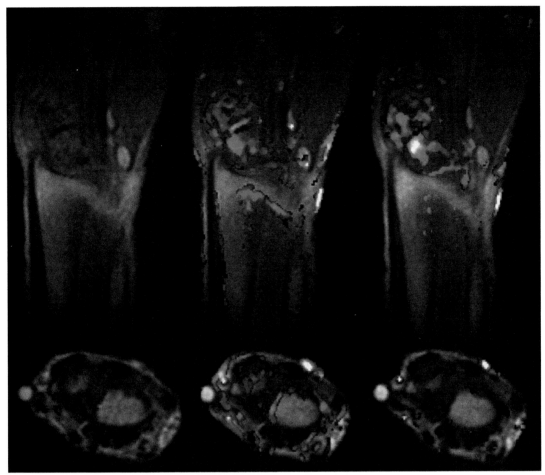

Fig. 12. Left: Coronal DCE-MR imaging of the wrist in a patient with RA (*top row*) and axial DCE-MR imaging of the wrist in a healthy control (*bottom row*). Center: Parametric map of inflammatory activity (ME) constructed before the application of patient motion correction. Right: Parametric map of activity (ME) constructed after the application of patient motion correction. On a visual scale, the dark-red colors in the map of ME indicate the lower degree of activity and the white-yellow indicate higher degree of activity. The patient in the top of the figure has high degree of activity in the radial part of the wrist only depicted after motion correction (*right*), and not clearly visible before the motion correction (*center*). The healthy control at the bottom of the figure will, due to the motion of the hand during the acquisition, have erroneously classification of moderate inflammatory activity. This activity is removed after motion correction (*right*), leaving only the physiologic blood vessels in the subcutaneous tissue color-coded/perfused as they should.

bony cysts, and erosions related to the localization of crystals.[46]

Clinically and biochemically, it can be challenging to distinguish between various inflammatory joint diseases, especially in the early stages, as they all present with joint pain, joint swelling, and often limited range of motion. Radiographs and ultrasound may be negative or nonspecific. Although ultrasound allows for detailed evaluation of articular and periarticular soft tissues of peripheral joints, standardized quantitative ultrasound-based measures of joint inflammation, such as the Doppler signal, have considerable issues with high interobserver and intraobserver variability.[47]

Thus, most ultrasound studies are primarily based on qualitative or semiquantitative scoring methodologies.[48–50] MR imaging, and especially DCE-MR imaging, sequences may help in providing detailed quantitative information and superior potential to differentiate between distinct joint disease entities that require targeted treatment strategies.[48,49]

DYNAMIC CONTRAST-ENHANCED MR IMAGING IN INFLAMMATORY JOINT DISEASES

T1w DCE-MR imaging is a well-known instrument for staging and monitoring different malignant tumors.[19,51] The use of DCE-MR imaging within the field of musculoskeletal disease is increasing because all inflammatory diseases show abnormal vascularization due to development of neovessels, defined as formation of new capillaries under the influence of many different chemokines. Most of these neovessels are structurally immature, lacking pericytes to stabilize their vessel walls, which results in significant increased permeability that will lead to increased hypoxia in the inflamed tissue, and extravasation of leukocytes.[43]

DCE-MR imaging is the optimal method for comprehensive investigation of perfusion changes of all tissues affected by rheumatic diseases and can be performed on both high-field and low-field MR imaging scanners.[5,9–11,49,52] In the past decade, validation of the DCE-MR imaging technique to detect synovitis in patients with RA has been intensified,[5,15,29,53,54] but assessing wrist joint synovitis with DCE-MR imaging in the same patients with RA on 0.25-T and 3-T MR imaging found only fair correlation between slopes of the SI curves. This is probably due to the difference in protocol design and variation of temporal resolution, illustrating the influence of MR imaging field strength on the resulting SI curves. Another study using low-field 0.2-T MR imaging scanner and manual injection of Gd contrast could not find an association between the axial DCE-MR imaging data from the wrist and the static RAMRIS scores,[55] as shown in other studies.[56] The reason for this is not clear, but could be related to timing of the contrast injection and the initiation of the DCE-MR imaging sequence as well as the use of axial and not coronal DCE-MR imaging slices.

Regardless, DCE-MR imaging parameters and especially the slope of the SI curves on 1.0 to 3.0 T seem to correlate highly with the number of neovessels and degree of inflammatory cell infiltration in histologic biopsies.[57–61] Combining the volume of enhancing tissue and the slope of the SI curve in some articles referred to as DEMRIQ-Inflammation has shown potential to differentiate between healthy subjects and patients with RA.[62,63] Classification of various SI curve profiles from the DCE-MR imaging data have been used in early diagnosis to identify patients with unclassified arthritis from patients developing RA and SpA,[64] and both the slope and the height of the enhancement curves were significantly different between patients with RA and patients with PsA.[65]

Potential to identify different disease entities among a significant number of undifferentiated arthropathies is especially important, as this will enable early interventions and targeted treatment strategies that could improve long-term outcomes.

Figs. 13 and 14 illustrate DCE-MR imaging acquired from patients with various inflammatory diseases and processed using heuristic quantitative methodology described previously.

Several studies confirmed that the changes in SI curve shapes and the associated quantitative volume of inflammation, including DEMRIQ-Volume as well as the quantitative volume weighted by the IRE DEMRIQ-Inflammation, in many cases are more sensitive measures of treatment response compared with the static MR imaging–based scoring methods, such as RA MR imaging scores (RAMRIS) or MR imaging OA scores (ie,

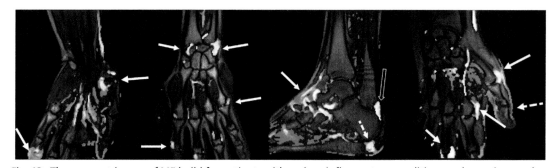

Fig. 13. The parametric map of ME build for patients with various inflammatory conditions and superimposed on MR image. On a visual scale, the dark-red colors in the map of ME indicate the lower degree of activity and the white-yellow indicate higher degree of activity. From the left to right: (1) patients with inflammatory osteoarthritis of the distal interphalangeal and first carpometacarpal joint; (2) inflammatory RA in the hand showing intracapsular synovitis in multiple joints (*arrows*); (3) inflammatory RA of hind foot and midfoot showing synovial inflammation in the midfoot (*closed arrow*) inflammation in the Achilles tendon bursa (*open arrow*), and inflammation in the rheumatoid nodule in the heel fat pad (*dotted arrow*); and (4) psoriatic arthritis showing entheseal and capsular inflammation in the first and second MCP and third proximal interphalangeal joint (*closed arrows*) and subcutaneous and nailbed enhancement in the 1 digit representing a sausage digit (*dotted arrow*).

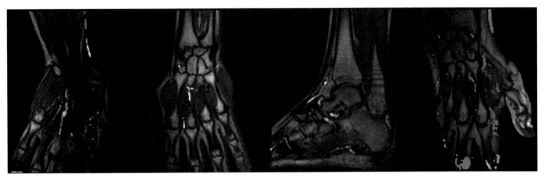

Fig. 14. The same patients as in Fig. 13 but using an IRE parametric map.

MOAKS).[56,66–73] Increased K^{trans} values in the synovitis of the MCP joints from patients with RA have also been linked to reduced glycose-aminoglycan values in the MCP joint cartilage measured by delayed Gd-enhanced MR imaging of cartilage (dGEMRIC).[74] Thus, DCE-MR imaging–based quantitative measures could be considered as one of the primary endpoints for assessment of the early synovitis responses in patients with RA and OA.[21,52] Clinically, longitudinally DCE-MR imaging–based quantitative measures also seem to follow the early clinical treatment effect after intra-articular steroid injections (Fig. 15)[56,66] or on initiation of biological therapy (Figs. 16

and 17).[75,76] One article has even linked the early synovitis responders on DCE-MR imaging (K^{trans}) following biological therapy to specific genetic pretreatment profiles.[77]

BME is considered to be highly predictive of future erosions in both early and established RA.[78–81] BME is seen in up to 75% of patients with early RA[78] and presence of BME in patients with anti-citrullinated protein antibodies in serum predicts a rapid development of RA.[82] The CIMESTRA trial has shown that BME is the strongest independent predictor of radiological progression in patients with RA within 1 year,[80] and biopsy studies from MCP joints with BME showed

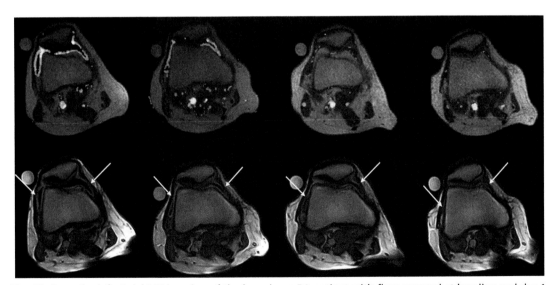

Fig. 15. From the left: Axial MR imaging of the knee in an RA patient with flare scanned at baseline and day 1, day 2, and day 7 after 40 mg intra-articular steroid injection and extraction of effusion ultrasound guided at baseline. Top: Axial DCE-MR imaging from 0.2-T scanner with the parametric map of ME. Bottom: Postcontrast 3-dimensional (3D) T1w GRE sequences acquired after the DCE-MR imaging sequence at the same location. Arrows indicate synovial enhancement on the postcontrast 3D T1w sequence as signs of synovitis. The 3D T1w GRE sequences show improvement in effusion and only marginal change in synovitis from baseline to day 7 with almost no change from day 1 to day 2. DCE-MR imaging shows partial remission on day 2 and complete DCE-MR imaging remission on day 7 following the clinical course of the patient.

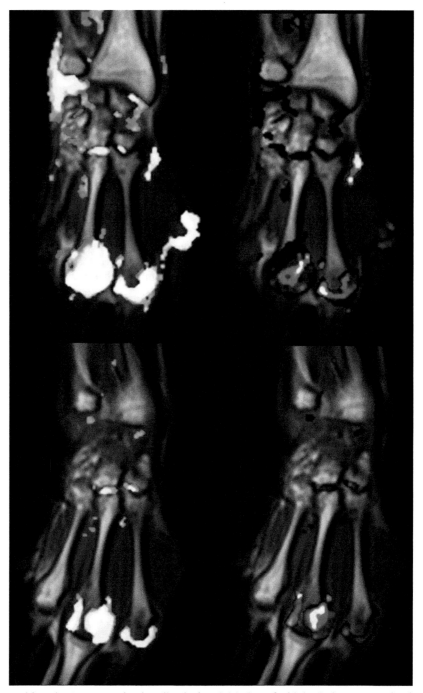

Fig. 16. Patient with active RA scanned at baseline before initiation of a biological treatment (*top*) and 3 months after (*bottom*). Left side of the figure shows maps of ME (*left*) and right side maps of IRE (*right*). The top row shows coronal DCE-MR images revealing high inflammatory activity in the second and third MCP joints as well as moderate synovitis in the wrist and tenosynovitis in ulnar side of the wrist. In the bottom row, the same patient had clinical remission and a moderate to good synovitis treatment response noted in both the wrist and 2nd MCP joint. Note that the third MCP joint shows continuous subclinical high inflammatory activity within newly developed erosion in the head of the MCP bone as further illustrated in **Fig. 17.**

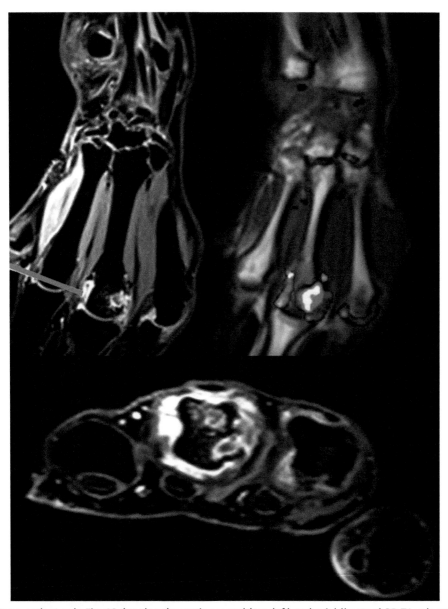

Fig. 17. Same patient as in **Fig. 16** showing the static coronal (*top left*) and axial (*bottom*) 3D T1 volumetric inter-polated breath-hold (VIBE) fat-saturated post-contrast images as well as the coronal DCE-MR imaging IRE map from the follow-up examination (**Fig. 16**) after initiation of biological treatment. Note the big erosion in the head of the third MCP joint with the surrounding enhancing synovitis and very high perfusion (*bright colors*) of the IRE map inside the erosion reflecting ongoing subclinical inflammatory activity. The blue line in the middle of the top left image indicates the slice plane and position of the axial image plane (*bottom*).

inflammatory infiltrates with neovessels in the area of BME.[83,84]

These findings have substantiated the use of DCE-MR imaging to quantify BME similar to syno-vitis quantification. DCE-MR imaging of BME in the wrist bones calculated as both DEMRIQ-Volume and DEMRIQ-Inflammation correlated highly with the static MR imaging RAMRIS bone edema scores in patients with RA.[56] Another study showed that the time intensity curves in wrist bone with BME and in the pannus within bony ero-sions have significantly higher perfusion patterns than normal bones, most likely reflecting ongoing inflammation.[85]

In addition, IRE has shown fast response to anti–tumor necrosis factor (TNF)-alpha therapy in the wrist bone of patients with RA with no concomitant change in the RAMRIS BME score, illustrating the advantage of DCE-MR imaging in BME for treatment monitoring.[86]

In SpA with predominant involvement of the SIJs and spine (axial SpA), the use of IV contrast for MR imaging is currently not recommended to diagnose sacroiliitis and/or spondylitis.[87] Nevertheless, spine DCE-MR imaging has been used to assess fractures, tumors, and bone marrow changes in osteoporosis and avascular necrosis.[88] In AS, DCE-MR imaging was used to monitor the treatment response[89] and differentiate between active and inactive sacroiliitis, concluding that the K^{trans} values from the SI joints had the highest correlation with the Bath Ankylosing Spondylitis Disease Activity Index, which on clinical evaluation reflects ongoing inflammation[87] (**Fig. 18**).

In JIA, several studies have been performed in the past decade on DCE-MR imaging. DCE-MR imaging proved to be feasible in wrists, hips, and knee joints in children with active disease.[90–93] Similar to the experiences from DCE-MR imaging analysis in RA, performing movement registration helps to improve image quality in JIA.[93] It also seems that broader usage of DCE-MR imaging is needed in JIA to enable more accurate assessment of disease activity and treatment monitoring compared with semiquantitative systems.[94] For instance, DCE-MR imaging is capable in differentiating patients with clinically active from inactive JIA with knee and wrist involvement by the difference in the relative number of SI curve shapes (see curve type 4 in **Fig. 4**), as well as with descriptive parameters of ME, maximal initial slope, and the initial area under the curve (AUC).[93,95] In the scope of further validation of DCE-MR imaging in JIA, a number of important steps were performed regarding the responsiveness and construct validity of this technique. It was found that DCE-MR imaging was sensitive to change in a longitudinal follow-up study as a decrease in pharmacokinetic parameter values corresponding to a decrease in clinical disease activity.[92] Moreover, it was shown that both the SI curve shape analysis and descriptive (semiquantitative) heuristic methods

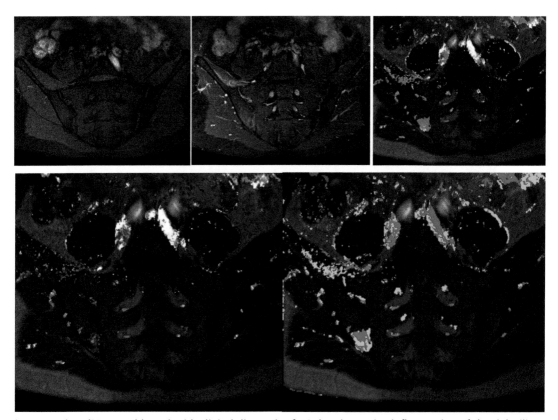

Fig. 18. Patient (35-year-old man) with clinical diagnosis of AS showing active inflammation of the right iliacus muscle and lower right part of the SI joint on MR imaging. Top row from left: Precontrast and postcontrast T1w para coronal static MR images and corresponding map of ME (*right*). Bottom row: Map of IRE and map of Gd Update. In ME and IRE maps, on the visual scale, white-yellow colors show higher degree of perfusion than darker red colors. In Gd Update map, tissues in which SI curves reached washout phase are in red, plateau in green, and wash-in in blue.

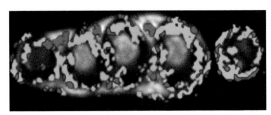

Fig. 19. Axial DCE-MR imaging from a 0.25-T MR imaging scanner of the MCP joint in a patient with JIA, and corresponding Gd map showing synovitis of all 5 MCP joints, which are thought of to be predictive clinical flares.

correlated moderately to substantially with conventional Juvenile Arthritis MRI Scores of disease activity[96,97] Recently, a study on the predictive value of DCE-MR imaging in JIA was performed, showing that the ME values of the synovium in knees of patients with clinically inactive JIA was able to predict clinical flares in children with JIA.[98] An example of DCE-MR imaging inflammation in the MCP joints of a patient with JIA is shown in **Fig. 19** and an example of knee inflammation is depicted in **Fig. 20**.

In psoriasis arthritis (PsA), the added value of using IV contrast is still debated.[99,100] Thus DCE-MR imaging results are scarce and less encouraging compared with patients with RA, possibly due to slow disease progression and primary involvement of the entheses and bone with lesser involvement of the synovium.

One study using a low-field MR imaging scanner showed higher slope and ME values in patients with PsA compared with patients with RA in the wrist,[65] whereas another study using 3T MR imaging showed similar early enhancement curves between both diseases at all time points but 15 minutes after IV injection.[101] A similar finding

with no significant differences in the early enhancement curves or kinetics until after 15 minutes was observed in the distal interphalangeal joints of patients with PsA or OA. In the only published study following biological treatment with conventional MR imaging and DCE-MR imaging parameters, both methods showed significant inflammatory reduction after 1 year with no progression in structural damage despite continuous signs of inflammatory activity on both MR imaging methods.[102]

In OA, DCE-MR imaging has not been evaluated as thoroughly as in inflammatory arthritis. However, a growing number of studies using DCE-MR imaging in OA are being published. DCE-MR imaging has demonstrated increases in enhancing synovial volume with advancing OA disease stages in the knee[103] and has shown increased K^{trans} values in the synovium adjacent hip implants,[104] suggesting altered tissue perfusion kinematics presumably reflecting greater inflammation and granuloma formation around the analyzed prosthesis. Similar to findings in RA, DCE-MR imaging quantitative parameters combining the volume of enhancing voxels (DEMRIQ-Volume), the volume weighted by the ME or IRE (DEMRIQ-Inflammation), significantly improved the correlation with the degree of neovessels and inflammatory cell infiltrate in biopsies from patients with end-stage knee OA.[59,105]

Similarly, DEMRIQ-Volume and DEMRIQ-Inflammation in both the synovium and Hoffa fat pad of obese patients with knee OA have demonstrated higher correlation with clinical symptoms than conventional static MR imaging scores[106,107] (**Fig. 21**).

K^{trans} values in the synovium have also been able to differentiate among healthy subjects, patients with RA, and patients with OA in the

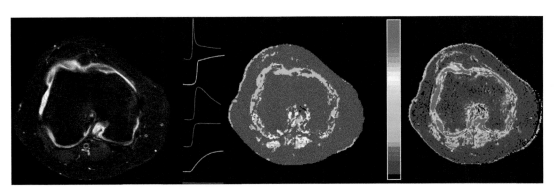

Fig. 20. Contrast-enhanced axial T1w fat-saturated image (*left*) of a 17-year-old girl with active polyarticular JIA showing an enhancing thickened synovial membrane. Corresponding DCE-MR images showing a color-coded SI curve-shape map (*middle*) and an ME map (*right*), clearly demonstrating the heterogeneous enhancement patterns of the inflamed synovial membrane.

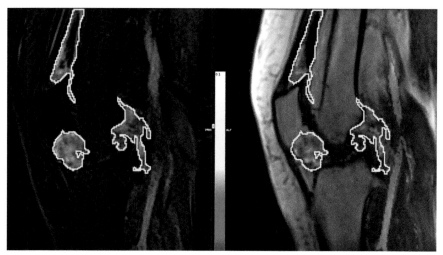

Fig. 21. Midsagittal DCE-MR images of a patient with knee OA and moderate synovitis. Example of how a subtraction image between the fist and the last temporal slice in the DCE-MR imaging data (*left*) can be used to capture enhancing synovium. This subtraction map was used to draw fast and reproducible ROIs around the enhancing synovium that are then automatically and simultaneously transferred to the temporal DCE-MR imaging data (*right*) for extraction of perfusion markers, here shown with the corresponding IRE map. (*Courtesy of* Robert Riis, MD, PhD, Parker Institute and Department of Radiology, Bispebjerg and Frederiksberg Hospital, Denmark from his PhD thesis Riis RG. Assessing synovitis with conventional static and dynamic contrast-enhanced magnetic resonance imaging in knee osteoarthritis. Dan Med J. 2018;65(4):B5464.)

assessment of finger joints.[108] K^{trans} values could also differentiate normal from pathologic cartilage lesions in the patellofemoral joint,[109] and similar K^{trans} values seemed to increase (improve) in the same cartilage region parallel to a clinical improvement after 6 months of oral glucosamine sulfate treatment[110]

DCE-MR imaging data at 3T have demonstrated significant reduction of the slope of enhancement in the synovium of patients with erosive OA of the interphalangeal joints following 12 months of anti–TNF-alpha treatment.[111] A similar pattern has been reported in 2 studies of knee OA showing the efficacy of intra-articular injection of 80 mg methylprednisolone after 2 weeks. Both studies concluded that DCE-MR imaging derived measures of synovial enhancement were more sensitive to the early response to treatment and more strongly associated with changes in pain than synovial volume[112] and static MR imaging scores.[113]

This observed treatment effect might be only short lived, because another large randomized controlled exercise trial could not detect differences in synovial volume or inflammation measures in the knee at 12 weeks after intra-articular injection of 40 mg methylprednisolone versus placebo (saline) preceding the exercise program.[114] Finally, a recent study found good clinical pain relief in patients with knee OA using a knee brace compared with a control group, but the pain reduction was not followed by a change in

perfusion markers of both K^{trans} and SI-curve parameters. Because pain reduction was not due to change in synovitis, other mechanisms may be causing the clinical effect.[115]

Bone marrow lesions (BMLs) also play a significant role in OA. BMLs in the knee have been associated with pain,[116] progressive cartilage and meniscal lesions,[117–119] and total knee joint replacement.[120] DCE-MR imaging has been used to study the volume of the enhancing BML voxels showing a positive association with clinical symptoms (WOMAC) cross-sectionally, but despite significant clinical improvement at 12-month follow-up, the BML volumes from both DCE-MR imaging and static conventional MR imaging remained unchanged[121] (**Fig. 22**).

Using K^{trans} values in BMLs from the tibia plateau in another knee OA cohort study, the investigators reported an association between the K^{trans} value and the size of the BMLs but no association with pain. Another recent study analyzed subchondral bone marrow perfusion in patients with knee OA by using K^{trans} values and found significantly higher AUC in regions with BML compared with areas without BMLs, as well as increased perfusion with advancing degree of OA measured on both radiographs and fat-saturated proton-density MR imaging sequences.[122] The observed higher AUC might reflect increased intravascular blood volume due to venous outflow obstruction or venous stasis as a consequence of

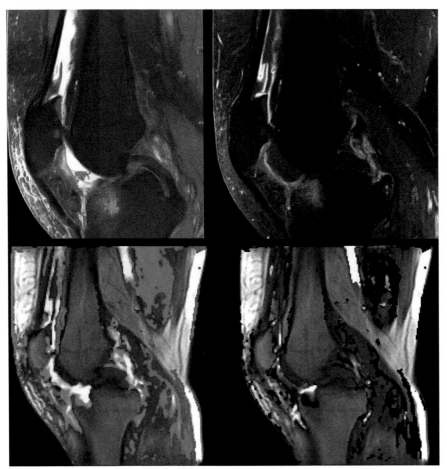

Fig. 22. Midsagittal MR imaging data from a patient with knee OA with high degree of synovitis and moderate effusion along with a BML in the anterior tibia. Top, left: Fat-saturated proton-density-weighted sequence showing water and synovium in bright white colors and fat and muscle in darker gray. Top, right: Postcontrast T1w 3D fat-saturated VIBE sequence showing the thickened synovium in bright white and water/effusion in dark enabling separation of the entities. Bottom left: map of ME; bottom right: map of IRE showing spotted high perfusion of both ME and IRE in the synovial lining in all compartments. Also note high IRE in the subchondral part of the BML in the anterior tibia.

the OA process. This hypothesis has emerged from recent DCE-MR imaging studies using DCE-MR imaging quantitative methodologies to assess the subchondral bone in animals with OA[122,123] (Fig. 23).

INFECTIOUS JOINT DISEASES

Infectious joint disease (IJD) or septic arthritis is less common than inflammatory joint disease. IJD is more often seen in elderly patients postsurgically after, for example, joint replacement or in immunocompromised individuals due to cancer or autoimmune or acquired immune deficiency syndromes.[124]

IJD can be transmitted by various routes, of which the most common is through indirect hematogenous spread from a distant source. The second most common cause is direct seeding from penetrating trauma, foreign bodies, iatrogenic surgical contamination (ie, arthroscopy), or more rarely from juxta articular infectious osteomyelitis, bursitis, or cellulitis.[124]

IJD is clinically divided into pyogenic and nonpyogenic courses. Patients with pyogenic arthritis often present with a severe progressive monoarthritic phenotype with rapid joint destruction, in most cases (up to 80%) due to *Staphylococcus aureus*, followed by other *Staphylococcus* species, streptococci, *Escherichia coli*, *Haemophilus influenzae*, or *Candida* species.[124] The nonpyogenic causes are often less aggressive clinically and caused by, for example, *Mycobacterium tuberculosis* or fungi.[124]

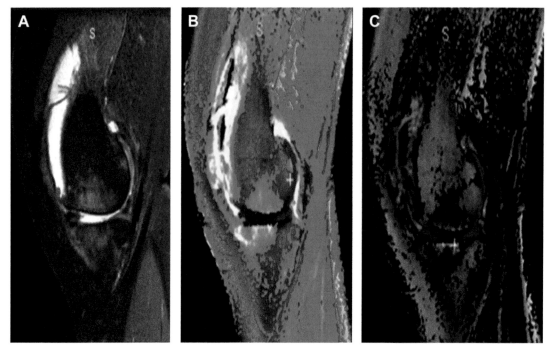

Fig. 23. From the left: (*A*) Sagittal fat-saturated proton-density MR imaging in the center of the medial compartment of the knee in a patient with severe OA showing severe synovitis, moderate effusion, severe cartilage delamination of both tibial and femoral weight-bearing surfaces replaced with effusion, as well as moderate BMLs in both femur and tibia (kissing lesion). (*B*) parametric map of ME and (*C*) IRE map showing high degree of synovitis on both the ME and IRE map. Also note that the BML has similar sizes in both tibia and femur (*A*) but has distinctly different IRE and ME values with higher values/brighter colors in the tibial BML.

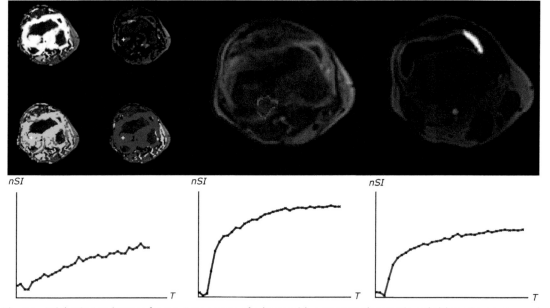

Fig. 24. Axial DCE-MR images from a 3-T scanner of a knee with postoperative septic arthritis and a corresponding acute osteomyelitis encircled by the red ROI in the center image. Top left: Parametric maps of ME, IRE, Gd Uptake, and Tonset (clockwise). Center: Postcontrast image of the knee with red ROI placed in the nidus of the osteomyelitis. Right: Postcontrast image of the knee with ROI placed within the inflamed synovial membrane. Bottom curves are normalized SI curves from the area of the surrounding reactive bone edema around the osteomyelitis (*left*), active osteomyelitis (*center*), and synovial inflammation (*right*), showing the difference of the degree of inflammatory perfusion for different types of tissue and pathologic processes.

DYNAMIC CONTRAST-ENHANCED MR IMAGING IN INFECTIOUS JOINT DISEASES

As inflammatory joint disease, IJD also leads to the development of neovessels and increased perfusion in the affected tissue due to the inflammatory reaction. Despite this, DCE-MR imaging has been used in only a few studies. Early research has stated that DCE-MR imaging parameters did not contribute to the description of septic sacroiliitis, but the method helped to detect differences between the vascularization patterns of neuropathic arthropathy and osteomyelitis.[112,125] In the spine, both IRE and ME of the SI curves and the K^{trans} values were the same in tuberculosis and metastatic cancer, but significantly higher K_{ep} values were reported in metastases compared with tuberculosis foci. AUC and dynamic contrast-enhanced ultrasound values (peek contrast uptake) showed higher perfusion in infected nonunion fracture cases compared with aseptic nonunion, with no significant differences between the methods, leading to the conclusion that both modalities can be use in this clinical dilemma.[126] Kim and colleagues[127] used SI curve shape analysis to differentiate between septic and transient synovitis in the hip joint and found that in the most of the septic hips, the contrast uptake and washout in the femoral head epiphysis was delayed compared with the contralateral hip, confirming earlier observations of lower contrast enhancement in the septic hips using static MR imaging. These results suggest that septic hip arthritis causes vessel constriction and venous obstruction, and may be similar to what is observed in the subchondral bone marrow of OA (**Fig. 24**).

SUMMARY

DCE-MR imaging is a powerful and widely available technique that ideally should be acquired and not left unexploited, if the use of contrast media is essential for patient examination or follow-up. DCE-MR imaging as opposed to the acquisition of static postcontrast images allows robust identification of the time point and speed of maximum contrast enhancement and enables extraction of quantitative information about the blood flow and capillary permeability. Despite the regulatory warning on the use of Gd-based imaging, the use of DCE-MR imaging in the field of musculoskeletal diseases is increasing, mainly due to its ability to provide comprehensive evaluation of perfusion and quantification of inflammation in the variety of joint tissues, which is essential for early diagnosis and assessment of rapid treatment responses.

In this context, it is critical to note that standardization of acquisitions, which includes protocol design, temporal resolution, use of consistent contrast media, and sometimes the use of power injectors, is paramount. It is also important to differentiate the scientific methodologies behind quantification of the postcontrast images and the DCE-MR imaging sequences and their reproducibility and sensitivity for the assessment of inflammation. With the use of appropriate software, DCE-MR imaging can yield robust and sensitive quantitative measures of perfusion in the synovium, bone, cartilage, muscle, and fat tissues to supplement morphologic measures from the static imaging sequences.

As this review describes, several studies have shown feasibility and validity of the DCE-MR imaging on both low-field and high-field MR imaging scanners, and DCE-MR imaging has primarily been applied in imaging of inflammatory arthritis, including RA, juvenile arthritis, and OA. Here the results have shown that various DCE-MR imaging–based parameters are more sensitive to treatment response and have better correlation to clinical scores and histologic grading of synovitis than static imaging–based measures. In other inflammatory diseases, such as AS, PsA, septic arthritis, and musculoskeletal infections in general, research studies using DCE-MR imaging are scarce, and the results are less conclusive. Finally, various DCE-MR imaging methodologies have been used to study the perfusion changes in the subchondral bone in inflammatory, degenerative, and septic arthritis, but in general more research and standardization of protocols and methods are required.

REFERENCES

1. Burge AJ, Nwawka OK, Berkowitz JL, et al. Imaging of inflammatory arthritis in adults: status and perspectives on the use of radiographs, ultrasound, and MRI. Rheum Dis Clin North Am 2016;42(4):561–85.
2. Math KR, Berkowitz JL, Paget SA, et al. Imaging of musculoskeletal infection. Rheum Dis Clin North Am 2016;42(4):769–84.
3. Rosenberg ZS, Shankman S, Steiner GC, et al. Rapid destructive osteoarthritis: clinical, radiographic, and pathologic features. Radiology 1992;182(1):213–6.
4. Turan A, Celtikci P, Tufan A, et al. Basic radiological assessment of synovial diseases: a pictorial essay. Eur J Rheumatol 2017;4(2):166–74.
5. Boesen M, Ostergaard M, Cimmino MA, et al. MRI quantification of rheumatoid arthritis: current knowledge and future perspectives. Eur J Radiol 2009; 71(2):189–96.
6. Weber U, Jurik AG, Lambert RG, et al. Imaging in spondyloarthritis: controversies in recognition of early disease. Curr Rheumatol Rep 2016;18(9):58.

7. Hayeri MR, Ziai P, Shehata ML, et al. Soft-tissue infections and their imaging mimics: from cellulitis to necrotizing fasciitis. Radiographics 2016;36(6): 1888–910.

8. Browne LP, Guillerman RP, Orth RC, et al. Community-acquired staphylococcal musculoskeletal infection in infants and young children: necessity of contrast-enhanced MRI for the diagnosis of growth cartilage involvement. AJR Am J Roentgenol 2012;198(1):194–9.

9. O'Connor JPB, Tofts PS, Miles KA, et al. Dynamic contrast-enhanced imaging techniques: CT and MRI. Br J Radiol 2011;84(Spec Iss 2): S112–20.

10. Cimmino MA, Innocenti S, Livrone F, et al. Dynamic gadolinium-enhanced magnetic resonance imaging of the wrist in patients with rheumatoid arthritis can discriminate active from inactive disease. Arthritis Rheum 2003;48(5):1207–13.

11. Lee RKL, Griffith JF, Wang DF, et al. Dynamic contrast-enhanced imaging of the wrist in rheumatoid arthritis: dedicated low-field (0.25-T) versus high-field (3.0-T) MRI. Skeletal Radiol 2015;44(8): 1095–101.

12. Boesen M, Kubassova O, Cimmino MA, et al. Dynamic contrast enhanced MRI can monitor the very early inflammatory treatment response upon intra-articular steroid injection in the knee joint: a case report with review of the literature. Arthritis 2011;2011:1–8.

13. Kubassova O, Boesen M, Boyle RD, et al. Fast and robust analysis of dynamic contrast enhanced MRI datasets. Med Image Comput Comput Assist Interv 2007;10(Pt 2):261–9.

14. Kubassova OA, Boyle RD, Radjenovic A. Quantitative analysis of dynamic contrast-enhanced MRI datasets of the metacarpophalangeal joints. Acad Radiol 2007;14(10):1189–200.

15. van de Sande MG, van der Leij C, Lavini C, et al. Characteristics of synovial inflammation in early arthritis analysed by pixel-by-pixel time-intensity curve shape analysis. Rheumatology (Oxford) 2012;51(7):1240–5.

16. Lavini C, de Jonge MC, van de Sande MG, et al. Pixel-by-pixel analysis of DCE MRI curve patterns and an illustration of its application to the imaging of the musculoskeletal system. Magn Reson Imaging 2007;25(5):604–12.

17. Cuenod CA, Balvay D. Perfusion and vascular permeability: basic concepts and measurement in DCE-CT and DCE-MRI. Diagn Interv Imaging 2013;94(12):1187–204.

18. Sourbron S. Technical aspects of MR perfusion. Eur J Radiol 2010;76(3):304–13.

19. Khalifa F, Soliman A, El-Baz A, et al. Models and methods for analyzing DCE-MRI: a review. Med Phys 2014;41(12):124301.

20. Kubassova O, Boesen M, Peloschek P, et al. Quantifying disease activity and damage by imaging in rheumatoid arthritis and osteoarthritis. Ann N Y Acad Sci 2009;1154:207–38.

21. Kubassova O, Boesen M, Cimmino MA, et al. A computer-aided detection system for rheumatoid arthritis MRI data interpretation and quantification of synovial activity. Eur J Radiol 2009. https://doi.org/10.1016/j.ejrad.2009.04.010.

22. Ostergaard M, Peterfy C, Conaghan P, et al. OMERACT rheumatoid arthritis magnetic resonance imaging studies. Core set of MRI acquisitions, joint pathology definitions, and the OMERACT RA-MRI scoring system. J Rheumatol 2003;30(6):1385–6.

23. Ostergaard M, McQueen F, Wiell C, et al. The OMERACT psoriatic arthritis magnetic resonance imaging scoring system (PsAMRIS): definitions of key pathologies, suggested MRI sequences, and preliminary scoring system for PsA hands. J Rheumatol 2009;36(8):1816–24.

24. Hunter DJ, Guermazi A, Lo GH, et al. Evolution of semi-quantitative whole joint assessment of knee OA: MOAKS (MRI osteoarthritis knee score). Osteoarthritis Cartilage 2011;19(8):990–1002.

25. Tofts PS, Kermode AG. Blood brain barrier permeability in multiple sclerosis using labelled DTPA with PET, CT and MRI. J Neurol Neurosurg Psychiatry 1989;52(8):1019–20.

26. O'Connor JP, Jackson A, Parker GJ, et al. Dynamic contrast-enhanced MRI in clinical trials of antivascular therapies. Nat Rev Clin Oncol 2012;9(3):167–77.

27. DCE-MRI Technical Committee. DCE-MRI quantification profile, quantitative imaging biomarkers alliance. Version 1.0. RSNA.org/QIBA; 2012. p. 1–46. Version 1. Available at: http://www.rsna.org/uploadedFiles/RSNA/Content/Science_and_Education/QIBA/DCE-MRI_Quantification_Profile_v1%200-ReviewedDraft%208-8-12.pdf. Accessed June 29, 2018.

28. Boesen M, Kubassova O, Parodi M, et al. Comparison of the manual and computer-aided techniques for evaluation of wrist synovitis using dynamic contrast-enhanced MRI on a dedicated scanner. Eur J Radiol 2011;77(2):202–6.

29. van der Leij C, van de Sande MG, Lavini C, et al. Rheumatoid synovial inflammation: pixel-by-pixel dynamic contrast-enhanced MR imaging time-intensity curve shape analysis—a feasibility study. Radiology 2009;253(1):234–40.

30. Peloschek P, Boesen M, Donner R, et al. Assessment of rheumatic diseases with computational radiology: current status and future potential. Eur J Radiol 2009. https://doi.org/10.1016/j.ejrad.2009.04.046.

31. Kubassova O, Boyle R, Boesen M. Registration of dynamic MRI data and its impact on diagnostic process. In: Hamarneh G, Abugharbieh R, editors.

Proceedings of the First Workshop on Analysis of Functional Medical Images. New York: 11th International Conference on Medical Image Computing & Computer Assisted Intervention, September 10th 2008; 2008. p. 57–64.

32. van der Leij C, Lavini C, van de Sande MG, et al. Reproducibility of DCE-MRI time-intensity curve-shape analysis in patients with knee arthritis: a comparison with qualitative and pharmacokinetic analyses. J Magn Reson Imaging 2015;42(6):1497–506.

33. Decker JL. American Rheumatism Association nomenclature and classification of arthritis and rheumatism (1983). Arthritis Rheum 1983;26(8):1029–32.

34. Savolainen E, Kaipiainen-Seppanen O, Kroger L, et al. Total incidence and distribution of inflammatory joint diseases in a defined population: results from the Kuopio 2000 arthritis survey. J Rheumatol 2003;30(11):2460–8.

35. Sellam J, Berenbaum F. The role of synovitis in pathophysiology and clinical symptoms of osteoarthritis. Nat Rev Rheumatol 2010;6(11):625–35.

36. Sofat N, Ejindu V, Kiely P. What makes osteoarthritis painful? The evidence for local and central pain processing. Rheumatology (Oxford) 2011;50(12):2157–65.

37. Gandhi R, Takahashi M, Virtanen C, et al. Microarray analysis of the infrapatellar fat pad in knee osteoarthritis: relationship with joint inflammation. J Rheumatol 2011;38(9):1966–72.

38. Lindblad S, Hedfors E. Arthroscopic and immunohistologic characterization of knee joint synovitis in osteoarthritis. Arthritis Rheum 1987;30(10):1081–8.

39. Ushiyama T, Chano T, Inoue K, et al. Cytokine production in the infrapatellar fat pad: another source of cytokines in knee synovial fluids. Ann Rheum Dis 2003;62(2):108–12.

40. Sokolove J, Lepus CM. Role of inflammation in the pathogenesis of osteoarthritis: latest findings and interpretations. Ther Adv Musculoskelet Dis 2013. https://doi.org/10.1177/1759720X12467868.

41. Clockaerts S, Bastiaansen-Jenniskens YM, Runhaar J, et al. The infrapatellar fat pad should be considered as an active osteoarthritic joint tissue: a narrative review. Osteoarthritis Cartilage 2010;18(7):876–82.

42. Grainger AJ, McGonagle D. Imaging in rheumatology. Imaging 2007;19(3):310–23.

43. Sudol-Szopinska I, Kontny E, Maslinski W, et al. The pathogenesis of rheumatoid arthritis in radiological studies. Part I: formation of inflammatory infiltrates within the synovial membrane. J Ultrason 2012;12(49):202–13.

44. Sieper J, Rudwaleit MF, Baraliakos XF, et al. The assessment of spondyloarthritis international Society (ASAS) handbook: a guide to assess spondyloarthritis. Ann Rheum Dis 2009. https://doi.org/10.1136/ard.2008.104018.

45. Sudol-Szopinska I, Matuszewska G, Kwiatkowska B, et al. Diagnostic imaging of psoriatic arthritis. Part I: etiopathogenesis, classifications and radiographic features. J Ultrason 2016;16(64):65–77.

46. McQueen FM, Doyle A, Dalbeth N. Imaging in gout—what can we learn from MRI, CT, DECT and US? Arthritis Res Ther 2011;13(6):246.

47. Torp-Pedersen S, Christensen RF, Szkudlarek MF, et al. Power and color Doppler ultrasound settings for inflammatory flow: impact on scoring of disease activity in patients with rheumatoid arthritis. Arthritis Rheumatol 2015. https://doi.org/10.1002/art.38940.

48. Boutry N, Morel M, Flipo RM, et al. Early rheumatoid arthritis: a review of MRI and sonographic findings. AJR Am J Roentgenol 2007;189(6):1502–9.

49. Bliddal H, Boesen M, Christensen R, et al. Imaging as a follow-up tool in clinical trials and clinical practice. Best Pract Res Clin Rheumatol 2008;22(6):1109–26.

50. Ellegaard K, Torp-Pedersen S, Terslev L, et al. Ultrasound colour Doppler measurements in a single joint as measure of disease activity in patients with rheumatoid arthritis–assessment of concurrent validity. Rheumatology (Oxford) 2009;48(3):254–7.

51. Garcia-Figueiras R, Padhani AR, Baleato-Gonzalez S. Therapy monitoring with functional and molecular MR imaging. Magn Reson Imaging Clin N Am 2016;24(1):261–88.

52. Sujlana P, Skrok J, Fayad LM. Review of dynamic contrast-enhanced MRI: technical aspects and applications in the musculoskeletal system. J Magn Reson Imaging 2018. https://doi.org/10.1002/jmri.25810.

53. Borrero CG, Mountz JM, Mountz JD. Emerging MRI methods in rheumatoid arthritis. Nat Rev Rheumatol 2011;7:85.

54. Zierhut ML, Gardner JC, Spilker ME, et al. Kinetic modeling of contrast-enhanced MRI: an automated technique for assessing inflammation in the rheumatoid arthritis wrist. Ann Biomed Eng 2007;35(5):781–95.

55. Wojciechowski W, Tabor Z, Urbanik A. Assessing synovitis based on dynamic gadolinium-enhanced MRI and EULAR-OMERACT scores of the wrist in patients with rheumatoid arthritis. Clin Exp Rheumatol 2013;31(6):850–6.

56. Boesen M, Kubassova O, Bouert R, et al. Correlation between computer-aided dynamic gadolinium-enhanced MRI assessment of inflammation and semi-quantitative synovitis and bone marrow oedema scores of the wrist in patients with rheumatoid arthritis–a cohort study. Rheumatology (Oxford) 2012;51(1):134–43.

57. Gaffney K, Cookson J, Blake D, et al. Quantification of rheumatoid synovitis by magnetic resonance imaging. Arthritis Rheum 1995;38(11):1610–7.

58. Tamai K, Yamato M, Yamaguchi T, et al. Dynamic magnetic resonance imaging for the evaluation of

synovitis in patients with rheumatoid arthritis. Arthritis Rheum 1994;37(8):1151–7.

59. Ostergaard M, Stoltenberg M, Lovgreen-Nielsen P, et al. Quantification of synovitis by MRI: correlation between dynamic and static gadolinium-enhanced magnetic resonance imaging and microscopic and macroscopic signs of synovial inflammation. Magn Reson Imaging 1998;16(7):743–54.

60. Axelsen MB, Stoltenberg M, Poggenborg RP, et al. Dynamic gadolinium-enhanced magnetic resonance imaging allows accurate assessment of the synovial inflammatory activity in rheumatoid arthritis knee joints: a comparison with synovial histology. Scand J Rheumatol 2012;41(2):89–94.

61. Vordenbäume S, Schleich C, Lögters M, et al. Dynamic contrast-enhanced magnetic resonance imaging of metacarpophalangeal joints reflects histological signs of synovitis in rheumatoid arthritis. Arthritis Res Ther 2014;16(5):452.

62. Axelsen MB, Ejbjerg BJ, Hetland ML, et al. Differentiation between early rheumatoid arthritis patients and healthy persons by conventional and dynamic contrast-enhanced magnetic resonance imaging. Scand J Rheumatol 2014;43(2):109–18.

63. Rastogi A, Kubassova O, Krasnosselskaia LV, et al. Evaluating automated dynamic contrast enhanced wrist 3T MRI in healthy volunteers: one-year longitudinal observational study. Eur J Radiol 2013. https://doi.org/10.1016/j.ejrad.2013.02.041.

64. Maijer KI, van der Leij C, de Hair MJ, et al. Dynamic contrast-enhanced magnetic resonance imaging using pharmacokinetic modeling: initial experience in patients with early arthritis. Arthritis Rheumatol 2016;68(3):587–96.

65. Cimmino MA, Barbieri F, Boesen M, et al. Dynamic contrast-enhanced magnetic resonance imaging of articular and extraarticular synovial structures of the hands in patients with psoriatic arthritis. J Rheumatol Suppl 2012;89:44–8.

66. Axelsen MB, Poggenborg RP, Stoltenberg M, et al. Reliability and responsiveness of dynamic contrast-enhanced magnetic resonance imaging in rheumatoid arthritis. Scand J Rheumatol 2013; 42(2):115–22.

67. Reece RJ, Kraan MC, Radjenovic A, et al. Comparative assessment of leflunomide and methotrexate for the treatment of rheumatoid arthritis, by dynamic enhanced magnetic resonance imaging. Arthritis Rheum 2002;46(2):366–72.

68. Hodgson RJ, O'Connor P, Moots R. MRI of rheumatoid arthritis image quantitation for the assessment of disease activity, progression and response to therapy. Rheumatology (Oxford) 2008;47(1):13–21.

69. Hodgson RJ, Connolly S, Barnes T, et al. Pharmacokinetic modeling of dynamic contrast-enhanced MRI of the hand and wrist in rheumatoid arthritis and the response to anti-tumor necrosis factor-alpha therapy. Magn Reson Med 2007; 58(3):482–9.

70. Hodgson RJ, Barnes T, Connolly S, et al. Changes underlying the dynamic contrast-enhanced MRI response to treatment in rheumatoid arthritis. Skeletal Radiol 2008;37(3):201–7.

71. Axelsen MB, Eshed I, Horslev-Petersen K, et al. A treat-to-target strategy with methotrexate and intra-articular triamcinolone with or without adalimumab effectively reduces MRI synovitis, osteitis and tenosynovitis and halts structural damage progression in early rheumatoid arthritis: results from the OPERA randomised controlled trial. Ann Rheum Dis 2015. https://doi.org/10.1136/annrheumdis-2013-204537.

72. Meier R, Thuermel K, Noel PB, et al. Synovitis in patients with early inflammatory arthritis monitored with quantitative analysis of dynamic contrast-enhanced optical imaging and MR imaging. Radiology 2014;270(1):176–85.

73. Conaghan PG, Ostergaard M, Bowes MA, et al. Comparing the effects of tofacitinib, methotrexate and the combination, on bone marrow oedema, synovitis and bone erosion in methotrexate-naive, early active rheumatoid arthritis: results of an exploratory randomised MRI study incorporating semiquantitative and quantitative techniques. Ann Rheum Dis 2016;75(6):1024–33.

74. Müller-Lutz A, Schleich C, Sewerin P, et al. Comparison of quantitative and semiquantitative dynamic contrast-enhanced MRI with respect to their correlation to delayed gadolinium-enhanced MRI of the cartilage in patients with early rheumatoid arthritis. J Comput Assist Tomogr 2015;39(1): 64–9.

75. Cimmino MA, Parodi M, Zampogna G, et al. Dynamic contrast-enhanced, extremity-dedicated MRI identifies synovitis changes in the follow-up of rheumatoid arthritis patients treated with rituximab. Clin Exp Rheumatol 2014;32(5):647–52.

76. Waterton JC, Ho M, Nordenmark LH, et al. Repeatability and response to therapy of dynamic contrast-enhanced magnetic resonance imaging biomarkers in rheumatoid arthritis in a large multicentre trial setting. Eur Radiol 2017;27(9):3662–8.

77. MacIsaac KD, Baumgartner R, Kang J, et al. Pretreatment whole blood gene expression is associated with 14-week response assessed by dynamic contrast enhanced magnetic resonance imaging in infliximab-treated rheumatoid arthritis patients. PLoS One 2014;9(12):e113937.

78. McQueen FM, Benton N, Perry D, et al. Bone edema scored on magnetic resonance imaging scans of the dominant carpus at presentation predicts radiographic joint damage of the hands and feet six years later in patients with rheumatoid arthritis. Arthritis Rheum 2003;48(7):1814–27.

79. Haavardsholm EA, Boyesen P, Ostergaard M, et al. Magnetic resonance imaging findings in 84 patients with early rheumatoid arthritis: bone marrow oedema predicts erosive progression. Ann Rheum Dis 2008;67(6):794–800.

80. Hetland ML, Ejbjerg BJ, Horslev-Petersen K, et al. MRI bone oedema is the strongest predictor of subsequent radiographic progression in early rheumatoid arthritis. Results from a 2 year randomized controlled trial (CIMESTRA). Ann Rheum Dis 2009. https://doi.org/10.1136/ard.2008.088245.

81. McQueen FM. Bone marrow edema and osteitis in rheumatoid arthritis: the imaging perspective. Arthritis Res Ther 2012;14(5):224.

82. Tamai M, Kawakami A, Uetani M, et al. A prediction rule for disease outcome in patients with undifferentiated arthritis using magnetic resonance imaging of the wrists and finger joints and serologic autoantibodies. Arthritis Care Res 2009;61(6):772–8.

83. McQueen FM, Gao A, Ostergaard M, et al. High-grade MRI bone oedema is common within the surgical field in rheumatoid arthritis patients undergoing joint replacement and is associated with osteitis in subchondral bone. Ann Rheum Dis 2007;66(12):1581–7.

84. Jimenez-Boj E, Nobauer-Huhmann I, Hanslik-Schnabel B, et al. Bone erosions and bone marrow edema as defined by magnetic resonance imaging reflect true bone marrow inflammation in rheumatoid arthritis. Arthritis Rheum 2007;56(4):1118–24.

85. Teruel JR, Burghardt AJ, Rivoire J, et al. Bone structure and perfusion quantification of bone marrow edema pattern in the wrist of patients with rheumatoid arthritis: a multimodality study. J Rheumatol 2014;41(9):1766–73.

86. Hodgson R, Grainger A, O'Connor P, et al. Dynamic contrast enhanced MRI of bone marrow oedema in rheumatoid arthritis. Ann Rheum Dis 2008;67(2):270–2.

87. Herregods N, Jaremko JL, Baraliakos X, et al. Limited role of gadolinium to detect active sacroiliitis on MRI in juvenile spondyloarthritis. Skeletal Radiol 2015;44(11):1637–46.

88. Biffar A, Dietrich O, Sourbron S, et al. Diffusion and perfusion imaging of bone marrow. Eur J Radiol 2010;76(3):323–8.

89. Gašperšič N, Serša I, Jevtič V, et al. Monitoring ankylosing spondylitis therapy by dynamic contrast-enhanced and diffusion-weighted magnetic resonance imaging. Skeletal Radiol 2008;37(2):123–31.

90. Malattia C, Damasio MB, Basso C, et al. Dynamic contrast-enhanced magnetic resonance imaging in the assessment of disease activity in patients with juvenile idiopathic arthritis. Rheumatology 2010;49(1):178–85.

91. Workie DW, Dardzinski BJ, Graham TB, et al. Quantification of dynamic contrast-enhanced MR imaging of the knee in children with juvenile rheumatoid arthritis based on pharmacokinetic modeling. Magn Reson Imaging 2004;22(9):1201–10.

92. Workie DW, Graham TB, Laor T, et al. Quantitative MR characterization of disease activity in the knee in children with juvenile idiopathic arthritis: a longitudinal pilot study. Pediatr Radiol 2007;37(6):535–43.

93. Nusman CM, Lavini C, Hemke R, et al. Dynamic contrast-enhanced magnetic resonance imaging of the wrist in children with juvenile idiopathic arthritis. Pediatr Radiol 2017;47(2):205–13.

94. Sudol-Szopinska I, Matuszewska G, Gietka P, et al. Imaging of juvenile idiopathic arthritis. Part II: ultrasonography and MRI. J Ultrason 2016;16(66): 237–51.

95. Hemke R, Lavini C, Nusman CM, et al. Pixel-by-pixel analysis of DCE-MRI curve shape patterns in knees of active and inactive juvenile idiopathic arthritis patients. Eur Radiol 2014;24(7):1686–93.

96. Hemke R, Nusman CM, van den Berg JM, et al. Construct validity of pixel-by-pixel DCE-MRI: correlation with conventional MRI scores in juvenile idiopathic arthritis. Eur J Radiol 2017; 94(Supplement C):1–5.

97. Hemke R, van Rossum MA, van Veenendaal M, et al. Reliability and responsiveness of the juvenile arthritis MRI Scoring (JAMRIS) system for the knee. Eur Radiol 2013;23(4):1075–83.

98. Nusman CM, Hemke R, Lavini C, et al. Dynamic contrast-enhanced magnetic resonance imaging can play a role in predicting flare in juvenile idiopathic arthritis. Eur J Radiol 2017;88:77–81.

99. Sudol-Szopinska I, Pracoń G. Diagnostic imaging of psoriatic arthritis. Part II: magnetic resonance imaging and ultrasonography. J Ultrason 2016;16(65):163–74.

100. Poggenborg RP, Østergaard M, Terslev L. Imaging in psoriatic arthritis. Rheum Dis Clin North Am 2015;41(4):593–613.

101. Schwenzer N, Kotter I, Henes J, et al. The role of dynamic contrast-enhanced MRI in the differential diagnosis of psoriatic and rheumatoid arthritis. AJR Am J Roentgenol 2010;194(3):715–20.

102. Poggenborg RP, Wiell C, Bøyesen P, et al. No overall damage progression despite persistent inflammation in adalimumab-treated psoriatic arthritis patients: results from an investigator-initiated 48-week comparative magnetic resonance imaging, computed tomography and radiography trial. Rheumatology (Oxford) 2014;53(4):746–56.

103. Krasnokutsky S, Belitskaya-Lévy I, Bencardino J, et al. Quantitative magnetic resonance imaging evidence of synovial proliferation is associated with radiographic severity of knee osteoarthritis. Arthritis Rheum 2011;63(10):2983–91.

104. Anwander H, Cron GO, Rakhra K, et al. Perfusion MRI in hips with metal-on-metal and metal-on-polyethylene total hip arthroplasty: a pilot study. Bone Joint Res 2016;5(3):73–9.

105. Riis RG, Gudbergsen H, Simonsen O, et al. The association between histological, macroscopic and magnetic resonance imaging assessed synovitis in end-stage knee osteoarthritis: a cross-sectional study. Osteoarthritis Cartilage 2017;25(2):272–80.

106. Ballegaard C, Riis RG, Bliddal H, et al. Knee pain and inflammation in the infrapatellar fat pad estimated by conventional and dynamic contrast-enhanced magnetic resonance imaging in obese patients with osteoarthritis: a cross-sectional study. Osteoarthritis Cartilage 2014;22(7):933–40.

107. Riis RG, Gudbergsen H, Henriksen M, et al. Synovitis assessed on static and dynamic contrast-enhanced magnetic resonance imaging and its association with pain in knee osteoarthritis: a cross-sectional study. Eur J Radiol 2016;85(6):1099–108.

108. Kirkhus E, Bjornerud A, Thoen J, et al. Contrast-enhanced dynamic magnetic resonance imaging of finger joints in osteoarthritis and rheumatoid arthritis: an analysis based on pharmacokinetic modeling. Acta Radiol 2006;47(8):845–51.

109. Sanz R, Marti-Bonmati L, Rodrigo JL, et al. MR pharmacokinetic modeling of the patellar cartilage differentiates normal from pathological conditions. J Magn Reson Imaging 2008;27(1):171–7.

110. Marti-Bonmati L, Sanz-Requena R, Rodrigo JL, et al. Glucosamine sulfate effect on the degenerated patellar cartilage: preliminary findings by pharmacokinetic magnetic resonance modeling. Eur Radiol 2009;19(6):1512–8.

111. Jans L, De Coninck T, Wittoek R, et al. 3 T DCE-MRI assessment of synovitis of the interphalangeal joints in patients with erosive osteoarthritis for treatment response monitoring. Skeletal Radiol 2013;42(2):255–60.

112. Gait AD, Hodgson R, Parkes MJ, et al. Synovial volume vs synovial measurements from dynamic contrast enhanced MRI as measures of response in osteoarthritis. Osteoarthritis Cartilage 2016;24(8):6.

113. Wenham CY, Balamoody S, Grainger AJ, et al. The responsiveness of novel, dynamic, contrast-enhanced magnetic resonance measures of total knee synovitis after intra-articular corticosteroid for painful osteoarthritis. Osteoarthritis Cartilage 2014;22(10):1614–8.

114. Riis RGC, Henriksen M, Klokker L, et al. The effects of intra-articular glucocorticoids and exercise on pain and synovitis assessed on static and dynamic magnetic resonance imaging in knee osteoarthritis: exploratory outcomes from a randomized controlled trial. Osteoarthritis Cartilage 2017;25(4):481–91.

115. Swaminathan V, Parkes MJ, Callaghan MJ, et al. With a biomechanical treatment in knee osteoarthritis, less knee pain did not correlate with synovitis reduction. BMC Musculoskelet Disord 2017;18(1):347.

116. Kim IJ, Kim DH, Jung JY, et al. Association between bone marrow lesions detected by magnetic resonance imaging and knee pain in community residents in Korea. Osteoarthritis Cartilage 2013;21(9):1207–13.

117. Koster IM, Oei EH, Hensen JH, et al. Predictive factors for new onset or progression of knee osteoarthritis one year after trauma: MRI follow-up in general practice. Eur Radiol 2011;21(7):1509–16.

118. Tanamas SK, Wluka AE, Pelletier JP, et al. Bone marrow lesions in people with knee osteoarthritis predict progression of disease and joint replacement: a longitudinal study. Rheumatology (Oxford) 2010;49(12):2413–9.

119. Lim YZ, Wang Y, Wluka A, et al. Are biomechanical factors, meniscal pathology, and physical activity risk factors for bone marrow lesions at the knee? A systematic review. Semin Arthritis Rheum 2013;43(2):187–94.

120. Roemer FW, Kwoh C, Hannon M, et al. Can structural joint damage measured with MR imaging be used to predict knee replacement in the following year? Radiology 2015;274(3):810–20.

121. Nielsen FK, Egund N, Jorgensen A, et al. Assessment of subchondral bone marrow lesions in knee osteoarthritis by MRI: a comparison of fluid sensitive and contrast enhanced sequences. BMC Musculoskelet Disord 2016;17(1):479.

122. Budzik JF, Ding J, Norberciak L, et al. Perfusion of subchondral bone marrow in knee osteoarthritis: a dynamic contrast-enhanced magnetic resonance imaging preliminary study. Eur J Radiol 2017;88:129–34.

123. Dyke JP, Synan M, Ezell P, et al. Characterization of bone perfusion by dynamic contrast-enhanced magnetic resonance imaging and positron emission tomography in the Dunkin-Hartley Guinea pig model of advanced osteoarthritis. J Orthop Res 2015;33(3):366–72.

124. Carpenter CR, Schuur JD, Everett WW, et al. Evidence-based diagnostics: adult septic arthritis. Acad Emerg Med 2011;18(8):781–96.

125. Martin NT, Luna AA, Beltran LS, et al. Advanced MR imaging techniques for differentiation of neuropathic arthropathy and osteomyelitis in the diabetic foot. Radiographics 2017;37(4):1161–80.

126. Fischer C, Preuss EM, Tanner M, et al. Dynamic contrast-enhanced sonography and dynamic contrast-enhanced magnetic resonance imaging for preoperative diagnosis of infected nonunions. J Ultrasound Med 2016;35(5):933–42.

127. Kim EY, Kwack KS, Cho JH, et al. Usefulness of dynamic contrast-enhanced MRI in differentiating between septic arthritis and transient synovitis in the hip joint. AJR Am J Roentgenol 2012. https://doi.org/10.2214/AJR.11.6937.

MR Imaging of the Musculoskeletal System Using Ultrahigh Field (7T) MR Imaging

Hamza Alizai, MD*, Gregory Chang, MD, Ravinder R. Regatte, PhD

KEYWORDS

• MR imaging • 7T • Bone • Muscle • Cartilage

KEY POINTS

- The signal-to-noise ratio gain of 7T MR imaging benefits both clinical and research musculoskeletal imaging.
- RF and B_0 inhomogeneity and coil design are the major challenges of MR imaging at 7T.
- Future musculoskeletal imaging protocols will likely be a hybrid of morphologic, compositional, and functional MR imaging sequences.

INTRODUCTION

In vivo musculoskeletal MR imaging plays a critical role in the modern medical practice. The excellent soft tissue contrast and multiplanar and multiparametric capabilities of MR imaging contribute to an unparalleled evaluation of all musculoskeletal tissues. Since the advent of diagnostic MR imaging, one of the most significant technological advancements has been the progressive increase in field strength (B_0) of the clinical MR imaging systems. MR imaging at higher field strength offers several advantages, including increased signal-to-noise ratio (SNR), higher spatial resolution, improved spectral resolution, improved sensitivity for X-nucleus imaging, and decreased image acquisition times.[1] The physics of imaging at higher field strengths also, however, poses technical challenges, some of which include radiofrequency (RF) coil design, increased chemical shift and susceptibility artifacts, increased RF energy deposition (specific absorption rate [SAR]), and changes in relaxation times compared with the lower field strength scanners.

In October 2017, the US Food and Drug Administration (FDA) approved the first 7T-Magnetom Terra (Siemens, Munich, Germany) MR imaging system for clinical diagnostic imaging of the head and the extremities. In this timely narrative review, we discuss the many potential opportunities as well as the challenges presented by 7T MR imaging systems. We also highlight recent developments in in vivo imaging of musculoskeletal tissues, including anatomic, structural, compositional, and functional imaging of cartilage, bone, and skeletal muscle, using these systems.

Conflict of Interest Statement: The authors certify that they have no affiliations with or involvement in any organization or entity with any financial interest or nonfinancial interest in the subject matter or materials discussed in this article.

Department of Radiology, New York University Langone Medical Center, 660 First Avenue, New York, NY 10016, USA

* Corresponding author.

E-mail address: Hamza.Alizai@nyumc.org

PET Clin 13 (2018) 551–565
https://doi.org/10.1016/j.cpet.2018.05.008

TECHNICAL ADVANTAGES AT HIGHER FIELD STRENGTHS

The SNR is often referred to as the "currency" of MR imaging and is an objective measure of image quality. Increasing SNR has been the primary driving force behind the development of higher field strength MR systems. Increasing field strength results in increased magnetization (also referred to as spin polarization), which provides a higher SNR and improved resolution.[2] Magnetization can be expressed by the following formula:

$$M_0 = B_0 \left(\gamma^2 \hbar^2 / 4 \kappa T \right) P_D$$

where P_D is proton spin density, γ represents the gyromagnetic ratio, $\hbar$ is Plank constant divided by 2π, k is the Boltzmann constant, T is the absolute temperature (Kelvin), and B_0 is the static magnetic field strength. The importance of field strength for magnetization can be easily delineated from the described formula. The calculation of SNR increase with increasing field strengths is, however, quite complicated and a detailed discussion can be found in the chapter by Collins[1] titled "Radio-frequency field calculations for high-field MR imaging." For those of us who prefer a simple statistic, moving from 3T to 7T results in a gain of SNR by a factor of approximately 2.3.[3] This SNR gain translates to greater spatial resolution as well as reduced scan times, because SNR scales with square root of acquisition time.[3] Additionally, higher field strength allows parallel imaging to be performed with higher speed reduction factors, which can further reduce acquisition time.[4]

The SNR gain at 7T also improves the spectral resolution of (^{1}H) magnetic resonance spectroscopy (MRS), allowing identification of biological molecules that would not be possible at lower field strengths.[5] Furthermore, there are many biologically relevant nuclei besides ^{1}H, such as sodium and phosphorous, which occur in lower concentrations and are therefore difficult to image at conventional clinical field strengths. The utility of 7T in evaluating these nuclei has already been shown. Sodium is closely associated with the glycosaminoglycan, an important component of the cartilage extracellular matrix. Sodium (^{23}Na) MR imaging of cartilage at 7T has been used to map the sodium distribution and therefore indirectly detects early cartilage damage.[6] Phosphorous (^{31}P) is an important skeletal muscle metabolite and localized dynamic (^{31}P) MRS at 7T has been used to study mitochondrial oxidative metabolism in vivo.[7]

TECHNICAL CHALLENGES AT HIGHER FIELD STRENGTHS

Besides the enormous cost of acquiring and operating a 7T MR imaging system, there are technical challenges that need to be overcome for it to be routinely used in clinical imaging. Five of these are described. First, inhomogeneous tissue excitation is a problem at 7T and RF-related artifacts have been described in multiple in vivo studies.[8] At 7T, RF frequencies are higher, and wavelengths may be shorter than the object of interest, resulting in decreased penetration and inhomogeneous excitation. Artifacts may result with the B_1 magnitude and signal intensity much higher in the center of the field than at the periphery, therefore distorting the image.[8] These effects are more likely to be seen in the head or body than the extremities, which on average have smaller dimensions. RF coils for 7T MR imaging must be designed to control RF field propagation and minimize energy deposition.[9] RF shimming and parallel RF transmission techniques may be used to improve image quality at 7T.[10,11]

Second, increasing field strength leads to changes in relaxation times; T_1 values increase[12] while T_2 values decrease.[13] Pulse sequences, therefore, need to be optimized to produce images with the contrast necessary to answer the diagnostic inquiry. Third, there is an increased sensitivity to susceptibility effects (decreased T_2^*) at higher field strengths.[13] Although this may be beneficial for susceptibility-weighted imaging, susceptibility artifact related to orthopedic hardware can hinder interpretation of clinical MR imaging. Both conventional static B_0 and dynamic shimming[14] can be used to reduce susceptibility effects.

Fourth, there is a substantial increase in chemical shift artifact in the frequency-encoded direction at 7T.[15] The chemical shift difference between water and fat resonance is 1040 Hz at 7T compared with 440 Hz at 3T, which at a bandwidth of 130 Hz/pixel amounts to a chemical shift of 8 pixels at 7T versus 3.4 pixels at 3T.[15] The increase in chemical shift improves spectral resolution of MRS; however, chemical shift artifact may hinder interpretation of clinical images. Several techniques, such as using adiabatic refocusing pulses[16] have been used to reduce chemical shift displacement artifacts, but resulting in increases in SAR.

Last, but most importantly, patient safety is paramount. Increased RF at 7T results in higher energy (heat) deposition in tissues. SAR is the measure of RF absorption and scales with essentially the square of the magnetic field. At 7T, SAR needs close monitoring to avoid tissue heating. The FDA has established limits for SAR for both pediatric and adult patients.[17] Although the FDA considers MR imaging under 8T to pose no health risk to adults and children older than 1 month, minor side effects have been reported at high field strengths.[18,19] **Table 1** provides a brief summary of some of the advantages and disadvantages of imaging at higher field strengths.

CARTILAGE
Cartilage Microarchitecture

Cartilage is composed of 70% to 80% fluid. The remainder is the extracellular matrix (ECM), a network of collagen fibrils and proteoglycan molecules. Proteoglycans consist of negatively charged glycosaminoglycan (GAGs) attached to protein core.[20] Cations such as sodium (Na^+) counter the negative charge of GAGs and maintain neutrality. The flow of water within the ECM provides the known biomechanical properties of cartilage.[21] In osteoarthritis (OA), the initial histologic changes include cartilage breakdown with proteoglycan loss and disorganization and/or loss of the collagen fiber network.[22]

Morphologic Imaging of Cartilage

Standard protocols for imaging cartilage morphology at 7T are yet to be established; however, will foreseeably follow the techniques used with 3T MR imaging systems. Springer and

colleagues[23] recently performed comparable routine knee imaging at 3T and 7T and found diagnostic confidence of radiologists for cartilage defects to be higher with 7T. The turbo spin echo (TSE) pulse sequence used in this study is the workhorse for the clinical musculoskeletal imaging due to its excellent soft tissue contrast and rapid acquisition. Fast Spin Echo and TSE are also part of the International Cartilage Repair Society's cartilage imaging protocol.[24] Fat saturation is also essential for clinical musculoskeletal imaging and chemical shift selective fat saturation is easier to perform at 7T.

An in-plane resolution of 0.3 mm resolves the earliest fraying of the cartilage surface.[25] Jin and colleagues[26] acquired high-resolution 2-dimensional (2D) and 3D image of the knee and ankle joints at 7T with a 0.3 mm in-plane resolution for TSE and 0.47 mm for isotropic sequences, such as dual echo steady state (3D-DESS). The open architecture 8-channel transmit-receive coil in this study even allowed dynamic imaging during continuous knee and ankle flexion-extension cycles. Regatte and Schweitzer[15] previously described the acquisition of sagittal knee images with a resolution of 0.25 mm using a gradient-based isotropic fast low-angle shot pulse sequence (3D-FLASH) with fat suppression.

Isotropic sequences obviate the need for multiplanar acquisition and reduce acquisition time.[27] The diagnostic accuracy of isotropic fast spin echo (FSE) for cartilage morphology is similar to

---

Table 1
A summary of potential advantages and disadvantages of high and ultrahigh field systems in musculoskeletal imaging

Characteristic	Trend	Positive	Negative
SNR	↑	Higher resolution, shorter scan time, X-nuclei	NA
SAR	↑	NA	Fewer slices, smaller flip angles
Physiologic side effects (7T)	↑	NA	Dizziness, nausea, metallic taste
Relaxation times	T_1 ↑		Scan time increase,
	T_2 ↓		DWI/DTI
	T_2^* ↓	Facilitates BOLD, SWI at 7T	
RF homogeneity	↓	Parallel reception, parallel transmission	Poor inversion, poor contrast
Susceptibility effects	↑	T_2^*	Geometric distortions Metal artifact
Chemical shift	↑	Fat saturation, spectral resolution	Fat/water Misregistration

Abbreviations: BOLD, Blood Oxygen Level Dependent contrast; DTI, diffusion tensor imaging; DWI, diffusion-weighted imaging; NA, not applicable; SAR, specific absorption rate; SNR, signal-to-noise ratio; SWI, Susceptibility weighted imaging; ↑, Increase; ↓, Decrease.

Adapted from Moser E, Stahlberg F, Ladd ME, et al. 7-T MR—from research to clinical applications? NMR Biomed 2012;25(5):695–716; with permission.

2D FSE at 3T; however, this remains to be studied for images obtained at 7T.[28] Other isotropic sequences, including 3D spoiled gradient recoiled echo (SPGR) and 3D-FLASH produce images with cartilage signal more intense than the surrounding tissues[26] and may be better suited for quantitative analysis of cartilage rather than morphologic assessment (**Fig. 1**).[29–31]

Compositional Imaging of Cartilage

By the time morphologic changes in cartilage are evident on clinical MR imaging, cartilage degeneration is in its advanced stages. Compositional imaging techniques have primarily been used in few research centers; however, allow detection of biochemical and microstructural changes in the cartilage ECM. These methods can, therefore, help identify cartilage breakdown at its earliest stages. We briefly describe some of these techniques and related recent developments at 7T.

T_2 Mapping and T_2* Mapping

T_2 mapping has been the most widely studied of all compositional imaging techniques and was an integral part of the knee imaging protocol in the large multicenter osteoarthritis initiative cohort study.[32]

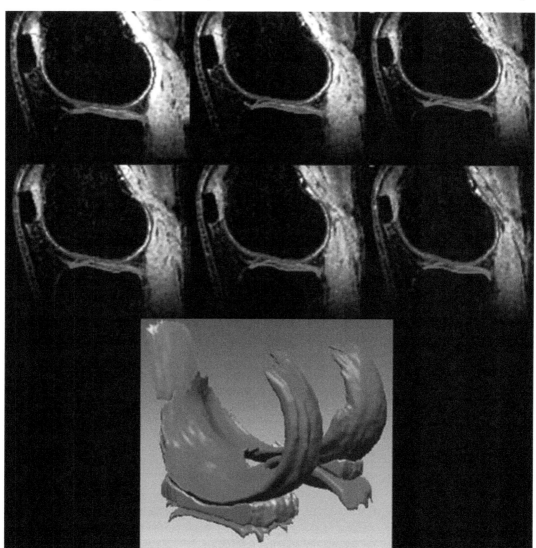

Fig. 1. Representative high-resolution (3D fast low-angle shot) sagittal knee images with fat suppression were acquired on a healthy volunteer at 7T for better visualization of cartilage and surrounding structures. Three-dimensional cartilage and menisci volume were reconstructed from corresponding segmented regions; 160 slices were acquired in approximately 13 minutes with 500 μm × 500 μm × 500 μm isotropic resolution. (*From* Regatte RR, Schweitzer ME. Novel contrast mechanisms at 3 T and 7 T. Semin Musculoskelet Radiol 2008;12(3):266–80; with permission.)

After application of an RF pulse, the rate constant of dephasing in the transverse plane equates to T_2 relaxation time. This value measured in milliseconds reflects water content and indirectly the collagen content in the cartilage ECM.[33] There is a laminar variation of T_2 values in cartilage with higher values at the articular surface compared with the bone interface.[34] Higher cartilage T_2 values have been shown to be predictive of the development of morphologic changes of cartilage deterioration.[35]

Welsch and colleagues[36] found less variation in T_2 measurements performed at 7T. This study reported cartilage T_2 values to be intrinsically lower compared with 3T and the laminar variation to be less pronounced. T_2 mapping at 7T has been shown to be able to discriminate between repaired knee cartilage and adjacent healthy cartilage (**Fig. 2**).[37–39] It has also been shown to detect maturation of reparative tissue after autologous chondrocyte transplantation.[40] Additionally, the increased resolution and decreased partial volume effects at 7T may allow T_2 and T_2^* mapping of thinner cartilage in the hips and ankles.[41] Juras and colleagues[42] have compared within-subject T2 values in the knee and ankle cartilage at 7T and found these to be significantly different owing to their varying biomechanical and biochemical properties.

T_2^* mapping measures transverse-plane dephasing using multi-echo gradient echo techniques, which are faster to acquire than T_2 but are also more vulnerable to local field inhomogeneity.[36,43] T_2^* values are also lower at 7T than at 3T.[36] Both T_2 and T_2^* are affected by magic angle effect; that is, the values increase as the angle between collagen fibers and B_0 approaches 55°.

T1rho Mapping

T1rho evaluates the spin-lattice (T_1) relaxation in the rotating frame.[44] It can evaluate the interaction between free (bulk) water and adjacent molecules and is understood to reflect particularly the proteoglycan content of the ECM.[45] T1rho, like T_2, predicts morphologic deterioration of articular cartilage.[46] T1rho imaging is more challenging to perform due to B_0 and B_1 inhomogeneity, specialized RF pulse sequence requirements, and long acquisition times. The long scan time is particularly a concern at 7T due to increased SAR. A recent study, however, leveraged the SNR advantage of 7T to acquire high-resolution T1rho images (0.2 mm^2 in-plane resolution) in reasonable acquisition times (<30 minutes) and within SAR constraints.[47] This study reported T1rho times lower at 7T than at 3T. It also found T1rho values to be higher in the medial femoral condyles of volunteers with meniscal tears compared with those without tears. Wyatt and colleagues[48] found T1rho values to be higher in patients with OA compared with healthy subjects, with the differences being higher and statistically significant in more regions at 7T than at 3T. Kogan and colleagues[49] compared T1-rho at 7T to the gagCEST sequence (described later in this article) and reported good agreement between the 2 techniques. The same investigators have also described combining the 2 methods at 7T to form a CESTrho sequence, which can quantify proton exchange at intermediate exchange

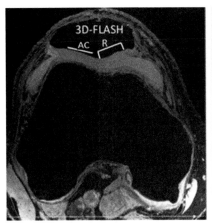 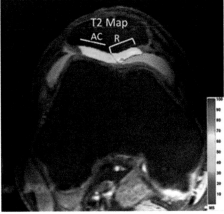

Fig. 2. Juvenile cartilage cell implantation. High-resolution 7T 3D-FLASH image (*left panel*, repetition time/echo time [TR/TE] = 20 ms/5.1 ms, 0.234 mm × 0.234 mm × 1 mm) and T2 map (*right panel*, TR/TE = 3000 ms/15, 30, 45, 60, 75, 90 ms, 0.586 mm × 0.586 mm × 2 mm) demonstrate close to normal thickness, but higher T2 values in the repair (R) tissue compared with adjacent cartilage (AC). (*From* Chang G, Xia D, Sherman O, et al. High resolution morphologic imaging and T2 mapping of cartilage at 7 T: comparison of cartilage repair patients and healthy controls. MAGMA 2013;26(6):539–48; with permission.)

rates, without being affected by confounding factors, which can affect proton exchange rates.[50]

Ultrashort Echo Time and Zero Echo Time Imaging

Musculoskeletal tissues such as cortical bone, tendon, ligaments, and the deep calcified part of cartilage contain a high fraction of components with "ultrashort" transverse relaxation times and therefore produce no signal on standard MR images as their signal decays before it can be acquired.[51] Ultrashort echo time (UTE) and zero echo time use specialized acquisition and reconstruction techniques to capture these ultrashort components before signal decay. The application of these techniques at 7T has primarily focused on tendons and cortical bone. At lower field strengths, UTE has been used to delineate the calcified deepest cartilage layer[52] and has also been used to evaluate the integrity of this layer in osteochondral allografts.[53] UTE also enables T_2 and T_2^* mapping of tissues with a high fraction of ultrashort components. Chu and colleagues[54] reported UTE T_2^* to be helpful in evaluating cartilage healing after anterior cruciate ligament reconstruction.

Delayed Gadolinium-Enhanced MR Imaging of Cartilage

Gadopentetate dimeglumine (Gd-DTPA^{2-}), the commonly used MR imaging contrast, is an anion and therefore repelled by the negatively charged GAGs. dGEMRIC takes advantage of this to map GAG content within cartilage. An area of damaged cartilage will accumulate Gd-DTPA^{2-} and therefore have a shorter T_1 relaxation time. In vivo delayed gadolinium-enhanced MR imaging of cartilage (dGEMRIC) studies at 7T are scarce. A feasibility study by Welsch and colleagues[39] found dGEMRIC to be promising at 7T. In this study of 5 healthy volunteers, T1 values differed between tibial and femoral cartilage.

At lower field strengths, dGEMRIC has been used for a wide range of musculoskeletal conditions, including cartilage repair,[55,56] tibial osteotomy,[57] inflammatory arthritis,[58] and chronic joint unloading.[59]

The disadvantages of dGEMRIC include the large doses of Gd-DTPA^{2-} required. There is also the delay between injection, joint exercise for efficient diffusion into the joint, and long acquisition times.[60] There is, however, a possibility of obtaining an indirect MR arthrogram during this delay, which can aid morphologic evaluation of intra-articular structures, particularly the hip labrum. A recent study by Lazik-Palm and colleagues[61] found that gadolinium administration at

7T did not significantly impact either T_2 or T_2^* relaxation times and improved morphologic image quality. The investigators suggest morphologic and quantitative analysis including dGEMRIC can, therefore, be combined to perform a comprehensive examination during a single visit.

Sodium (^{23}Na) Imaging

The negatively charged GAGs in cartilage ECM attract positive ^{23}Na$^+$ counter-ions, the distribution of which reflect local GAG concentration. Loss of GAG content with cartilage degeneration will result in a lower concentration of ^{23}Na$^+$ ions.[62] ^{23}Na has a spin magnetic moment; however, its concentration is only 0.08% that of ^{1}H, which makes it difficult to elicit signal, resulting in noisy MR images and long acquisition times. The SNR gain at 7T MR imaging is hence particularly useful for ^{23}Na imaging, as it increases its sensitivity[63] and improves resolution. ^{23}Na imaging has been shown to correlate well with dGEMRIC.[64] Unlike dGEMRIC, ^{23}Na imaging can assess cartilage proteoglycan without intravenous contrast injection. The Larmor frequency of ^{23}Na$^+$ is much lower than that of ^{1}H, so specialized transmit-receive coils are, however, required.[65] SAR is also a concern with sodium imaging at long acquisition times; however, Medelin and colleagues[66] have demonstrated that compressed sensing image reconstruction can reduce scan times to less than 10 minutes without losing sodium quantification accuracy. Additionally, sodium inversion recovery pulse sequences can be designed to mitigate RF absorption while improving quality through suppression of free sodium in the synovial fluid.[67,68] As with T_2 Mapping, sodium imaging has been shown to be able to discriminate between cartilage repair tissue and healthy cartilage (**Fig. 3**).[68,69] The investigators of this study reported lower sodium signal intensity in repair tissue after microfracture surgery or matrix autologous chondrocyte transplantation (MACT) compared with healthy cartilage, suggesting diminished GAG content. A different study by the same group found repair tissue after MACT to have higher sodium signal intensity than after bone marrow stimulation, leading them to imply that MACT repair is of better quality.[70]

Diffusion Tensor Imaging

The cartilage collagen network is highly organized resulting in anisotropic water diffusion within the ECM. Diffusion tensor imaging (DTI) can assess both proteoglycan content through mean apparent diffusion coefficient (ADC) and collagen microarchitecture through fractional anisotropy (FA).

7T ¹H MRI   7T [²³Na] map   7T [²³Na]-IR map

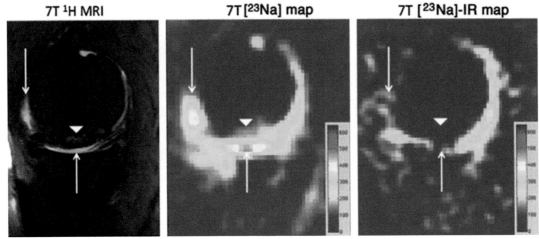

Fig. 3. Sagittal T2-weighted 7T MR image (*left panel*) of the right knee demonstrating an osteochondral allograft (*arrowhead*) at the weight-bearing aspect of the medial femoral condyle. There is synovial fluid at the articular surface (*arrows*). On the conventional ^{23}Na concentration map (*middle panel*), hyperintense signal is seen from synovial fluid at the articular surface (*arrows*) and to a lesser extent in a subchondral location at the repair site (*arrowhead*). On the sodium concentration map generated from ^{23}Na-IR MR imaging (*right panel*), there is suppression of signal from free sodium within synovial fluid (*arrows*) and also in the subchondral location (*arrowhead*). The sodium images represent concentration maps, with colored bars indicating range of [Na⁺] in mM (*red* = 600 mM, *blue* = 0 mM). The larger apparent joint space size on sodium maps compared with proton images is likely due to partial volume averaging from the lower resolution of the sodium maps (2 mm × 2 mm × 2 mm vs 0.546 mm × 0.546 mm × 2 mm). (*Reprinted from* Chang G, Madelin G, Sherman OH, et al. Improved assessment of cartilage repair tissue using fluid-suppressed ^{23}Na inversion recovery MR imaging at 7 T: preliminary results. Eur Radiol 2012;22:1341–9; with permission.)

Raya and colleagues[71] used a line-scan DTI imaging sequence at 7T to compare articular cartilage of healthy subjects with cartilage in subjects with osteoarthritis. They found that both mean ADC and FA values to be good discriminators between the groups, with FA having higher specificity. Ex vivo imaging performed by the same group at 17.6 T found DTI to be excellent for detecting cartilage damage (95% accuracy) and demonstrate good performance for grading cartilage damage (75% accuracy).[72] DTI imaging of cartilage is overall challenging to perform in vivo owing to the short T2 of articular cartilage and the high resolution needed to depict the cartilage anatomy.

Glycosaminoglycan Chemical Exchange Saturation Transfer Imaging

Water protons bound to macromolecules exchange their magnetization with free water protons within the ECM. Water protons bound to macromolecules have unique RF frequency and can be saturated using off-resonance RF pulses. Subsequently, the magnetization exchange with free water results in a loss of image signal intensity, and this effect can be measured to estimate local macromolecule content. With GAG chemical exchange saturation transfer imaging (gagCEST), GAGs are the macromolecules being evaluated with the off-resonance

RF saturation pulses applied to saturate exchangeable protons residing on the hydroxyl groups of cartilage GAGs (**Fig. 4**).[73] gagCEST has been shown to be sensitive to cartilage proteoglycan content.[73] It also correlates well with ^{23}Na⁺ imaging and feasible at 7T.[74] Singh and colleagues[75] compared CEST in knee cartilage at 3T and 7T and found CEST measurements to be negligible at 3T, whereas the results were more promising at 7T. Kogan and colleagues[49] recently described a volumetric multislice gagCEST technique, which can reduce acquisition time.

SKELETAL MUSCLE
Morphologic Images of Skeletal Muscle

Morphologic imaging of skeletal muscle at 7T is similar to imaging at lower field strengths. Routine clinical protocols will need to be optimized to maintain contrast desired by the radiologists to respond to the diagnostic inquiries.

Chemical-Shift-Encoded Water-Fat Separation MR Imaging

As previously described, chemical shift is increased at 7T resulting in improved spectral resolution. Chemical-shift-encoded water-fat separation (WFI) techniques have been used for

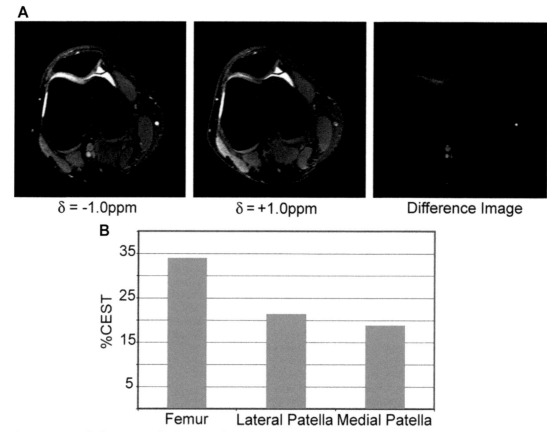

A

δ = −1.0ppm   δ = +1.0ppm   Difference Image

B

Fig. 4. Images of a human patella in vivo with irradiation at δ = −1.0 ppm, δ = +1.0 ppm, and the difference image (A) along with the extracted CEST contrast from the femur and the lateral and medial sides of the patella (B). The total duration of the presaturation pulse sequence was 320 ms at an average rf power of 42 Hz. (*From* Ling W, Regatte RR, Navon G, et al. Assessment of glycosaminoglycan concentration in vivo by chemical exchange-dependent saturation transfer (gagCEST). Proc Natl Acad Sci U S A 2008;105(7):2266–70; © 2008 National Academy of Sciences, U.S.A. with permission.)

intramuscular adipose tissue quantification. WFI captures the phase difference between water and fat protons by acquiring ≥2 echoes and can provide high-resolution 3D imaging of fat composition.[76] This technique is yet to be applied in vivo in human subjects at 7T. At lower field strengths, fat-fraction (FF) estimated using WFI is reliable in comparison with biopsy[77] and more accurate than visual fat grading.[78] The distribution of MR imaging measured intramuscular fat is different in type 2 diabetes compared with healthy subjects[79] and intramuscular FF also progressively increases in patients with neuromuscular disorders. Quadriceps muscle FF is associated with osteoarthritis,[80] whereas shoulder rotator cuff muscle FF correlates with the success of repair as well with pain and range of motion.[81]

MR Spectroscopy

Glycogen, intramyocellular lipid (IMCL), and extramyocellular lipid (EMCL) and phosphocreatine (PCr) are all sources of energy for skeletal muscle, which can be measured in vivo using ^{13}C, ^{1}H, and ^{31}P MR spectroscopy (MRS).[82] The frequency difference between IMCL and EMCL is too small to delineate with chemical-shift imaging but can be assessed with ^{1}H MRS.[83] At 7T, the increased resolution of lipid spectra allows identification of additional lipid peaks, which are not visible at lower field strengths.[84] Compared with 3T, the T_1 relaxation times of skeletal muscle metabolites are increased at 7T, whereas T_2 relaxation times are decreased.[84] MRS is particularly of interest to endocrinologists, as IMCL levels are elevated in subjects with insulin resistance.[83]

^{31}P MRS provides information about skeletal muscle bioenergetics. It can detect phosphorylated compounds including phosphocreatine (PCr), inorganic phosphates (Pi), the phosphate groups in ATP, and phosphomonoesters (**Fig. 5**). The advantages of performing this technique at 7T are clear. Bogner and colleagues[85] found 7T

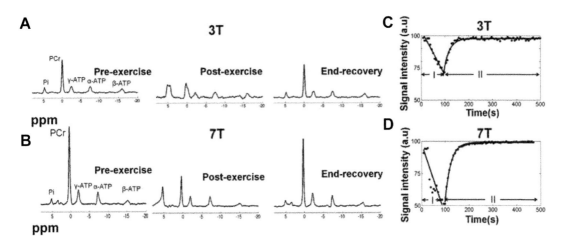

Fig. 5. MR spectra of the same volunteer before and after exercise, and at the end of the recovery period (*A*) at 3T and (*B*) at 7T. We have normalized the amplitude of all postexercise spectra to the preexercise ones. We observed an almost threefold increase of SNR at 7T relative to 3T. Evolution of the phosphocreatine (PCr) MRS signal intensity during the execution of the exercise (I) and the recovery period (II) from the same volunteer. PCr depletion rates were estimated by fitting a linear function to phase I, whereas the PCr recovery kinetics were characterized by fitting a mono-exponential growth function to phase II of the exercise. (*C*) At 3T, the PCr depletion rate is 0.35 s^{-1} (estimated from the slope of the fitted line, $r = 0.997$) and the recovery rate constant is 22.4 s ($r = 0.981$). (*D*) At 7T, the PCr depletion rate is 0.49 s^{-1} ($r = 0.945$) and the recovery rate constant is 23.89 s ($r = 0.998$). (*From* Parasoglou P, Xia D, Chang G, et al. Dynamic three-dimensional imaging of phosphocreatine recovery kinetics in the human lower leg muscles at 3T and 7T: a preliminary study. NMR Biomed 2013;26(3):348–56; with permission.)

^{31}P MRS in the human calf muscle has shorter measurement times with increased SNR and improved temporal resolution in dynamic studies. Parasoglou and colleagues[86] developed a spectrally selective 3D TSE sequence, which can provide simultaneous measurement of PCr resynthesis rates in several muscles of the exercising body part. ^{31}P MRS has shown that athletes have higher PCr/Pi ratios for a given workload and a faster recovery of PCr.[87] Both of these measurements have been proposed to provide MR-based functional measures of mitochondrial density.[88] ^{31}P MRS has also been used as a tool to study several diseases, including peripheral arterial disease[89] and type 2 diabetes.[90]

T_2 Mapping

The advantages of skeletal muscle T_2 mapping at 7T remain to be determined. Preliminary work, including optimization of sequence parameters and the determination of how perfusion and oxygenation might affect T_2 mapping at 7T, is ongoing.[91] Theoretically, the higher spatial resolution would allow more accurate and more automated for quantitative analysis. A preliminary study at New York University performed T2 mapping in a small cohort of volunteers after plantar flexion exercises and found T2 values to decrease after exercise. The calculated T2 values for skeletal muscle and the time course of recovery for T2 values after exercise were similar to those described at lower field strength.[9]

At lower field strengths, T2 mapping has been shown to correlate with nonquantitative MR scores for fatty infiltration and proposed as a potential imaging biomarker for neuromuscular disorders, such as Duchene muscular dystrophy[92] and Pompe disease.[93] It also may be valuable for measuring therapeutic effects of corticosteroids on the skeletal muscle in these patients.[94]

^{23}Na MR Imaging

Sodium concentration gradients across the cell membrane contribute to the resting membrane potential and help generate action potentials leading to muscle contraction.[9] The general challenges of sodium imaging, as well as advantages of 7T sodium MR imaging, were previously discussed in the cartilage section. The feasibility of 23Na MR imaging at 7T was demonstrated by Chang and colleagues[95] in a study comparing the effect of exercise on skeletal muscle sodium concentrations in healthy subjects and diabetic individuals. Sodium signal intensity increased within the

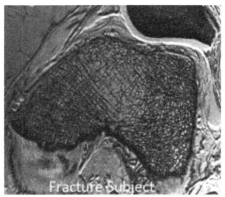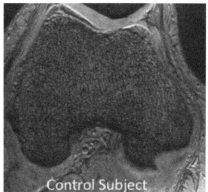

Fig. 6. MR imaging at 7T reveals deterioration in distal femur trabecular bone microarchitecture in a fragility fracture subject (*left*) compared with a control subject (*right*). The fracture subject demonstrates fewer trabeculae, which are disconnected, and more widely spaced apart. (*From* Chang G, Boone S, Martel D, et al. MR imaging assessment of bone structure and microarchitecture. J Magn Reson Imaging 2017;46(2):323–37; with permission.)

muscle in both groups after exercise; however, the diabetic individuals demonstrated a delayed return to preexercise sodium signal intensity.

At lower field strengths, ^{23}Na MR imaging has been used to study skeletal muscle in health volunteers as well as patients with neuromuscular disorders such as Duchenne muscular dystrophy[96] and paramyotonia congentia.[97] Increased sodium signal intensity in the skeletal muscle of patients with the neuromuscular disorder has been proposed as being a contributor to the pathogenesis via intracellular muscle edema.

BONE

Osteoporosis is characterized by a decrease in bone mineral density (BMD) resulting in susceptibility to fragility fractures.[98] Dual-energy x-ray absorptiometry (DXA), the current screening standard for osteoporosis, may artificially underestimate or overestimate fracture risk.[99] A big component of bone imaging research, therefore, focuses on establishing better measures of bone quality and strength and improving prediction of fragility fractures. Normal bone is composed of an outer compact cortical component, internal trabecular component, and bone marrow. The SNR gain and increased resolution of 7T makes it easier to quantify apparent trabecular structural parameters. MR imaging of trabecular bone has been validated via comparisons with micro–computed tomography and histology,[100,101] and these measurements have also been shown to be reproducible.[102] Chang and colleagues[103] demonstrated the feasibility of performing a comprehensive hip MR imaging protocol at 7T that included high-resolution imaging of bone microarchitecture and cartilage, as well as clinical

imaging. They also found that same 7T MR imaging of bone microarchitecture can discriminate between women without and with fragility fractures who do not differ by DXA-derived BMD (**Fig. 6**).[104,105] On the other hand, a study of bone microarchitecture in Olympic fencing athletes found them to have better bone quality than controls.[106] Micro–finite element analysis (FEA), traditionally an engineering tool, has also been performed on 7T high-resolution MR imaging of the distal tibia and proximal femur. MR imaging–based FEA provides bone stiffness measures as a potential imaging marker for bone strength.[107] Professional dancers, for example, were found to have increased bone stiffness in comparison with inactive controls.[108] Feasibility of performing these bone MR imaging techniques at 7T in smaller joints such as the wrist has been demonstrated.[109]

Due to its short T_2 components, cortical bone demonstrates low signal on routine MR imaging. UTE can, however, improve assessment of cortical bone and at lower field strengths has been successfully applied to study cortical water content, which is related to cortical porosity.[110,111] A feasibility study by Krug and colleagues[3] used an isotropic UTE sequence at 7T and 3T. The investigators reported an SNR gain by a factor of 1.7 (from 3T to 7T) and significantly shorter T_2 values. Further studies are needed to fully explore the potential of UHF MR imaging for imaging cortical bone.

SUMMARY

The recent approval of 7T MR imaging for clinical use is a major advancement that will drive the development of both clinical and research applications for musculoskeletal imaging. The SNR gain at

7T is an irrefutable advantage. The technical challenges are plentiful but RF inhomogeneity and coil design are the 2 that are underlined. Future musculoskeletal imaging protocols will likely include a combination of clinical morphologic and compositional imaging sequences. Advancement of compositional imaging techniques at 7T will likely be rapid. Further development of CEST techniques will enable high-resolution imaging of organic molecules, such as glucose and proteins, which play critical roles in disease pathogenesis. Higher SNR will permit X-nuclei MRS, including ^{23}Na, ^{39}K, ^{31}P, ^{13}C, ^{17}O, and so on, which will provide vital information regarding cellular processes, metabolic turnovers, energy metabolism, and oxygen consumption rate. MR imaging at 7T is another big step in the continued drive toward precision personalized medicine.

REFERENCES

1. Collins C. Radiofrequency field calculations for high field MRI. In: Robitaille PM, Berliner LJ, editors. Ultra High Field Magnetic Resonance Imaging. New York: Springer; 2006. p. 209–48.
2. Moser E, Stahlberg F, Ladd ME, et al. 7-T MR—from research to clinical applications? NMR Biomed 2012;25(5):695–716.
3. Krug R, Stehling C, Kelley DA, et al. Imaging of the musculoskeletal system in vivo using ultra-high field magnetic resonance at 7 T. Invest Radiol 2009;44(9):613–8.
4. Wiesinger F, Van de Moortele P-F, Adriany G, et al. Potential and feasibility of parallel MRI at high field. NMR Biomed 2006;19(3):368–78.
5. Scheenen TW, Heerschap A, Klomp DW. Towards 1H-MRSI of the human brain at 7T with slice-selective adiabatic refocusing pulses. MAGMA 2008;21(1–2):95–101.
6. Staroswiecki E, Bangerter NK, Gurney PT, et al. In vivo sodium imaging of human patellar cartilage with a 3D cones sequence at 3 T and 7 T. J Magn Reson Imaging 2010;32(2):446–51.
7. Meyerspeer M, Robinson S, Nabuurs CI, et al. Comparing localized and nonlocalized dynamic 31P magnetic resonance spectroscopy in exercising muscle at 7 T. Magn Reson Med 2012;68(6):1713–23.
8. Van de Moortele P-F, Akgun C, Adriany G, et al. B1 destructive interferences and spatial phase patterns at 7 T with a head transceiver array coil. Magn Reson Med 2005;54(6):1503–18.
9. Chang G, Wang L, Cardenas-Blanco A, et al. Biochemical and physiological MR imaging of skeletal muscle at 7 tesla and above. Semin Musculoskelet Radiol 2010;14(2):269–78.
10. Setsompop K, Alagappan V, Zelinski AC, et al. High-flip-angle slice-selective parallel RF transmission with 8 channels at 7 T. J Magn Reson 2008;195(1):76–84.
11. Hsu YC, Chu YH, Chern IL, et al. Mitigate B(1)(+) inhomogeneity by nonlinear gradients and RF shimming. Conf Proc IEEE Eng Med Biol Soc 2013;2013:1085–8.
12. Jordan CD, Saranathan M, Bangerter NK, et al. Musculoskeletal MRI at 3.0 T and 7.0 T: a comparison of relaxation times and image contrast. Eur J Radiol 2013;82(5):734–9.
13. Pruessmann KP. Parallel imaging at high field strength: synergies and joint potential. Top Magn Reson Imaging 2004;15(4):237–44.
14. Sengupta S, Welch EB, Zhao Y, et al. Dynamic B0 shimming at 7 T. Magn Reson Imaging 2011;29(4):483–96.
15. Regatte RR, Schweitzer ME. Ultra-high-field MRI of the musculoskeletal system at 7.0T. J Magn Reson Imaging 2007;25(2):262–9.
16. Balchandani P, Spielman D. Fat suppression for 1H MRSI at 7T using spectrally selective adiabatic inversion recovery. Magn Reson Med 2008;59(5):980–8.
17. U.S. Department of Health and Human Services, Food and Drug Administration, Center for Devices and Radiological Health, Guidance for Industry and FDA Staff. Criteria for significant risk investigations of magnetic resonance diagnostic devices, June 20, 2014.
18. Chakeres DW, Kangarlu A, Boudoulas H, et al. Effect of static magnetic field exposure of up to 8 Tesla on sequential human vital sign measurements. J Magn Reson Imaging 2003;18(3):346–52.
19. de Vocht F, Stevens T, Glover P, et al. Cognitive effects of head-movements in stray fields generated by a 7 Tesla whole-body MRI magnet. Bioelectromagnetics 2007;28(4):247–55.
20. Binks DA, Hodgson RJ, Ries ME, et al. Quantitative parametric MRI of articular cartilage: a review of progress and open challenges. Br J Radiol 2013;86(1023):20120163.
21. Sophia Fox AJ, Bedi A, Rodeo SA. The basic science of articular cartilage: structure, composition, and function. Sports Health 2009;1(6):461–8.
22. Buckwalter JA, Mankin HJ. Articular cartilage: degeneration and osteoarthritis, repair, regeneration, and transplantation. Instr Course Lect 1998;47:487–504.
23. Springer E, Bohndorf K, Juras V, et al. Comparison of routine knee magnetic resonance imaging at 3 T and 7 T. Invest Radiol 2017;52(1):42–54.
24. Bobic V. ICRS articular cartilage imaging committee. ICRS MR imaging protocol for knee articular cartilage. 2000;12.
25. Rubenstein JD, Li JG, Majumdar S, et al. Image resolution and signal-to-noise ratio requirements for MR imaging of degenerative cartilage. AJR Am J Roentgenol 1997;169(4):1089–96.

26. Jin J, Weber E, Destruel A, et al. An open 8-channel parallel transmission coil for static and dynamic 7T MRI of the knee and ankle joints at multiple postures. Magn Reson Med 2018;79(3):1804–16.

27. Mugler JP 3rd. Optimized three-dimensional fast-spin-echo MRI. J Magn Reson Imaging 2014; 39(4):745–67.

28. Kijowski R, Davis KW, Woods MA, et al. Knee joint: comprehensive assessment with 3D isotropic resolution fast spin-echo MR imaging–diagnostic performance compared with that of conventional MR imaging at 3.0 T. Radiology 2009;252(2):486–95.

29. Mohr A. The value of water-excitation 3D FLASH and fat-saturated PDw TSE MR imaging for detecting and grading articular cartilage lesions of the knee. Skeletal Radiol 2003;32(7):396–402.

30. Blankenbaker DG, Ullrick SR, Kijowski R, et al. MR arthrography of the hip: comparison of IDEAL-SPGR volume sequence to standard MR sequences in the detection and grading of cartilage lesions. Radiology 2011;261(3):863–71.

31. Regatte RR, Schweitzer ME. Novel contrast mechanisms at 3 tesla and 7 tesla. Semin Musculoskelet Radiol 2008;12(3):266–80.

32. Peterfy CG, Schneider E, Nevitt M. The osteoarthritis initiative: report on the design rationale for the magnetic resonance imaging protocol for the knee. Osteoarthritis Cartilage 2008;16(12):1433–41.

33. Liess C, Lusse S, Karger N, et al. Detection of changes in cartilage water content using MRI T2-mapping in vivo. Osteoarthritis Cartilage 2002; 10(12):907–13.

34. Carballido-Gamio J, Blumenkrantz G, Lynch JA, et al. Longitudinal analysis of MRI T(2) knee cartilage laminar organization in a subset of patients from the osteoarthritis initiative. Magn Reson Med 2010;63(2):465–72.

35. Joseph GB, Baum T, Alizai H, et al. Baseline mean and heterogeneity of MR cartilage T2 are associated with morphologic degeneration of cartilage, meniscus, and bone marrow over 3 years–data from the Osteoarthritis Initiative. Osteoarthritis Cartilage 2012;20(7):727–35.

36. Welsch GH, Apprich S, Zbyn S, et al. Biochemical (T2, T2* and magnetisation transfer ratio) MRI of knee cartilage: feasibility at ultra-high field (7T) compared with high field (3T) strength. Eur Radiol 2011;21(6):1136–43.

37. Chang G, Xia D, Sherman O, et al. High resolution morphologic imaging and T2 mapping of cartilage at 7 Tesla: comparison of cartilage repair patients and healthy controls. MAGMA 2013;26(6):539–48.

38. Domayer SE, Apprich S, Stelzeneder D, et al. Cartilage repair of the ankle: first results of T2 mapping at 7.0 T after microfracture and matrix associated autologous cartilage transplantation. Osteoarthritis Cartilage 2012;20(8):829–36.

39. Welsch GH, Mamisch TC, Hughes T, et al. In vivo biochemical 7.0 Tesla magnetic resonance: preliminary results of dGEMRIC, zonal T2, and T2* mapping of articular cartilage. Invest Radiol 2008;43(9): 619–26.

40. Welsch GH, Mamisch TC, Marlovits S, et al. Quantitative T2 mapping during follow-up after matrix-associated autologous chondrocyte transplantation (MACT): full-thickness and zonal evaluation to visualize the maturation of cartilage repair tissue. J Orthop Res 2009;27(7):957–63.

41. Lazik A, Theysohn JM, Geis C, et al. 7 Tesla quantitative hip MRI: T1, T2 and T2* mapping of hip cartilage in healthy volunteers. Eur Radiol 2016; 26(5):1245–53.

42. Juras V, Zbyn S, Mlynarik V, et al. The compositional difference between ankle and knee cartilage demonstrated by T2 mapping at 7 Tesla MR. Eur J Radiol 2016;85(4):771–7.

43. Mamisch TC, Hughes T, Mosher TJ, et al. T2 star relaxation times for assessment of articular cartilage at 3 T: a feasibility study. Skeletal Radiol 2012;41(3):287–92.

44. Sepponen RE, Pohjonen JA, Sipponen JT, et al. A method for T1 rho imaging. J Comput Assist Tomogr 1985;9(6):1007–11.

45. Keenan KE, Besier TF, Pauly JM, et al. Prediction of glycosaminoglycan content in human cartilage by age, T1rho and T2 MRI. Osteoarthritis Cartilage 2011;19(2):171–9.

46. Prasad AP, Nardo L, Schooler J, et al. T(1)rho and T(2) relaxation times predict progression of knee osteoarthritis. Osteoarthritis Cartilage 2013;21(1): 69–76.

47. Singh A, Haris M, Cai K, et al. High resolution T1rho mapping of in vivo human knee cartilage at 7T. PLoS One 2014;9(5):e97486.

48. Wyatt C, Guha A, Venkatachari A, et al. Improved differentiation between knees with cartilage lesions and controls using 7T relaxation time mapping. J Orthop Translat 2015;3(4):197–204.

49. Kogan F, Hargreaves BA, Gold GE. Volumetric multislice gagCEST imaging of articular cartilage: optimization and comparison with T1rho. Magn Reson Med 2017;77(3):1134–41.

50. Kogan F, Singh A, Cai K, et al. Investigation of chemical exchange at intermediate exchange rates using a combination of chemical exchange saturation transfer (CEST) and spin-locking methods (CESTrho). Magn Reson Med 2012;68(1):107–19.

51. Bae WC, Du J, Bydder GM, et al. Conventional and ultrashort time-to-echo magnetic resonance imaging of articular cartilage, meniscus, and intervertebral disk. Top Magn Reson Imaging 2010;21(5): 275–89.

52. Bae WC, Dwek JR, Znamirowski R, et al. Ultrashort echo time MR imaging of osteochondral junction of

the knee at 3 T: identification of anatomic structures contributing to signal intensity. Radiology 2010; 254(3):837–45.

53. Chang EY, Pallante-Kichura AL, Bae WC, et al. Development of a Comprehensive Osteochondral Allograft MRI Scoring System (OCAMRISS) with histopathologic, micro-computed tomography, and biomechanical validation. Cartilage 2014;5(1):16–27.

54. Chu CR, Williams AA, West RV, et al. Quantitative magnetic resonance imaging UTE-T2* mapping of cartilage and meniscus healing after anatomic anterior cruciate ligament reconstruction. Am J Sports Med 2014;42(8):1847–56.

55. Lazik A, Korsmeier K, Classen T, et al. 3 Tesla high-resolution and delayed gadolinium enhanced MR imaging of cartilage (dGEMRIC) after autologous chondrocyte transplantation in the hip. J Magn Reson Imaging 2015;42(3):624–33.

56. Watanabe A, Wada Y, Obata T, et al. Delayed gadolinium-enhanced MR to determine glycosaminoglycan concentration in reparative cartilage after autologous chondrocyte implantation: preliminary results. Radiology 2006;239(1):201–8.

57. d'Entremont AG, McCormack RG, Agbanlog K, et al. Cartilage health in high tibial osteotomy using dGEMRIC: relationships with joint kinematics. Knee 2015;22(3):156–62.

58. Schleich C, Muller-Lutz A, Sewerin P, et al. Intra-individual assessment of inflammatory severity and cartilage composition of finger joints in rheumatoid arthritis. Skeletal Radiol 2015;44(4):513–8.

59. Owman H, Tiderius CJ, Ericsson YB, et al. Long-term effect of removal of knee joint loading on cartilage quality evaluated by delayed gadolinium-enhanced magnetic resonance imaging of cartilage. Osteoarthritis Cartilage 2014;22(7):928–32.

60. Burstein D, Velyvis J, Scott KT, et al. Protocol issues for delayed Gd(DTPA)(2-)-enhanced MRI (dGEMRIC) for clinical evaluation of articular cartilage. Magn Reson Med 2001;45(1):36–41.

61. Lazik-Palm A, Kraff O, Geis C, et al. Morphological imaging and T2 and T2* mapping of hip cartilage at 7 Tesla MRI under the influence of intravenous gadolinium. Eur Radiol 2016;26(11):3923–31.

62. Madelin G, Lee JS, Regatte RR, et al. Methods and applications. Prog Nucl Magn Reson Spectrosc 2014;79:14–47.

63. Madelin G, Babb J, Xia D, et al. Articular cartilage: evaluation with fluid-suppressed 7.0-T sodium MR imaging in subjects with and subjects without osteoarthritis. Radiology 2013;268(2):481–91.

64. Trattnig S, Welsch GH, Juras V, et al. 23Na MR imaging at 7 T after knee matrix-associated autologous chondrocyte transplantation preliminary results. Radiology 2010;257(1):175–84.

65. Wiggins GC, Brown R, Lakshmanan K. High-performance radiofrequency coils for (23)Na MRI: brain and musculoskeletal applications. NMR Biomed 2016;29(2):96–106.

66. Madelin G, Chang G, Otazo R, et al. Compressed sensing sodium MRI of cartilage at 7T: preliminary study. J Magn Reson 2012;214(1):360–5.

67. Lee JS, Xia D, Madelin G, et al. Sodium inversion recovery MRI on the knee joint at 7 T with an optimal control pulse. J Magn Reson 2016;262:33–41.

68. Chang G, Madelin G, Sherman OH, et al. Improved assessment of cartilage repair tissue using fluid-suppressed (2)(3)Na inversion recovery MRI at 7 Tesla: preliminary results. Eur Radiol 2012;22(6):1341–9.

69. Zbyn S, Brix MO, Juras V, et al. Sodium magnetic resonance imaging of ankle joint in cadaver specimens, volunteers, and patients after different cartilage repair techniques at 7 T: initial results. Invest Radiol 2015;50(4):246–54.

70. Zbyn S, Stelzeneder D, Welsch GH, et al. Evaluation of native hyaline cartilage and repair tissue after two cartilage repair surgery techniques with 23Na MR imaging at 7 T: initial experience. Osteoarthritis Cartilage 2012;20(8):837–45.

71. Raya JG, Horng A, Dietrich O, et al. Articular cartilage: in vivo diffusion-tensor imaging. Radiology 2012;262(2):550–9.

72. Raya JG, Melkus G, Adam-Neumair S, et al. Diffusion-tensor imaging of human articular cartilage specimens with early signs of cartilage damage. Radiology 2013;266(3):831–41.

73. Ling W, Regatte RR, Navon G, et al. Assessment of glycosaminoglycan concentration in vivo by chemical exchange-dependent saturation transfer (gagCEST). Proc Natl Acad Sci U S A 2008;105(7):2266–70.

74. Schmitt B, Zbyn S, Stelzeneder D, et al. Cartilage quality assessment by using glycosaminoglycan chemical exchange saturation transfer and (23)Na MR imaging at 7 T. Radiology 2011;260(1):257–64.

75. Singh A, Haris M, Cai K, et al. Chemical exchange saturation transfer magnetic resonance imaging of human knee cartilage at 3 T and 7 T. Magn Reson Med 2012;68(2):588–94.

76. Eggers H, Bornert P. Chemical shift encoding-based water-fat separation methods. J Magn Reson Imaging 2014;40(2):251–68.

77. Gaeta M, Scribano E, Mileto A, et al. Muscle fat fraction in neuromuscular disorders: dual-echo dual-flip-angle spoiled gradient-recalled MR imaging technique for quantification–a feasibility study. Radiology 2011;259(2):487–94.

78. Alizai H, Nardo L, Karampinos DC, et al. Comparison of clinical semi-quantitative assessment of muscle fat infiltration with quantitative assessment using chemical shift-based water/fat separation in

MR studies of the calf of post-menopausal women. Eur Radiol 2012;22(7):1592–600.

79. Karampinos DC, Baum T, Nardo L, et al. Characterization of the regional distribution of skeletal muscle adipose tissue in type 2 diabetes using chemical shift-based water/fat separation. J Magn Reson Imaging 2012;35(4):899–907.

80. Kumar D, Karampinos DC, MacLeod TD, et al. Quadriceps intramuscular fat fraction rather than muscle size is associated with knee osteoarthritis. Osteoarthritis Cartilage 2014;22(2): 226–34.

81. Nardo L, Karampinos DC, Lansdown DA, et al. Quantitative assessment of fat infiltration in the rotator cuff muscles using water-fat MRI. J Magn Reson Imaging 2014;39(5):1178–85.

82. Stephenson MC, Gunner F, Napolitano A, et al. Applications of multi-nuclear magnetic resonance spectroscopy at 7T. World J Radiol 2011;3(4): 105–13.

83. Boesch C. Musculoskeletal spectroscopy. J Magn Reson Imaging 2007;25(2):321–38.

84. Wang L, Salibi N, Wu Y, et al. Relaxation times of skeletal muscle metabolites at 7T. J Magn Reson Imaging 2009;29(6):1457–64.

85. Bogner W, Chmelik M, Schmid AI, et al. Assessment of (31)P relaxation times in the human calf muscle: a comparison between 3 T and 7 T in vivo. Magn Reson Med 2009;62(3):574–82.

86. Parasoglou P, Xia D, Chang G, et al. Dynamic three-dimensional imaging of phosphocreatine recovery kinetics in the human lower leg muscles at 3T and 7T: a preliminary study. NMR Biomed 2013;26(3):348–56.

87. Minotti JR, Johnson EC, Hudson TL, et al. Training-induced skeletal muscle adaptations are independent of systemic adaptations. J Appl Physiol (1985) 1990;68(1):289–94.

88. van Oorschot JW, Schmitz JP, Webb A, et al. 31P MR spectroscopy and computational modeling identify a direct relation between Pi content of an alkaline compartment in resting muscle and phosphocreatine resynthesis kinetics in active muscle in humans. PLoS One 2013;8(9):e76628.

89. Schunk K, Romaneehsen B, Rieker O, et al. Dynamic phosphorus-31 magnetic resonance spectroscopy in arterial occlusive disease: effects of vascular therapy on spectroscopic results. Invest Radiol 1998;33(6):329–35.

90. Scheuermann-Freestone M, Madsen PL, Manners D, et al. Abnormal cardiac and skeletal muscle energy metabolism in patients with type 2 diabetes. Circulation 2003;107(24):3040–6.

91. Towse TF, Childs BT, Sabin SA, et al. Comparison of muscle BOLD responses to arterial occlusion at 3 and 7 Tesla. Magn Reson Med 2016;75(3): 1333–40.

92. Kim HK, Laor T, Horn PS, et al. T2 mapping in Duchenne muscular dystrophy: distribution of disease activity and correlation with clinical assessments. Radiology 2010;255(3):899–908.

93. Carlier PG, Azzabou N, de Sousa PL, et al. Skeletal muscle quantitative nuclear magnetic resonance imaging follow-up of adult Pompe patients. J Inherit Metab Dis 2015;38(3):565–72.

94. Arpan I, Willcocks RJ, Forbes SC, et al. Examination of effects of corticosteroids on skeletal muscles of boys with DMD using MRI and MRS. Neurology 2014;83(11):974–80.

95. Chang G, Wang L, Schweitzer ME, et al. 3D 23Na MRI of human skeletal muscle at 7 Tesla: initial experience. Eur Radiol 2010;20(8):2039–46.

96. Weber MA, Nagel AM, Jurkat-Rott K, et al. Sodium (23Na) MRI detects elevated muscular sodium concentration in Duchenne muscular dystrophy. Neurology 2011;77(23):2017–24.

97. Weber MA, Nielles-Vallespin S, Huttner HB, et al. Evaluation of patients with paramyotonia at 23Na MR imaging during cold-induced weakness. Radiology 2006;240(2):489–500.

98. Johnell O, Kanis JA. An estimate of the worldwide prevalence and disability associated with osteoporotic fractures. Osteoporos Int 2006;17(12): 1726–33.

99. Link TM. Osteoporosis imaging: state of the art and advanced imaging. Radiology 2012;263(1):3–17.

100. Sell CA, Masi JN, Burghardt A, et al. Quantification of trabecular bone structure using magnetic resonance imaging at 3 tesla—calibration studies using microcomputed tomography as a standard of reference. Calcif Tissue Int 2005;76(5):355–64.

101. Driban JB, Barbe MF, Amin M, et al. Validation of quantitative magnetic resonance imaging-based apparent bone volume fraction in peri-articular tibial bone of cadaveric knees. BMC Musculoskelet Disord 2014;15:143.

102. Chang G, Wang L, Liang G, et al. Reproducibility of subregional trabecular bone micro-architectural measures derived from 7-Tesla magnetic resonance images. MAGMA 2011;24(3):121–5.

103. Chang G, Deniz CM, Honig S, et al. MRI of the hip at 7T: feasibility of bone microarchitecture, high-resolution cartilage, and clinical imaging. J Magn Reson Imaging 2014;39(6):1384–93.

104. Chang G, Honig S, Liu Y, et al. 7 Tesla MRI of bone microarchitecture discriminates between women without and with fragility fractures who do not differ by bone mineral density. J Bone Miner Metab 2015; 33(3):285–93.

105. Chang G, Boone S, Martel D, et al. MRI assessment of bone structure and microarchitecture. J Magn Reson Imaging 2017;46(2):323–37.

106. Chang G, Pakin SK, Schweitzer ME, et al. Adaptations in trabecular bone microarchitecture in

Olympic athletes determined by 7T MRI. J Magn Reson Imaging 2008;27(5):1089–95.

107. Chang G, Rajapakse CS, Babb JS, et al. In vivo estimation of bone stiffness at the distal femur and proximal tibia using ultra-high-field 7-Tesla magnetic resonance imaging and micro-finite element analysis. J Bone Miner Metab 2012; 30(2):243–51.

108. Chang G, Rajapakse CS, Diamond M, et al. Micro-finite element analysis applied to high-resolution MRI reveals improved bone mechanical competence in the distal femur of female pre-professional dancers. Osteoporos Int 2013;24(4): 1407–17.

109. Chang G, Wang L, Liang G, et al. Quantitative assessment of trabecular bone micro-architecture of the wrist via 7 Tesla MRI: preliminary results. MAGMA 2011;24(4):191–9.

110. Techawiboonwong A, Song HK, Wehrli FW. In vivo MRI of submillisecond T2 species with two-dimensional and three-dimensional radial sequences and applications to the measurement of cortical bone water. NMR Biomed 2008;21(1): 59–70.

111. Du J, Hamilton G, Takahashi A, et al. Ultrashort echo time spectroscopic imaging (UTESI) of cortical bone. Magn Reson Med 2007;58(5): 1001–9.

The Role of Dual-Energy Computed Tomography in Musculoskeletal Imaging

Takeshi Fukuda, MD[a,b,*], Kunihiko Fukuda, MD, PhD[c]

KEYWORDS

- Dual energy • Spectral • Computed tomography • DECT • Musculoskeletal

KEY POINTS

- Dual-energy computed tomography (DECT) can reduce beam hardening artifacts by synthesizing a virtual monochromatic image and enables detailed evaluation of prosthetic complications.
- DECT can display monosodium urate crystal deposition, which helps to make a correct diagnosis in atypical gout and precise therapeutic assessment.
- DECT iodine maps can delineate soft tissue inflammation of arthritis and may be beneficial for evaluating peripheral joints because of its high spatial resolution.

INTRODUCTION

Dual-energy computed tomography (DECT) enables material decomposition and acquisition of virtual monochromatic images by performing 2 exposures at different energy levels. Its development has led to several interesting image processing applications that have been applied to a range of clinical entities. Bone removal in DECT angiography may be useful for detecting aneurysms adjacent to the skull base.[1] Iodine maps for pulmonary embolism have shown perfusion defects in areas of vascular occlusion.[2] For musculoskeletal imaging, DECT has been used to create virtual noncalcium images, to diagnose and follow the progression of gout, to create iodine maps, and to examine tendons through material decomposition techniques. Furthermore, virtual monochromatic images have also been used in musculoskeletal imaging to reduce metal artifacts when imaging patients with arthroplasty. In this article, the authors review these musculoskeletal imaging techniques with some representative cases.

All subjects were examined in the authors' institution with dual-source DECT (SOMATOM Definition Flash; Siemens Healthineers, Forchheim, Germany), and all images were created on a commercial workstation (Syngo Dual Energy; Siemens Healthineers Erlangen, Germany).

VARIETY OF DUAL-ENERGY COMPUTED TOMOGRAPHY IMAGE ACQUISITION TECHNIQUES

There are several ways to acquire DECT data, including sequential acquisition, dual source, rapid kilovoltage switching, and double layer technology.[3–5]

Sequential acquisition requires 2 separate sequential scans at different energy levels. It needs only the most basic hardware, but the high radiation dose, long acquisition time, and misregistration limit its utility.[3,5]

Dual-source DECT carries 2 independent X-ray tubes orthogonally in one unit so that data from the 2 different energy levels can be obtained at

Disclosure Statement: All authors have nothing to disclose.
[a] Department of Radiology, The Jikei University School of Medicine, 3-19-18, Nishi-Shimbashi, Minato-ku, Tokyo 105-8471, Japan; [b] Department of Radiology, Stony Brook Medicine, HSC Level 4, Room 120, Stony Brook, NY 11794, USA; [c] Centre for International Affairs, The Jikei University, 3-25-8, Nishi-Shimbashi, Minato-ku, Tokyo 105-8461, Japan
* Corresponding author. Department of Radiology, The Jikei University School of Medicine, 3-19-18, Nishi-Shimbashi, Minato-ku, Tokyo 105-8471, Japan.
E-mail address: takenet616@gmail.com

PET Clin 13 (2018) 567–578
https://doi.org/10.1016/j.cpet.2018.05.009
1556-8598/18/© 2018 Elsevier Inc. All rights reserved.

the same time. This technology allows the current modulation in each tube and tin filter usage. Tin filter reduces unnecessary radiation exposure and emphasizes spectral separation between low- and high-energy X-ray beams. However, the cross-scatter radiation that occurs with 2 simultaneous radiographs may cause deterioration of the data.[5]

Rapid kilovoltage switching uses a single X-ray tube that switches rapidly between 2 different energy settings. The high temporal resolution limits motion artifacts, but adapting the tube current is difficult.[3] The radiation dose and long scanning time are the main disadvantages.[5]

Last, double layer technology uses 2 detector layers: lower-energy radiographs are absorbed by the superficial detector layer and higher-energy radiographs are absorbed by the deeper detector layer. This technology provides temporospatially matched dual-energy data while preserving a full field of view. However, a high radiation dose is required to compensate for poor soft tissue contrast.[3,5]

Currently, dual source (Siemens Healthineers) and fast kilovoltage switching (GE Healthcare) are the market-leading technologies, and most of the available clinical data related to DECT have been obtained using these techniques.

VIRTUAL MONOCHROMATIC IMAGES

For musculoskeletal radiologists, interpreting the images of patients with metallic prostheses for surgical and postsurgical complications, such as infection, metallic prosthesis loosening, and fracture, is a daily task. Recently, the importance of early diagnosis of adverse local tissue reactions in arthroplasty has been recognized.[6] MR imaging is ideal for detecting soft tissue pathologic condition, but higher magnetic field makes the effect of magnetic susceptibility of metal increased. Recently, advanced techniques, such as slice encoding for metal artifact correction and multiacquisition with variable-resonance image combination, have been available for metallic artifact reduction and dedicated to the better image quality.[7,8] Conventional CT also suffers image deterioration from beam hardening artifacts. Polychromatic radiographs from conventional CT include low-energy radiographs, which are responsible for beam hardening artifacts.[9] On the other hand, DECT allows creation of a virtual monochromatic energy image from which complications adjacent to metallic implants can be evaluated with less artifact (Fig. 1). Beam hardening can be eliminated by increasing X-ray energy, with the optimal virtual monochromatic energy reported as between 105 and 150 keV.[10–14] However, increasing the X-ray energy

diminishes the soft tissue contrast that is important for evaluating soft tissue complications around surgical devices. Bamberg and colleagues[11] suggested that 105 keV may be the ideal energy for the evaluation of bone and soft tissue surrounding prostheses. If applicable, metal artifact reduction software added to DECT monochromatic images further reduces metallic artifacts.[10,15,16] Recently tailoring the monochromatic energy to the implant type has been recommended by Wellenberg and colleagues.[17] They suggested that stainless steel implants produced more severe artifacts and needed higher monochromatic energy settings for optimal artifact reduction than titanium implants.

VIRTUAL NONCALCIUM IMAGES

DECT virtual noncalcium (VNCa) images are an image processing technique that subtracts high-attenuation calcium from cancellous bone to depict several bone marrow lesions. As the representative lesion, bone marrow edema is a common pathologic condition in clinical usage. On MR imaging, bone marrow edema is detected as hypointensity on T1-weighted images and ill-defined hyperintensity on fluid-sensitive sequences. Although CT has high spatial resolution and allows retrospective reconstruction of images, MR imaging can diagnose occult or nondisplaced fractures more precisely by delineating the fracture line and surrounding bone marrow edema.[18,19] With the DECT VNCa technique, edema in bone marrow can be detected on grayscale or color-coded images. It is thought that color-coded maps are better for detecting attenuation changes in bone marrow edema.[20] Because Pache and colleagues[21] used VNCa images for acute knee trauma in 2010, several other studies have reported the validity of VNCa images for detecting bone marrow edema in subjects with trauma or fracture[21–28] (Table 1), particularly in vertebral fractures. The sensitivity and specificity of VNCa images for detecting bone marrow edema were acceptable except for the low specificity from a study of nondisplaced hip fractures.[25] In that study there were 3 false-positive cases, but their reference was not MR imaging, which is sensitive to bone marrow edema. Because of the visibility of bone marrow edema, a recent article showed that adding DECT VNCa to conventional bone reconstruction increased diagnostic sensitivity, specificity, and confidence in images of patients with fracture[29,30] (Fig. 2). Some limitations have also been reported. Bone marrow lesions adjacent to cortical bone could not be detected with VNCa images due to spatial averaging effects.[21] Wang and colleagues[23] also suggested that gas and

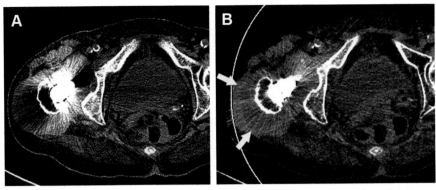

Fig. 1. An 84-year-old woman with right hip pain status post total hip arthroplasty. Although (A) conventional CT suffered from severe beam hardening artifacts, (B) DECT virtual monochromatic image showed reduction of beam hardening, and abnormal fluid collection could be visualized with more confidence (arrows).

sclerosis of bone decreased the attenuation values of bone marrow edema and resulted in false negatives (see **Table 1**).

Many disorders cause bone marrow edema other than bone contusions and fractures. Osteoarthritis is a common disease, mainly among obese and elderly people worldwide. Bone marrow edema is frequently found in patients with osteoarthritis and is associated with pain[31] and worsening of radiographic joint space narrowing.[32] Again, MR imaging is ideal for understanding the cause of pain and predicting the progression of OA.[33] However, CT has advantages when investigating cortical bone and osteophytes, and visualization of bone marrow edema with VNCa should be an interesting topic for future research

Table 1
Summary of the literature regarding the dual-energy computed tomography virtual noncalcium technique applied to bone marrow edema

Author, Year	Trauma/ Fracture Site	No. of Patients	Mean Age ± SD	Gold Standard of Bone Marrow Edema	DECT Sensitivity	DECT Specificity	DECT Interobserver Reliability (κ)
Pache et al,[21] 2010	Knee	21	35.9 ± 14.3	MRI	0.86	0.94–0.96	0.78 for femoral lesion 0.87 for tibial lesion
Guggenberger et al,[22] 2012	Ankle	30	34 ± 11.8	MRI	0.9	0.81–0.82	0.66
Wang et al,[23] 2013	Spine	63	71.6 ± 10.3	MRI	0.63 0.96[a]	0.99 0.98[a]	NA
Bierry et al,[24] 2014	Spine	20	69 ± 14	MRI	0.84	0.97	0.75
Reddy et al,[25] 2015	Hip	21	77	Radiologic or clinical diagnosis at 30-d follow-up	0.9	0.4	NA
Karaca et al,[26] 2016	Spine	23	61 ± 15	MRI	0.89	0.99	0.82
Diekhoff et al,[27] 2017	Spine	9	75 ± 8.7	MRI	0.88	1	0.63–0.89
Petritsch et al,[28] 2017	Spine	22	60 ± 23	MRI	0.64	0.99	0.85

Abbreviation: SD, standard deviation.
[a] In the group of vertebral bodies with less than 50% sclerosis and/or air.

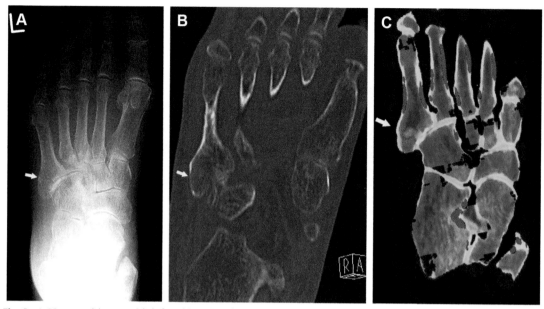

Fig. 2. A 93-year-old man with left ankle pain after a sprain injury. (*A*) Radiograph and (*B*) CT show nondisplaced fracture of the fifth metatarsal base (*arrow*). It is not so obvious because of background osteoporosis and nondisplaced nature. (*C*) VNCa image shows color-coded bone marrow edema along the fracture site (*arrow*) and makes an easier detection.

(**Fig. 3**). Rheumatoid arthritis is one of the most common arthritides in clinical rheumatology. Bone marrow edema has been recently recognized as an independent predictor for bone erosion.[34] However, little has been reported on the use of VNCa in peripheral bones,[35] and prospective studies with large numbers are needed to verify this application of VNCa.

Tumor infiltration is also a relevant and important topic in VNCa imaging and had been studied in patients with multiple myeloma.[36,37] Kosmala and colleagues[37] showed that both sensitivity and specificity of VNCa images to multiple myeloma lesions were 0.91 when compared with MR imaging. The authors experienced a case in which adding VNCa images to a conventional CT image improved the detectability of bone metastases (**Fig. 4**). Even though CT is regarded as the most common modality for follow-up of patients with cancer, it has the lowest sensitivity for detecting bone metastases compared with other modalities, such as MR imaging, FDG-PET, and bone scintigraphy.[38] If VNCa images can compensate for this shortcoming, CT could become even more useful.

GOUT

Gout is a common inflammatory arthritis caused by the deposition of monosodium urate (MSU) crystals

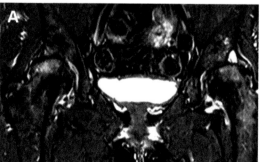
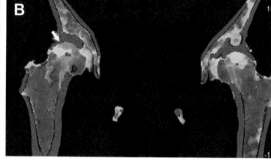

Fig. 3. A 63-year-old woman with bilateral hip osteoarthritis. (*A*) Short-tau inversion recovery MR imaging shows bilateral bone-on-bone osteoarthritis and bone marrow edema in both acetabular and femoral head. (*B*) DECT VNCa image also detected bone marrow edema in a comparable way, but subarticular sclerosis may interrupt precise detection of subarticular bone marrow edema in the right femoral head (*arrow*).

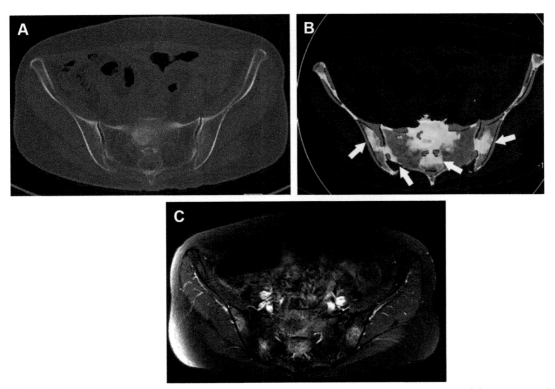

Fig. 4. A 66-year-old woman with lung cancer and bone metastasis undergoing chemotherapy. (A) Conventional CT shows sclerotic bone metastasis in the sacral bone. (B) DECT VNCa image (without intravenous contrast) detects more bone marrow lesions than conventional display (arrows), and (C) a contrast-enhanced fat-suppressed T1-weighted MR imaging confirms these are metastatic lesions.

in synovial fluid and other soft tissues. Untreated hyperuricemia passes through several stages: asymptomatic hyperuricemia, acute gouty arthritis, intercritical gout, and tophaceous gout.[39] Gout is usually diagnosed with swelling and redness of peripheral joints, frequently monoarticular, typically the first metatarsophalangeal joint.[40] However, it is true that there are cases with unusual presentation (eg, atypical site, polyarticular, or indolent course) that can make the diagnosis challenging.[41] Joint fluid aspiration is regarded as the gold standard for diagnosis, but it is not always possible to obtain joint fluid because of insufficient fluid or inaccessibility. Furthermore, joint fluid analysis can be negative in 25% of acute gouty arthritis patients regardless of its invasiveness.[42] Serum urate level varies among acute gouty arthritis patients, and gout should not be excluded even when serum urate levels are normal.[43] Imaging modalities, such as X-ray, ultrasound, conventional CT, and MR imaging, have been used as aids to diagnosis. Although ultrasound and MR imaging can detect joint effusion or synovitis, which are signs of acute arthritis, they have been used mainly for evaluating or detecting tophus in the chronic stage.[44,45] Ultrasound can detect MSU deposition on hyaline cartilage as a hyperechoic

line parallel to the subchondral bone plate (double contour sign)[46] in the early phase, but it is limited by the inaccessibility of deep structures and its dependence on the examiner.

On the other hand, by use of material decomposition techniques, DECT can distinguish MSU from calcific mineralization and delineate MSU deposition itself as a color-coded structure[47,48] (Fig. 5). DECT detectability of tophus was significantly higher than physical examination,[49] and sensitivity, specificity, and interobserver reliability of DECT in detection of MSU deposition were 1.0, 0.79 to 0.89, and κ = 0.87, respectively, using joint aspiration as reference.[50] One of the most important advantages of DECT over other imaging modalities is that DECT has the potential to diagnose gout by displaying MSU deposition regardless of the deposition site and the phase of disease.[51] Therefore, DECT is a suitable method for any practitioner to make a diagnosis with confidence and without joint aspiration. Because DECT has been applied to the diagnosis of gout, it has been recognized that MSU can accumulate anywhere in the body, including the spine,[52] tendons, and ligaments[53] (Fig. 6). In fact, the presence of MSU deposition on DECT

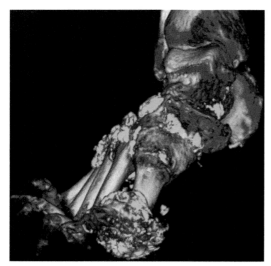

Fig. 5. A 33-year-old man with gout. Tophaceous MSU deposits are clearly visualized with DECT as green masses around the joints, mainly the first metatarsophalangeal joint.

has been newly included as one of the important factors in the latest classification criteria for gout.[54]

DECT is also highly reproducible when quantifying the volume of deposited MSU.[55] The amount of MSU deposition is automatically calculated if the images are displayed with a commercial workstation (see **Fig. 6**). Automatic quantification of MSU deposition should be a useful tool for monitoring therapeutic effects and to educate patients for better compliance.

There are several fascinating future possibilities for DECT and gout. Because acute gouty attacks typically follow years of asymptomatic hyperuricemia, there must be subclinical MSU deposition in patients with hyperuricemia before the attack.

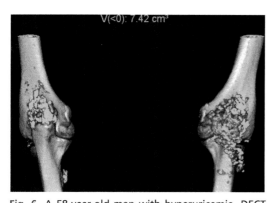

Fig. 6. A 58-year-old man with hyperuricemia. DECT of the extensor side of the elbow joint shows MSU deposition along the bilateral triceps brachii tendon. The accumulated MSU is automatically quantified as 7.42 cm³.

Although serum urate levels higher than 6.8 mg/dL are above saturation and may lead to MSU deposition in the body,[56] the reported normal range varies among laboratories, and elevated serum urate levels do not always lead to deposition of MSU.[57] However, DECT can calculate the amount of MSU deposition independently. From this point of view, there are advantages over conventional images. First, identification of MSU deposition in asymptomatic patients may lead to earlier recognition and treatment of hyperuricemia.[48] Second, more accurate and objective assessment of therapeutic effects with DECT MSU quantification may help one to understand how drugs affect tophus.[58]

IODINE MAPS

With DECT, iodine can be subtracted from contrast-enhanced images to create virtual noncontrast images. Afterward, by overlaying subtracted iodine as color on the virtual noncontrast image, an iodine map can be created.[59] Iodine maps have been used for many clinical entities, but its use is still limited in musculoskeletal imaging.[60,61]

Current treatment of inflammatory arthritis has been greatly changed by the development of biological agents. Biological agents are so effective that progression of structural change can be halted and pain may be relieved. An early diagnosis is the key to receiving the maximum benefit from biologic agents and for a better prognosis.[62–65] Images are regarded as more sensitive to inflammatory lesions than physical examination, with several studies suggesting they can help with an early diagnosis.[66,67] At the same time, biological agents are expensive, and some of them increase the risk of infectious disease[68]; objective monitoring for inflammatory status is necessary to reduce or stop biologics with appropriate timing. Again, imaging is expected to be one of the methods to monitor inflammation.[66,67] MR imaging and ultrasound are widely used for these purposes, but use of CT has been rare. The contrast resolution of CT is not sufficient to delineate joint inflammation, even with contrast enhancement. CT does, however, have obvious advantages over other modalities especially for evaluation of peripheral arthritis. First, it has high spatial resolution, and images can be reconstructed retrospectively in any section without deterioration. An entire small joint can be evaluated with few artifacts even when there is severe dislocation or deformity. Second, CT is the most reliable modality for assessing bone structure, which is important for both diagnosis and prognosis.[69] Third, a CT examination is patient friendly;

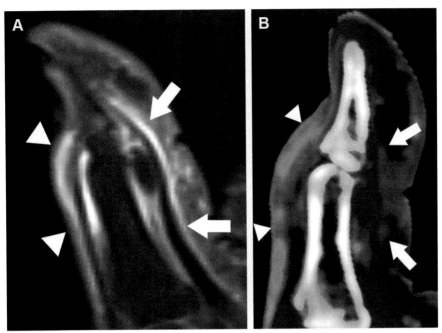

Fig. 7. Sagittal image of a thumb in a 56-year-old man with PsA. (*A*) Fat-saturated contrast-enhanced MR imaging and (*B*) DECT iodine map show compatible flexor tenosynovitis (*arrows*) and extensor peritendinitis (*arrowheads*) as prominent enhancement along the flexor tendon sheath and extensor tendon, respectively. (*Data from* Fukuda T, Umezawa Y, Tojo S, et al. Initial experience of using dual-energy CT with iodine overlay image for hand psoriatic arthritis: comparison study with contrast-enhanced MR imaging. Radiology 2017;284(1):138. Fig. 1.)

it is fast (about 10 seconds) and not noisy. Last, CT is usually more widely available than MR imaging. Easy access to the technology is important for making an early diagnosis.

Recently, the authors have tried to compensate for the poor contrast resolution of CT with a DECT iodine map technique to see if it can delineate inflammatory lesions of arthritis. When the authors included patients with psoriasis or psoriatic arthritis (PsA) as the subjects, the sensitivity and specificity of the DECT iodine map in delineating inflammatory lesions were 0.78 and 0.87, respectively, using contrast-enhanced MR imaging as reference (**Fig. 7**). DECT, however, detected significantly

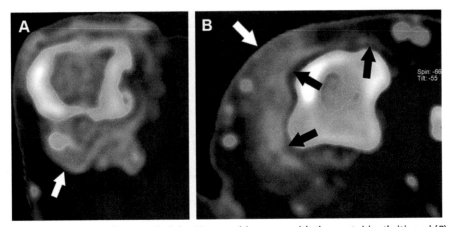

Fig. 8. Axial image of a DECT iodine map in (*A*) a 69-year-old woman with rheumatoid arthritis and (*B*) a 43-year-old woman with PsA. (*A*) Pannus formation is apparent inside the joint capsule between bone and linear inflamed synovium (*arrow*) in rheumatoid arthritis. (*B*) Besides the linear inflamed synovium (*black arrows*), extra-articular inflammation (*white arrow*) is more prominent in PsA due to enthesitis. (*From* Fukuda T, Umezawa Y, Asahina A, et al. Dual energy CT iodine map for delineating inflammation of inflammatory arthritis. Eur Radiol 2017;27(12):5036. Fig. 1; with permission.)

more inflammatory lesions, mainly in the distal interphalangeal (DIP) joints, than MR imaging. Although there was no histopathological correlation, the advantages of DECT, such as high spatial resolution and image reconstruction technology, may improve the detectability of inflammatory lesions. Recent development of disease-specific biologics requires differentiating rheumatoid arthritis from PsA before their characteristic bone changes occur. High spatial resolution and image reconstruction technology may make DECT a suitable tool for differentiating these 2 disorders even in peripheral joints because it may enable to reflect different inflammatory targets: synovium for rheumatoid arthritis and

enthesis for PsA[61,70–72] (**Fig. 8**). In PsA, nail deformity has been recognized as a predictor for DIP arthritis.[73] McGonagle and colleagues[74] reported there is a close relationship between the extensor tendon enthesis and the nail, and the entheseal complex is likely to be an inflammatory target in DIP-involved PsA. DECT can show prominent enhancement in thickened nail beds in the DIP joint in patients with PsA, which is consistent with a previous high-resolution MR imaging study[75] (**Fig. 9**). When the authors used DECT in an early-stage patient with PsA, due to the high spatial resolution, they could observe local abnormal enhancement from the extensor tendon enthesis to the nail bed without obvious DIP joint inflammation.[76] DECT also has the potential to assess therapeutic effects objectively (**Fig. 10**). Since the Outcome Measures in Rheumatology Clinical Trial (OMERACT) working group issued an MR imaging scoring system for

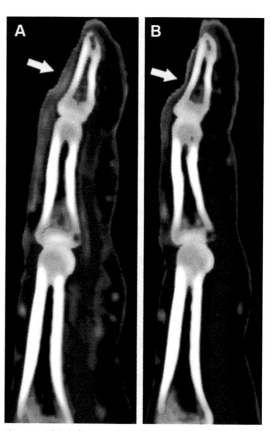

Fig. 9. Second finger of a 40-year-old man with PsA. DECT iodine map delineates prominent swelling and enhancement around the DIP joint. On the extensor side, inflammation along the extensor tendon and enthesis continuously spreads to the thickened nail bed (*arrow*). Flexor tenosynovitis is also noted (*arrowhead*).

Fig. 10. Third finger of a 43-year-old with PsA. (*A*) DECT iodine map shows abnormal enhancement along the extensor tendon and flexor tendon sheath with swelling of the DIP joint. Nail bed is also thickened and enhanced (*arrow*). (*B*) After therapy with a biologic agent, even though some slight enhancement of the extensor side of the DIP joint remains, the obvious decrease of abnormal enhancement and thickness of the nail is clear (*arrow*).

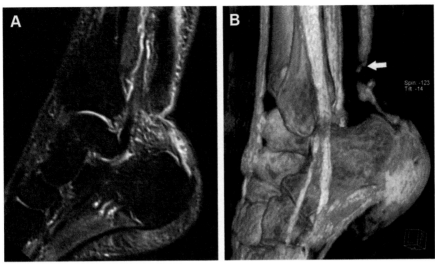

Fig. 11. A 77-year-old woman with a tear of the Achilles tendon. (*A*) Short-tau inversion recovery MR imaging shows the Achilles tendon with a portion retracted proximally. (*B*) DECT also shows a complete tear of the tendon. Calcification at the proximal tendon stump is more clearly visualized than on the MR imaging (*arrow*).

rheumatoid arthritis and PsA,[77,78] the system has been validated.[79,80] The scoring system is applicable to DECT assessment, and the iodine in a DECT iodine map is quantifiable; this means that DECT can assess therapeutic change quantitatively and objectively.

TENDON

The short acquisition time and easy access of CT are ideal features for evaluating trauma patients. However, the ability to evaluate collagenous structures, such as ligaments and tendons, is limited in CT. MR imaging is commonly used to diagnose ligament or tendon injuries, but the availability of MR imaging varies among institutions, especially in emergency situations or at night. Furthermore, the long acquisition time requires acute trauma patients to keep still for a long time. A widely available technique that can detect collagenous structures might well increase the role of CT in trauma cases. An initial study of DECT applied to knee ligaments showed that DECT displayed some knee ligaments, including the anterior cruciate ligament and posterior cruciate ligament, but not others, such as the tibial collateral ligament and transverse ligament.[81] On the other hand, tendons of the hand and foot were clearly visualized with DECT[82] (**Fig. 11**). A comparison study between DECT and MR imaging for detecting iatrogenic anterior cruciate ligament injury in a porcine model showed that MR imaging had higher sensitivity and specificity than DECT for complete tears (1.0 and 0.75, for MR imaging and 0.75 and 0.69, for DECT).[83]

SUMMARY

DECT has several useful applications for musculoskeletal imaging. Even though the evidence for some of them is still limited, it is true that DECT can display what conventional CT cannot and which normally requires MR imaging. Virtual monochromatic images are a promising technique to reduce metallic artifacts, and DECT have been embedded in the latest classification criteria for gout. VNCa images have the potential to detect bone marrow lesions and may be applicable to various pathologic conditions other than fracture, which has been its main focus. Iodine maps may become beneficial for evaluating peripheral arthritis with high spatial resolution and quantification of iodine.

REFERENCES

1. Postma AA, Hofman PA, Stadler AA, et al. Dual-energy CT of the brain and intracranial vessels. AJR Am J Roentgenol 2012;199(5 Suppl):S26–33.
2. Kang M-J, Park CM, Lee C-H, et al. Dual-energy CT: clinical applications in various pulmonary diseases. Radiographics 2010;30(3):685–98.
3. Johnson TR. Dual-energy CT: general principles. AJR Am J Roentgenol 2012;199(5 Suppl):S3–8.
4. Marin D, Boll DT, Mileto A, et al. State of the art: dual-energy CT of the abdomen. Radiology 2014;271(2): 327–42.
5. Mallinson PI, Coupal TM, McLaughlin PD, et al. Dual-energy CT for the musculoskeletal system. Radiology 2016;281(3):690–707.
6. Grammatopolous G, Pandit H, Kwon Y-M, et al. Hip resurfacings revised for inflammatory pseudotumour

have a poor outcome. J Bone Joint Surg Br 2009; 91(8):1019–24.

7. Gupta A, Subhas N, Primak AN, et al. Metal artifact reduction: standard and advanced magnetic resonance and computed tomography techniques. Radiol Clin North Am 2015;53(3):531–47.

8. Talbot BS, Weinberg EP. MR imaging with metal-suppression sequences for evaluation of total joint arthroplasty. RadioGraphics 2016;36(1):209–25.

9. Barrett JF, Keat N. Artifacts in CT: recognition and avoidance. RadioGraphics 2004;24(6):1679–91.

10. Wang F, Xue H, Yang X, et al. Reduction of metal artifacts from alloy hip prostheses in computer tomography. J Comput Assist Tomogr 2014;38(6): 828–33.

11. Bamberg F, Dierks A, Nikolaou K, et al. Metal artifact reduction by dual energy computed tomography using monoenergetic extrapolation. Eur Radiol 2011; 21(7):1424–9.

12. Lewis M, Reid K, Toms AP. Reducing the effects of metal artefact using high keV monoenergetic reconstruction of dual energy CT (DECT) in hip replacements. Skeletal Radiol 2013;42(2):275–82.

13. Huang JY, Kerns JR, Nute JL, et al. An evaluation of three commercially available metal artifact reduction methods for CT imaging. Phys Med Biol 2015;60(3): 1047–67.

14. Dong Y, Shi AJ, Wu JL, et al. Metal artifact reduction using virtual monochromatic images for patients with pedicle screws implants on CT. Eur Spine J 2016; 25(6):1754–63.

15. Lee YH, Park KK, Song HT, et al. Metal artefact reduction in gemstone spectral imaging dual-energy CT with and without metal artefact reduction software. Eur Radiol 2012;22(6):1331–40.

16. Cha J, Kim HJ, Kim ST, et al. Dual-energy CT with virtual monochromatic images and metal artifact reduction software for reducing metallic dental artifacts. Acta Radiol 2017;58(11):1312–9.

17. Wellenberg RHH, Donders JCE, Kloen P, et al. Exploring metal artifact reduction using dual-energy CT with pre-metal and post-metal implant cadaver comparison: are implant specific protocols needed? Skeletal Radiol 2018;47(6):839–45.

18. Deutsch AL, Mink JH, Waxman AD. Occult fractures of the proximal femur: MR imaging. Radiology 1989; 170(1):113–6.

19. Ahn JM, El-Khoury GY. Occult fractures of extremities. Radiol Clin North Am 2007;45(3):561–79, ix.

20. Pache G, Bulla S, Baumann T, et al. Dose reduction does not affect detection of bone marrow lesions with dual-energy CT virtual noncalcium technique. Acad Radiol 2012;19(12):1539–45.

21. Pache G, Krauss B, Strohm P, et al. Dual-Energy CT virtual noncalcium technique: detecting posttraumatic bone marrow lesions—feasibility study. Radiology 2010;256(2):617–24.

22. Guggenberger R, Gnannt R, Hodler J, et al. Diagnostic performance of dual-energy ct for the detection of traumatic bone marrow lesions in the ankle: comparison with MR imaging. Radiology 2012; 264(1):164–73.

23. Wang C-K, Tsai J-M, Chuang M-T, et al. Bone marrow edema in vertebral compression fractures: detection with dual-energy CT. Radiology 2013; 269(2):525–33.

24. Bierry G, Venkatasamy A, Kremer S, et al. Dual-energy CT in vertebral compression fractures: performance of visual and quantitative analysis for bone marrow edema demonstration with comparison to MRI. Skeletal Radiol 2014;43(4):485–92.

25. Reddy T, McLaughlin PD, Mallinson PI, et al. Detection of occult, undisplaced hip fractures with a dual-energy CT algorithm targeted to detection of bone marrow edema. Emerg Radiol 2015;22(1):25–9.

26. Karaca L, Yuceler Z, Kantarci M, et al. The feasibility of dual-energy CT in differentiation of vertebral compression fractures. Br J Radiol 2016;89(1057): 20150300.

27. Diekhoff T, Hermann KG, Pumberger M, et al. Dual-energy CT virtual non-calcium technique for detection of bone marrow edema in patients with vertebral fractures: a prospective feasibility study on a single-source volume CT scanner. Eur J Radiol 2017;87:59–65.

28. Petritsch B, Kosmala A, Weng AM, et al. Vertebral compression fractures: third-generation dual-energy CT for detection of bone marrow edema at visual and quantitative analyses. Radiology 2017;284(1): 161–8.

29. Kellock TT, Nicolaou S, Kim SSY, et al. Detection of bone marrow edema in nondisplaced hip fractures: utility of a virtual noncalcium dual-energy CT application. Radiology 2017;284(3):922.

30. Kaup M, Wichmann JL, Scholtz J-E, et al. Dual-energy CT–based display of bone marrow edema in osteoporotic vertebral compression fractures: impact on diagnostic accuracy of radiologists with varying levels of experience in correlation to MR imaging. Radiology 2016;280(2):510–9.

31. Zhang Y, Nevitt M, Niu J, et al. Fluctuation of knee pain and changes in bone marrow lesions, effusions, and synovitis on magnetic resonance imaging. Arthritis Rheum 2011;63(3):691–9.

32. Edwards MH, Parsons C, Bruyère O, et al. High kellgren-lawrence grade and bone marrow lesions predict worsening rates of radiographic joint space narrowing; the SEKOIA study. J Rheumatol 2016; 43(3):657–65.

33. Hayashi D, Roemer FW, Jarraya M, et al. Imaging in osteoarthritis. Radiol Clin North Am 2017;55(5): 1085–102.

34. Hetland ML, Ejbjerg B, Horslev-Petersen K, et al. MRI bone oedema is the strongest predictor of subsequent radiographic progression in early rheumatoid

arthritis. Results from a 2-year randomised controlled trial (CIMESTRA). Ann Rheum Dis 2009;68(3):384–90.

35. Diekhoff T, Scheel M, Hermann S, et al. Osteitis: a retrospective feasibility study comparing single-source dual-energy CT to MRI in selected patients with suspected acute gout. Skeletal Radiol 2017; 46(2):185–90.

36. Thomas C, Schabel C, Krauss B, et al. Dual-energy CT: virtual calcium subtraction for assessment of bone marrow involvement of the spine in multiple myeloma. AJR Am J Roentgenol 2015;204(3): W324–31.

37. Kosmala A, Weng AM, Heidemeier A, et al. Multiple myeloma and dual-energy CT: diagnostic accuracy of virtual noncalcium technique for detection of bone marrow infiltration of the spine and pelvis. Radiology 2018;286(1):205–13.

38. Yang HL, Liu T, Wang XM, et al. Diagnosis of bone metastases: a meta-analysis comparing (1)(8)FDG PET, CT, MRI and bone scintigraphy. Eur Radiol 2011;21(12):2604–17.

39. Gentili A. Advanced imaging of gout. Semin Musculoskelet Radiol 2003;7(03):165–74.

40. Hainer BL, Matheson E, Wilkes RT. Diagnosis, treatment, and prevention of gout. Am Fam Physician 2014;90(12):831–6.

41. Ning TC, Keenan RT. Unusual clinical presentations of gout. Curr Opin Rheumatol 2010;22(2):181–7.

42. Swan A, Amer H, Dieppe P. The value of synovial fluid assays in the diagnosis of joint disease: a literature survey. Ann Rheum Dis 2002;61(6):493–8.

43. Schlesinger N, Norquist JM, Watson DJ. Serum urate during acute gout. J Rheumatol 2009;36(6):1287–9.

44. McQueen FM, Doyle A, Dalbeth N. Imaging in gout– what can we learn from MRI, CT, DECT and US? Arthritis Res Ther 2011;13(6):246.

45. Girish G, Glazebrook KN, Jacobson JA. Advanced imaging in gout. AJR Am J Roentgenol 2013; 201(3):515–25.

46. Thiele RG, Schlesinger N. Diagnosis of gout by ultrasound. Rheumatology (Oxford) 2007;46(7):1116–21.

47. Johnson TR, Weckbach S, Kellner H, et al. Clinical image: dual-energy computed tomographic molecular imaging of gout. Arthritis Rheum 2007;56(8):2809.

48. Desai MA, Peterson JJ, Garner HW, et al. Clinical utility of dual-energy CT for evaluation of tophaceous gout. Radiographics 2011;31(5):1365–75 [discussion: 1376–7].

49. Choi HK, Al-Arfaj AM, Eftekhari A, et al. Dual energy computed tomography in tophaceous gout. Ann Rheum Dis 2009;68(10):1609–12.

50. Glazebrook KN, Guimaraes LS, Murthy NS, et al. Identification of intraarticular and periarticular uric acid crystals with dual-energy CT: initial evaluation. Radiology 2011;261(2):516–24.

51. Nicolaou S, Yong-Hing CJ, Galea-Soler S, et al. Dual-energy CT as a potential new diagnostic tool in the management of gout in the acute setting. AJR Am J Roentgenol 2010;194(4):1072–8.

52. Parikh P, Butendieck R, Kransdorf M, et al. Detection of lumbar facet joint gouty arthritis using dual-energy computed tomography. J Rheumatol 2010; 37(10):2190–1.

53. Dalbeth N, Kalluru R, Aati O, et al. Tendon involvement in the feet of patients with gout: a dual-energy CT study. Ann Rheum Dis 2013;72(9):1545–8.

54. Neogi T, Jansen TL, Dalbeth N, et al. 2015 gout classification criteria: an American College of Rheumatology/ European League against Rheumatism collaborative initiative. Ann Rheum Dis 2015;74(10):1789–98.

55. Choi HK, Burns LC, Shojania K, et al. Dual energy CT in gout: a prospective validation study. Ann Rheum Dis 2012;71(9):1466–71.

56. Schlesinger N. Diagnosis of gout: clinical, laboratory, and radiologic findings. Am J Manag Care 2005;11(15 Suppl):S443–50 [quiz: S465–48].

57. Roddy E, Choi HK. Epidemiology of gout. Rheum Dis Clin North Am 2014;40(2):155–75.

58. Dalbeth N, Nicolaou S, Baumgartner S, et al. Presence of monosodium urate crystal deposition by dual-energy CT in patients with gout treated with allopurinol. Ann Rheum Dis 2017. https://doi.org/ 10.1136/annrheumdis-2017-212046.

59. Heye T, Nelson RC, Ho LM, et al. Dual-energy CT applications in the abdomen. AJR Am J Roentgenol 2012;199(5 Suppl):S64–70.

60. Fukuda T, Umezawa Y, Tojo S, et al. Initial Experience of using dual-energy CT with an iodine overlay image for hand psoriatic arthritis: comparison study with contrast-enhanced MR imaging. Radiology 2017;284(1):134–42.

61. Fukuda T, Umezawa Y, Asahina A, et al. Dual energy CT iodine map for delineating inflammation of inflammatory arthritis. Eur Radiol 2017;27(12):5034–40.

62. Kyburz D, Gabay C, Michel BA, et al. The long-term impact of early treatment of rheumatoid arthritis on radiographic progression: a population-based cohort study. Rheumatology (Oxford) 2011;50(6): 1106–10.

63. Lukas C, Combe B, Ravaud P, et al. Favorable effect of very early disease-modifying antirheumatic drug treatment on radiographic progression in early inflammatory arthritis: data from the Etude et Suivi des polyarthrites indifferenciees recentes (study and followup of early undifferentiated polyarthritis). Arthritis Rheum 2011;63(7):1804–11.

64. Tillett W, Jadon D, Shaddick G, et al. Smoking and delay to diagnosis are associated with poorer functional outcome in psoriatic arthritis. Ann Rheum Dis 2013;72(8):1358–61.

65. Haroon M, Gallagher P, FitzGerald O. Diagnostic delay of more than 6 months contributes to poor radiographic and functional outcome in psoriatic arthritis. Ann Rheum Dis 2015;74(6):1045–50.

66. Colebatch AN, Edwards CJ, Ostergaard M, et al. EULAR recommendations for the use of imaging of the joints in the clinical management of rheumatoid arthritis. Ann Rheum Dis 2013;72(6):804–14.

67. Mandl P, Navarro-Compan V, Terslev L, et al. EULAR recommendations for the use of imaging in the diagnosis and management of spondyloarthritis in clinical practice. Ann Rheum Dis 2015;74(7):1327–39.

68. Kievit W, Adang EM, Fransen J, et al. The effectiveness and medication costs of three anti-tumour necrosis factor alpha agents in the treatment of rheumatoid arthritis from prospective clinical practice data. Ann Rheum Dis 2008;67(9):1229–34.

69. Dohn UM, Ejbjerg BJ, Court-Payen M, et al. Are bone erosions detected by magnetic resonance imaging and ultrasonography true erosions? A comparison with computed tomography in rheumatoid arthritis metacarpophalangeal joints. Arthritis Res Ther 2006;8(4):R110.

70. McGonagle D, Gibbon W, Emery P. Classification of inflammatory arthritis by enthesitis. Lancet 1998; 352(9134):1137–40.

71. Benjamin M, Moriggl B, Brenner E, et al. The "enthesis organ" concept: why enthesopathies may not present as focal insertional disorders. Arthritis Rheum 2004;50(10):3306–13.

72. Chang EY, Chen KC, Huang BK, et al. Adult inflammatory arthritides: what the radiologist should know. Radiographics 2016;36(6):1849–70.

73. Wilson FC, Icen M, Crowson CS, et al. Incidence and clinical predictors of psoriatic arthritis in patients with psoriasis: a population-based study. Arthritis Rheum 2009;61(2):233–9.

74. McGonagle D, Tan AL, Benjamin M. The nail as a musculoskeletal appendage–implications for an improved understanding of the link between psoriasis and arthritis. Dermatology 2009;218(2):97–102.

75. Tan AL, Grainger AJ, Tanner SF, et al. A high-resolution magnetic resonance imaging study of distal interphalangeal joint arthropathy in psoriatic arthritis and osteoarthritis: are they the same? Arthritis Rheum 2006;54(4):1328–33.

76. Asahina A, Fukuda T, Ishiuji Y, et al. Usefulness of dual-energy computed tomography for the evaluation of early-stage psoriatic arthritis only accompanied by nail psoriasis. J Dermatol 2017;44(12): e326–7.

77. Ostergaard M, McQueen F, Wiell C, et al. The OMERACT psoriatic arthritis magnetic resonance imaging scoring system (PsAMRIS): definitions of key pathologies, suggested MRI sequences, and preliminary scoring system for PsA hands. J Rheumatol 2009;36(8):1816–24.

78. Conaghan P, Bird P, Ejbjerg B, et al. The EULAR-OMERACT rheumatoid arthritis MRI reference image atlas: the metacarpophalangeal joints. Ann Rheum Dis 2005;64(Suppl 1). i11–21.

79. Peterfy C, Emery P, Tak PP, et al. MRI assessment of suppression of structural damage in patients with rheumatoid arthritis receiving rituximab: results from the randomised, placebo-controlled, double-blind RA-SCORE study. Ann Rheum Dis 2016; 75(1):170–7.

80. Glinatsi D, Bird P, Gandjbakhch F, et al. Validation of the OMERACT Psoriatic Arthritis Magnetic Resonance Imaging Score (PsAMRIS) for the hand and foot in a randomized placebo-controlled trial. J Rheumatol 2015;42(12):2473–9.

81. Sun C, Miao F, Wang XM, et al. An initial qualitative study of dual-energy CT in the knee ligaments. Surg Radiol Anat 2008;30(5):443–7.

82. Deng K, Sun C, Liu C, et al. Initial experience with visualizing hand and foot tendons by dual-energy computed tomography. Clin Imaging 2009;33(5): 384–9.

83. Fickert S, Niks M, Dinter DJ, et al. Assessment of the diagnostic value of dual-energy CT and MRI in the detection of iatrogenically induced injuries of anterior cruciate ligament in a porcine model. Skeletal Radiol 2013;42(3):411–7.

Percutaneous Minimally Invasive Thermal Ablation of Musculoskeletal Lesions
Usefulness of PET-Computed Tomography

Anderanik Tomasian, MD[a],*, Farrokh Dehdashti, MD[b],
Jack W. Jennings, MD, PhD[b]

KEYWORDS

• PET-CT • FDG • PET-MR • Musculoskeletal metastases • Thermal ablation • Local tumor control
• Pain palliation

KEY POINTS

- Bone is the third most common site of metastatic disease and percutaneous minimally invasive thermal ablation is becoming an important contributor to multidisciplinary treatment algorithms.
- PET-computed tomography scan has an integral role in preablation imaging and postablation follow-up in the musculoskeletal system, especially in the setting of local tumor control.
- Nuclear medicine physicians and radiologists interpreting postablation PET-computed tomography studies must be familiar with expected postablation findings as well as indicators of tumor recurrence/progression.

INTRODUCTION

Bone is the third most common site of metastatic disease; up to 85% of patients with breast, prostate, kidney, and lung cancers are found to have osseous metastases at autopsy.[1] Symptomatic patients most commonly present with pain, which is multifactorial owing to tumor-induced biochemical stimulation of periosteal and endosteal nociceptors, tumor mass effect on surrounding vital structures particularly nerves or spinal cord, or associated pathologic fracture.[1,2] In patients with painful osseous metastases, the goal of therapy is to achieve rapid and durable pain relief.[3] Radiation therapy is the standard of care for pain palliation secondary to metastases, but it has important limitations. First, certain tumor histologies respond variably to radiation therapy, particularly renal cell carcinoma, melanoma, and soft tissue sarcoma.[4–6] Second, radiation therapy may be limited by the cumulative radiation tolerance of nearby radiosensitive organs, such as the spinal cord or bowel. Third, some patients may not respond until 4 to 6 weeks after radiation therapy, which is suboptimal for patients with short life expectancies.[7] Finally, radiation therapy may exclude patients from certain clinical trials. Additionally, painful bone metastases are often refractory to systemic therapies such as chemotherapy, hormonal therapy, radiopharmaceuticals, and bisphosphonates.[8] Surgical intervention, including resection, cementation and internal fixation, and stabilization,

Disclosure Statement: A. Tomasian: Consultant, Medtronic Inc. J.W. Jennings: Consultant, Interventional Oncology Advisory Board, and Speaker Panel: Medtronic and BTG (Galil).
[a] Department of Radiology, University of Southern California, 1500 San Pablo Street, Los Angeles, CA 90095, USA; [b] Mallinckrodt Institute of Radiology, Washington University, 510 South Kingshighway Boulevard, St Louis, MO 63110, USA
* Corresponding author.
E-mail address: tomasianx@yahoo.com

PET Clin 13 (2018) 579–585
https://doi.org/10.1016/j.cpet.2018.05.010

is often of limited benefit in patients with osseous metastases because of its morbidity, patients' often poor functional status, and the short expected life span. These procedures are generally reserved for patients with neurologic compromise or osseous instability. Pain palliation with systemic analgesics remains the only alternative for many patients.[9]

Over the past few years, there has been growth in the use of minimally invasive percutaneous thermal ablation technologies for management of osseous metastases including radiofrequency ablation, cryoablation, microwave ablation, and high-intensity focused ultrasound treatment, which may be performed in an outpatient setting under conscious sedation.[10–19] There is typically rapid recovery and no hindrance or compromise of adjuvant radiation or chemotherapy. Percutaneous thermal ablation for osseous metastases is performed to achieve pain palliation, local tumor control, or both (often with cementation for pathologic fracture stabilization or prevention). In cases of osseous oligometastatic disease (<5 lesions), ablation may be performed with curative intent.[14,16]

PET-computed tomography (CT) scanning provides both anatomic and metabolic information and has an integral role in the minimally invasive percutaneous ablation of bone metastases. This article discusses the role of PET-CT scanning in percutaneous minimally invasive ablation of osseous metastases including diagnosis and preprocedural factors related to patient selection and procedure planning, intraprocedural imaging guidance, and posttreatment imaging assessment.

PREPROCEDURAL PET-COMPUTED TOMOGRAPHY SCANS

PET-CT scanning, along with MRI and routine CT scans, plays an important role in the initial diagnosis and staging of primary bone tumors and osseous metastases. In clinical practice, [18F]-fluoro-2-deoxy-D-glucose (FDG) is the most commonly used radiopharmaceutical for the PET-CT evaluation of osseous metastases. The expanding list of PET radiopharmaceuticals with the potential to target specific tumor types or specific biological characteristics of the tumors supports growing applications of PET-CT scanning and PET-MRI for preablation assessment of musculoskeletal lesions[20–22] (Fig. 1). Such radiopharmaceuticals include 18F- or 11C-acetate, 18F- or 11C-choline, and 18F-sodium fluoride.[20–22] The major advantages of PET-CT scans and PET-MRI include the ability to detect tumors that are occult on conventional anatomic cross-sectional

imaging and to identify metabolically active portions of tumors. This factor is particularly useful for the detection of tumor recurrence after ablation or other therapies to plan subsequent percutaneous ablation.[23]

Preablation PET-CT scanning provides information for preprocedural planning to support accurate placement of ablation probes, electrodes, or antennae to safely achieve the therapeutic goal. When treating with palliative intent, ablation of all bone–tumor and soft tissue–tumor interfaces is sufficient. However, to achieve local tumor control, the ablation zone must completely envelope the gross tumor volume plus an ablative margin of at least 5 mm.[24] In addition, preprocedural PET-CT scanning is important for the choice of ablation technology. For example, cryoablation is favored for osteoblastic lesions or larger bone tumors with soft tissue components and complex geometries, because multiple cryoprobes can be strategically arranged to produce a contiguous ice ball with a tailored configuration.[12,16] Radiofrequency ablation is favored for vertebral body osteolytic or mixed lesions as well as challenging-to-reach anatomic locations, such as the posterior vertebral body, where navigating tip of recently introduced electrodes can be articulated in different orientations through the same osseous access site.[25] Microwave ablation is most commonly used for musculoskeletal lesions where the surrounding vital structures are reasonably distant from the planned ablation zone.[25] Furthermore, when the planned ablation zone is in close proximity to structures at risk for ablation-induced injury, such as the spinal cord, spinal nerve roots, peripheral nerves, skin, and vital torso soft tissues including the bowel, precise assessment of the surrounding structures on preablation PET-CT scans helps the operator to develop appropriate passive and active thermal protection strategies to prevent undesired thermal injuries.

INTRAPROCEDURAL PET-COMPUTED TOMOGRAPHY SCANS

Investigators have successfully used PET-CT scans for percutaneous interventions, including needle biopsies and thermal ablations.[26–28] A variety of techniques have been described to incorporate PET imaging into intraprocedural guidance, including the fusion of PET images obtained at the beginning of the procedure with CT images obtained intermittently during the procedure, fusion of intraprocedural CT images with preablation PET, and direct use of PET images for needle guidance.[26–28] Fusion of CT and PET

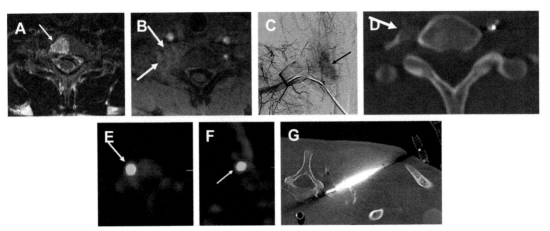

Fig. 1. A 15-year-old boy with neck pain for 3 months. The case demonstrates the usefulness of PET-computed tomography (CT) scanning to accurately identify a benign and treatable lesion. Axial T2-weighted MRI (*A*) and axial T1-weighted fat-saturated contrast-enhanced MRI (*B*) images obtained at slightly different levels show T2 hyperintensity and enhancement within the right C7 vertebral body and right superior articular process of C7 and extending to surrounding soft tissues (*A* and *B*, *arrows*). The MRI interpretation favored sarcoma. Conventional angiography (*C*) shows tumor blush (*C*, *arrow*). Based on clinical symptoms, osteoid osteoma was suspected and F18 sodium fluoride PET-CT scanning was performed. An axial CT image (*D*) shows a partly mineralized nidus within the right superior articular process of C7 (*D*, *arrow*) with focal, intense radiopharmaceutical uptake on PET-CT scanning confined to the lesion (*E* and *F*, *arrows*), most compatible with an osteoid osteoma. Prone axial CT image during radiofrequency ablation (*G*) shows placement of a radiofrequency ablation electrode within the nidus of the biopsy-proven osteoid osteoma with slight posterior articulation of the tip for optimal positioning.

images may be performed using visual or software co-registration, which can be combined with electromagnetic needle tracking.[29] In addition, split dose periprocedural PET/CT scanning has been performed to determine ablation adequacy.[30] In this technique, 4 mCi of FDG was administered before the procedure for localization and imaging guidance. At completion of the ablation, an additional 8 mCi of FDG was administered to assess ablation adequacy. Investigators reported that there was no evidence of viable tumor in 97% of cases.[30]

Furthermore, anatomic data provided by the CT component of a PET-CT scan allows for the accurate implementation of thermoprotective techniques, such as the precise placement of needles in close proximity to vital structures, such as nerves, spinal cord, and vital soft tissues of the torso such as the bladder and bowel, to inject carbon dioxide or cool/warm fluid for pneumodissection or hydrodissection, respectively.

POSTPROCEDURAL PET-COMPUTED TOMOGRAPHY SCANS

The vast majority of the literature to date addresses postablation PET-CT evaluation in nonmusculoskeletal tumors. Postablation PET-CT scanning has been used to evaluate treatment

adequacy, local tumor recurrence, and progression of musculoskeletal metastatic disease.[31]

Our practice is to perform a baseline study, most commonly MRI, 6 to 8 weeks after treatment to allow postablation inflammation to subside. However, in many cases standard of care PET-CT scanning is requested by the oncologists to evaluate systemic response, at which time evaluation of the ablated lesion can be performed. Subsequent imaging is obtained at the discretion of the treating medical or surgical oncologist to assess for local tumor control or when the patient complains of new or increasing pain at the site of ablation. Histopathologically, ablation creates a cavity of coagulation necrosis surrounded by an inner rim of hemorrhagic congestion and outer rim of granulation tissue.[32] Over time, the rim of granulation tissue evolves into vascular fibrosis.[33] Widely used methods for assessing treatment response, such as the Response Evaluation Criteria in Solid Tumors[34] and World Health Organization Handbook for Reporting Results of Cancer Treatment,[35] are not applicable to ablative therapies because these methods are based on maximum dimensional measurements that do not account for tumor necrosis. Therefore, treatment adequacy is mainly assessed by correlating the volume of the nonenhancing ablation cavity with tumor volume on pretreatment imaging, which demonstrates photopenia on PET-CT scans corresponding with tissue necrosis[25,31] (**Fig. 2**). During the early postablation period, and for up to 8 to 12 weeks after ablation, the metabolism within the inner rim of hemorrhagic congestion surrounding the ablation cavity is unaltered and normal radiopharmaceutical (FDG) uptake manifests as a thin rim of uniform low-grade uptake, which should not be mistaken for residual tumor.[25,31] It should be recognized that the outer rim of granulation tissue surrounding the ablation cavity often evolves into vascular fibrosis over time and may demonstrate variable degrees of both peripheral enhancement and increased FDG uptake.[36] Furthermore, vascular fibrosis can evolve for years after ablation, mimicking tumor progression.[25,37] In such cases, PET-CT may help to differentiate FDG-avid tumor from vascular fibrosis, which should not have increased FDG uptake (**Fig. 2**). As a PET-CT criterion for assessment of tumor recurrence or progression after percutaneous ablation in musculoskeletal system (**Fig. 3**), Packard and colleagues[31] have described the ratio of tumor maximum standardized uptake value to blood pool tumor maximum standardized uptake value using both ^{11}C-choline and ^{18}F-FDG, and demonstrated that the tumor maximum standardized uptake value ratio to be significantly higher in patients with tumor progression or recurrence.

When evaluating for local tumor recurrence or progression on postablation PET-CT scans, particular attention should be paid to the margins of the ablation zone located in close proximity to vital structure such the spinal cord, nerve roots, or peripheral nerves, where the risk of nerve injury often precludes aggressive ablation. Ultimately, when clinical findings do not corroborate imaging findings of tumor progression, biopsy is recommended before initiation of further radiation therapy, surgery, or a change in systemic chemotherapy. Additionally, in the setting of oligometastatic disease, where only a few lesions demonstrate progressive growth or metabolic hyperactivity on PET-CT scans while undergoing systemic therapy, local ablative therapies may be used for local tumor control.

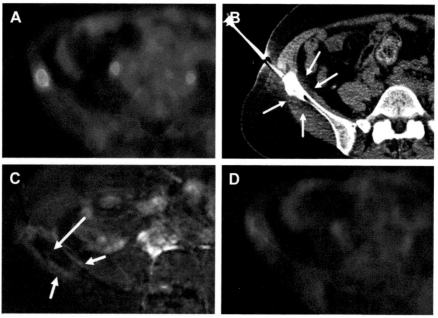

Fig. 2. A 61-year-old woman with oligometastatic breast cancer and enlarging painful right iliac lesion. Cryoablation was performed for pain palliation and local tumor control. Axial PET-computed tomography (CT) scan with fludeoxyglucose F 18 (FDG) image (*A*) shows a hypermetabolic metastatic lesion in the anterior right iliac bone. Axial CT image during cryoablation (*B*) shows 1 of the 2 cryoprobes placed within the lesion in a coaxial fashion with the hypoattenuating ice ball (*B, arrows*) encompassing the lesion and extending to surrounding musculature and adipose tissues. Axial T1-weighted contrast-enhanced MRI obtained 2 months after cryoablation (*C*) shows nonenhancing ablation cavity (*C, long white arrow*) with primarily thin peripheral enhancement (*C, short white arrows*). There is thick nodular enhancement along the anterior margin of the ablation cavity (*C, black arrow*) that was favored to reflect granulation tissue and vascular fibrosis. However, tumor recurrence remained a possibility. Axial FDG PET-CT image obtained 4 months after cryoablation (*D*), shows no evidence of residual or recurrent tumor with mild FDG uptake along the peripheral inflammatory zone (granulation tissue and vascular fibrosis), corresponding with the MRI findings.

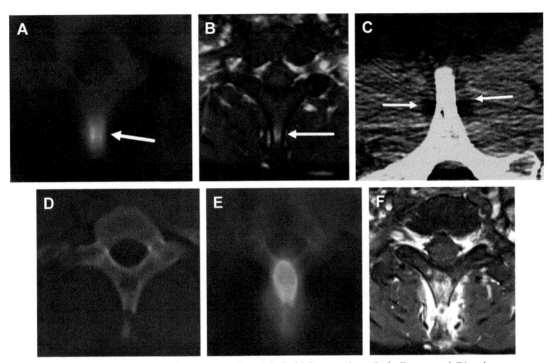

Fig. 3. A 22-year-old man with oligometastatic epithelioid hemangioendothelioma and T1 spinous process lesion. Cryoablation was performed for local tumor control. Axial PET-computed tomography (CT) scan with flu-deoxyglucose F 18 (FDG) (A) and axial T1-weighted fat-saturated contrast-enhanced MRI (B) show a hypermet-abolic enhancing T1 spinous process lesion (A and B, arrow). Prone axial CT scanning immediately after cryoablation (C) shows hypo-attenuating ice ball encompassing the lesion and extending to surrounding soft tissues (C, arrows). Axial CT (D), FDG PET-CT (E), and T1-weighted fat-saturated contrast-enhanced MRI (F) studies obtained 2 months after cryoablation show development of osteolytic hypermetabolic enhancing lesion extending from the anterior margin of the previously treated tumor to the spinolaminar junction, compatible with local tumor progression/recurrence.

LIMITATIONS OF PET-COMPUTED TOMOGRAPHY SCANS

The main limitation of PET-CT scans includes diminished sensitivity to detect tumor with decreasing metabolic activity and lesion size (particularly when <5 mm) owing to spatial resolu-tion of PET.[38] In addition, when superimposed infection is clinically suspected, PET-CT scans should be interpreted with caution.

FUTURE DIRECTIONS

The development of combined PET-MRI over the past several years has several clinical implications for percutaneous thermal ablation. The superior tissue contrast resolution of MRI compared with CT evaluation may result in increased sensitivity for tumor detection and improved accuracy for cancer staging. In addition, the technology allows for possible combined PET-MRI guidance during ablation procedures for the purpose of lesion tar-geting with MRI-compatible ablation probes (eg, cryoablation). Furthermore, after ablation, the combined imaging modalities could allow for earlier diagnosis and treatment of residual and recurrent tumor.[22]

SUMMARY

The combination of anatomic and metabolic data afforded by PET-CT imaging has proved instru-mental in interventional oncology for minimally invasive percutaneous tumor thermal ablation of musculoskeletal lesions.

REFERENCES

1. Mundy GR. Metastasis to bone: causes, conse-quences and therapeutic opportunities. Nat Rev Cancer 2002;2:584–93.
2. Urch C. The pathophysiology of cancer-induced bone pain: current understanding. Palliat Med 2004;18:267–74.
3. Wallace AN, Robinson CG, Meyer J, et al. The met-astatic spine disease multidisciplinary working group algorithms. Oncologist 2015;20:1205–15.

4. Deschavanne PJ, Fertil B. A review of human cell radiosensitivity in vitro. Int J Radiat Oncol Biol Phys 1996;34:251–66.

5. Rofstad EK. Radiation biology of malignant melanoma. Acta Radiol Oncol 1986;25:1–10.

6. Strander H, Turesson I, Cavallin-Stahl E. A systematic overview of radiation therapy effects in soft tissue sarcomas. Acta Oncol 2003;42:516–31.

7. van der Linden YM, Steenland E, van Houwelingen HC, et al. Patients with a favourable prognosis are equally palliated with single and multiple fraction radiotherapy: results on survival in the Dutch bone metastasis study. Radiother Oncol 2006;78:245–53.

8. Rosenthal D, Callstrom MR. Critical review and state of the art in interventional oncology: benign and metastatic disease involving bone. Radiology 2012;262: 765–80.

9. Hara S. Opioids for metastatic bone pain. Oncology 2008;74(suppl 1):52–4.

10. Dupuy DE, Liu D, Hartfeil D, et al. Percutaneous radiofrequency ablation of painful osseous metastases: a multicenter American College of Radiology Imaging Network trial. Cancer 2010;116:989–97.

11. Goetz MP, Callstrom MR, Charboneau JW, et al. Percutaneous image-guided radiofrequency ablation of painful metastases involving bone: a multicenter study. J Clin Oncol 2004;22:300–6.

12. Tomasian A, Wallace A, Northrup B, et al. Spine cryoablation: pain palliation and local tumor control for vertebral metastases. AJNR Am J Neuroradiol 2016;37(1):189–95.

13. Callstrom MR, Dupuy DE, Solomon SB, et al. Percutaneous image guided cryoablation of painful metastases involving bone: multicenter trial. Cancer 2013;119:1033–41.

14. McMenomy BP, Kurup AN, Johnson GB, et al. Percutaneous cryoablation of musculoskeletal oligometastatic disease for complete remission. J Vasc Interv Radiol 2013;24:207–13.

15. Prologo JD, Passalacqua M, Patel I, et al. Image-guided cryoablation for the treatment of painful musculoskeletal metastatic disease: a single-center experience. Skeletal Radiol 2014;43:1551–9.

16. Wallace AN, McWilliams SR, Connolly SE, et al. Percutaneous image-guided cryoablation of musculoskeletal metastases: pain palliation and local tumor control. J Vasc Interv Radiol 2016;27:1788–96.

17. Kastler A, Alnassan H, Aubry S, et al. Microwave thermal ablation of spinal metastatic bone tumors. J Vasc Interv Radiol 2014;25:1470–5.

18. Napoli A, Anzidei M, Marincola BC, et al. MR imaging-guided focused ultrasound for treatment of bone metastasis. Radiographics 2013;33(6):1555–68.

19. Napoli A, Anzidei M, Marincola BC, et al. Primary pain palliation and local tumor control in bone metastases treated with magnetic resonance-guided focused ultrasound. Invest Radiol 2013;48(6):351–8.

20. Nanni C, Fantini L, Nicolini S, et al. Non-FDG PET. Clin Radiol 2010;65:536e48.

21. Jadvar H. Prostate cancer: PET with 18F-FDG, 18F- or 11C-acetate, and 18F- or 11C-choline. J Nucl Med 2011;52:81–9.

22. Pichler BJ, Kolb A, Nägele T, et al. PET/MRI: paving the way for the next generation of clinical multimodality imaging applications. J Nucl Med 2010; 51(3):333–6.

23. Gallamini A, Zwarthoed C, Borra A. Positron emission tomography (PET) in oncology. Cancers (Basel) 2014;6:1821–89.

24. Wang X, Sofocleous CT, Erinjeri JP, et al. Margin size is an independent predictor of local tumor progression after ablation of colon cancer liver metastases. Cardiovasc Intervent Radiol 2013;36:166–75.

25. Tomasian A, Gangi A, Wallace AN, et al. Percutaneous thermal ablation of spinal metastases: recent advances and review. AJR Am J Roentgenol 2018; 210(1):142–52.

26. Cazzato RL, Garnon J, Shaygi B, et al. PET/CT-guided interventions: indications, advantages, disadvantages and the state of the art. Minim Invasive Ther Allied Technol 2017;23:1–6.

27. McLoney ED, Isaacson AJ, Keating P. The role of PET imaging before, during, and after percutaneous hepatic and pulmonary tumor ablation. Semin Intervent Radiol 2014;31(2):187–92.

28. El-Haddad G. PET-based percutaneous needle biopsy. PET Clin 2016;11(3):333–49.

29. Venkatesan AM, Kadoury S, Abi-Jaoudeh N, et al. Real-time FDG PET guidance during biopsies and radiofrequency ablation using multimodality fusion with electromagnetic navigation. Radiology 2011; 260(3):848–56.

30. Ryan ER, Sofocleous CT, Schöder H, et al. Split-dose technique for FDG PET/CT-guided percutaneous ablation: a method to facilitate lesion targeting and to provide immediate assessment of treatment effectiveness. Radiology 2013;268(1): 288–95.

31. Packard AT, Broski SM, Callstrom MR, et al. Utility of PET/CT after cryoablation for early identification of local tumor progression in osseous metastatic disease. AJR Am J Roentgenol 2017;208(6):1342–51.

32. Wallace AN, Hillen TJ, Friedman MV, et al. Percutaneous spinal ablation in a sheep model: protective capacity of an intact cortex, correlation of ablation parameters with ablation zone size, and correlation of postablation MRI and pathologic findings. AJNR Am J Neuroradiol 2017;38(8):1653–9.

33. Sainani NI, Gervais DA, Mueller PR, et al. Imaging after percutaneous radiofrequency ablation of hepatic tumors. Part 1. Normal findings. AJR Am J Roentgenol 2013;200:184–93.

34. Eisenhauer EA, Therasse P, Bogaerts J, et al. New response evaluation criteria in solid tumours: revised

RECIST guideline (version 1.1). Eur J Cancer 2009; 45:228–47.

35. World Health Organization. WHO handbook for reporting results of cancer treatment. WHO offset publication no. 48. Geneva (Switzerland): World Health Organization; 1979.

36. Vogt FM, Antoch G, Veit P, et al. Morphologic and functional changes in nontumorous liver tissue after radiofrequency ablation in an in vivo model: comparison of 18F-FDG PET/CT, MRI, ultrasound, and CT. J Nucl Med 2007;48(11):1836–44.

37. Al-Omair A, Smith R, Kiehl T, et al. Radiation-induced vertebral compression fracture following spine stereotactic radiosurgery: clinicopathological correlation. J Neurosurg Spine 2012;16:379–86.

38. Schmidt GP, Haug AR, Schoenberg SO, et al. Whole body MRI and PET-CT in the management of cancer patients. Eur Radiol 2006;16(6):1216–25.

Musculoskeletal Pitfalls on Fluorodeoxyglucose F 18 PET-Computed Tomography
Pictorial Review

Mariet Asadoorian, MD[a],*, George R. Matcuk Jr, MD[a],
Dakshesh B. Patel, MD[a], Anderanik Tomasian, MD[a],
Heidi R. Wassef, MD[a], Eric A. White, MD[a]

KEYWORDS

- PET-CT pitfalls • Musculoskeletal radiology • ^{18}F-FDG PET-CT • False positives
- Musculoskeletal lesions

KEY POINTS

- Cancer cells commonly demonstrate increased uptake on PET. However, increased fluorodeoxyglucose (FDG) uptake is nonspecific and does not equate to cancer.
- Several musculoskeletal entities including reactive, benign neoplastic, inflammatory, traumatic, posttreatment, and degenerative may demonstrate increased FDG uptake and mimic malignancy.
- Prior familiarity with these pitfalls as well as use of tools such as the unfused computed tomography (CT) portion of the PET-CT including the bone windows, multiple imaging planes, the nonattenuation-corrected PET images, radiographs, and the clinical picture are useful in avoiding these pitfalls.

INTRODUCTION

PET-computed tomography with fluorodeoxyglucose F 18 (^{18}F-FDG PET-CT) is a common practice in diagnosis, staging, and monitoring therapy in oncologic conditions, especially evaluation for metastases. FDG is a glucose analogue that is taken up by cell membrane glucose transporters and transported into the cells. After phosphorylation by hexokinase, the molecule is trapped in the cell as it cannot undergo glycolysis.[1] The accumulated intracellular glucose analogue is detected on PET and correlates with the metabolic activity.

Cancer cells commonly demonstrate increased uptake on PET; however, increased FDG uptake is nonspecific and does not always indicate malignancy. In traumatic and inflammatory conditions, there is an increase in expression of the cell membrane glucose transporters in macrophages, leading to increased FDG uptake in these conditions.[2] Similarly, in cases of malignant tumors, there is increased FDG uptake secondary to increased glucose transporters in the cancer cells, as well as surrounding inflammatory cells and granulation tissue,[3] leading to increased activity on PET. In

Presented at the *Annual RSNA Meeting 2016*, Chicago, IL. Exhibit Space #: MK184-ED-WEB7.
This study had no financial support and the authors have nothing to disclose.
[a] Department of Radiology, Keck School of Medicine, University of Southern California, 1500 San Pablo Street, 2nd Floor Imaging, Los Angeles, CA 90033-5313, USA
* Corresponding author. Department of Radiology, University of Southern California, 1200 North State Street, D&T 3D321, Los Angeles, CA 90033.
E-mail address: masadoor2012@gmail.com

PET Clin 13 (2018) 587–607
https://doi.org/10.1016/j.cpet.2018.06.001

pet.theclinics.com

this article, the authors present multiple cases of benign musculoskeletal conditions, including benign tumors that can demonstrate increased FDG uptake and may be misinterpreted as malignancy. Ways to avoid these pitfalls will also be discussed.

Arthropathies and Degenerative Disease

Synovitis in rheumatoid arthritis

Inflammatory arthropathies, such as rheumatoid arthritis, demonstrate increased FDG uptake during the active phase of disease (**Fig. 1**). It has been shown that PET can assess the metabolic activity of synovitis and measure disease activity in rheumatoid arthritis. In a study, assessing rheumatoid arthritis with ultrasound and PET, it was found that the maximum standardized uptake value (SUVmax) was significantly higher in joints demonstrating synovial thickening and power Doppler signal on ultrasound. Significantly higher SUVmax was also noted in clinically active cases with swollen and tender joints and cases with higher erythrocyte sedimentation rate and serum

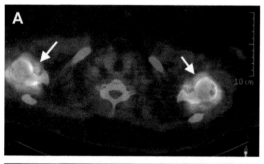

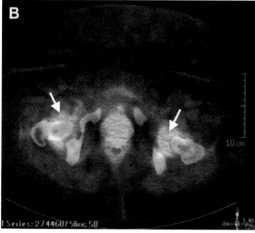

Fig. 1. A 65-year-old woman with rheumatoid arthritis. (*A, B*) Axial fused 18F-FDG PET/CT reconstructions at the level of the glenohumeral (*A*) and hip (*B*) joints show increased FDG uptake (*arrows*), representing active synovitis.

C-reactive protein levels. The study findings suggested that FDG-PET could be used in assessment of disease activity in patients with inflammatory arthropathies.[4] This may be explained by the leukocyte infiltrate and synovial membrane proliferation and neovascularization giving rise to synovial hypertrophy and pannus characteristic of rheumatoid arthritis, which is responsible for cartilage degradation, marginal erosions, and joint space narrowing.[4] In addition, other studies have documented correlative findings on contrast-enhanced MRI and PET for rheumatoid arthritis. Response to treatment can be monitored and comparison of drug efficacy can be made by contrast-enhanced MRI as well as PET by quantification of joint inflammation.[5]

Facet joint osteoarthritis and active osteophyte

Osteoarthritis may or may not be associated with increased FDG uptake depending on the presence or absence of active synovitis.[6] It has been found that abnormally increased FDG uptake has been seen in 22% of spine degenerative diseases. Osteophytes and facet arthropathy can give rise to increased FDG uptake (**Figs. 2** and **3**). In the spine, they can mimic metastases. Because the spine is a common site for skeletal metastases as well as degenerative disease, the CT portion of PET-CT is crucial in differentiating a metastatic lesion from degenerative disease because they are typically located at different sites and have different morphology. It is worth mentioning that there is weak correlation between the severity of degenerative disease involving the spine on CT and the severity of FDG uptake, which is likely related to the stage of disease and presence of inflammation. CT shows the end morphologic result of prior inflammation, and as such, FDG uptake may be minimal in a patient with severe degenerative changes on CT because inflammation may have already subsided by the time severe morphologic abnormalities have resulted.[7]

Baastrup syndrome

Also known as kissing spine syndrome, Baastrup syndrome (or disease) is a benign condition that can be a cause of low back pain on extension, which is relieved by flexion, and can be treated by local anesthetic/steroid injection or excision of the involved spinous processes.[8] It commonly affects the lumbar spine and is characterized by close approximation of adjacent spinous processes with reactive sclerosis and inflammation.[9] Baastrup disease can demonstrate increased FDG uptake between the spinous processes (**Fig. 4**), and knowledge of the PET-CT appearance of this condition is important to avoid misdiagnosis

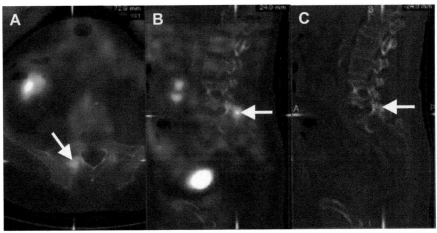

Fig. 2. A 74-year-old man with prostate carcinoma demonstrating facet arthropathy. (*A–C*) Axial (*A*) and sagittal (*B*) fused 18F-FDG PET/CT reconstructions and sagittal CT reformation (*C*) show joint space narrowing and osteophyte formation (*arrows*).

as a malignant condition. The characteristic CT appearance of enlargement, sclerosis, and flattening of the spinous processes is helpful in diagnosis.[10] The location of metastatic disease is typically different than the distribution of findings demonstrated in Basstrup syndrome, with metastases commonly involving the body and pedicle of the vertebral bodies. In addition, PET can be helpful in pinpointing the site of inflammation where steroid and anesthetic injection can be performed to treat Basstrup syndrome–related pain, especially with multilevel vertebral involvement.[9]

Traumatic Pathologies

Fractures

Fractures can mimic osseous metastases, as both can present as foci of increased FDG uptake on PET-CT (**Fig. 5**). An additional level of challenge is added because fused PET-CT images can obscure details of osseous anatomy. This pitfall can be avoided by evaluating the bones on bone windows of unfused CT images. An additional level of complexity is added when attempting to differentiate between fractures of benign and malignant cause. In a study evaluating 34 fractures, it was shown that higher FDG uptake was noted in malignant fractures compared with fractures of benign cause, with an SUVmax of 12 compared with 2.9 in malignant versus benign fractures, respectively.[11] In addition, the timing of fracture onset can be helpful in evaluation of fractures. In a retrospective study of 1517 consecutive patients who underwent whole-body FDG-PET, it was shown that FDG uptake was normalized within 3 months of fracture incident unless the process

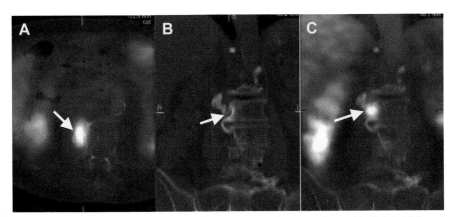

Fig. 3. 72-year-old man with history of lymphoma showing an active osteophyte. (*A–C*) Axial (*A*) and coronal (*C*) CT fused 18F-FDG PET/CT reconstruction and coronal CT (*B*) images show multilevel degenerative disc disease, with a prominent osteophyte (*arrows*) extending adjacent to the L2 vertebral body.

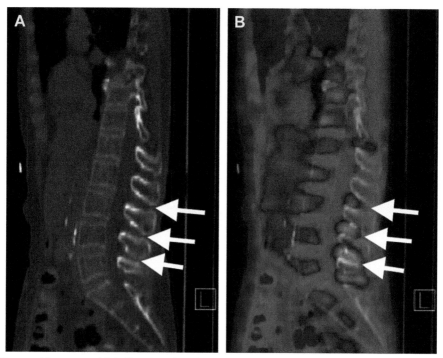

Fig. 4. A 59-year-old woman with infiltrating ductal carcinoma of the breast demonstrating Baastrup disease. (*A, B*) Sagittal CT (*A*) and fused 18F-FDG PET/CT (*B*) reconstructions show close approximation between the spinous processes from L2 to L5, with corresponding intense activity (*arrows*).

was complicated by infection or malignancy.[12] As such, follow-up PET-CT can be helpful, because uptake associated with simple fractures is expected to normalize within 3 months. In addition to FDG-PET, PET-CT with sodium fluoride F 18 (^{18}F-NaF PET-CT), which is used for evaluation of metastatic bone disease, has also been found useful in detection of fractures. In contrast to FDG, where the uptake reflects lesion metabolic activity, ^{18}F-NaF is a bone-specific agent, the uptake of which reflects increased blood flow and underlying osteoblastic activity in response to osteoclastic activity and bone destruction.[13] In a study involving a pediatric population, the sensitivity for fractures was found to be 85% using ^{18}F-NaF PET.[14]

Sacral insufficiency fractures

Sacral insufficiency fractures are a type of stress fracture. These insufficiency fractures are

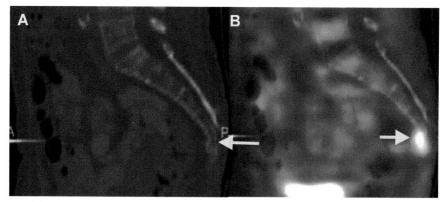

Fig. 5. 56-year-old woman with history of breast cancer and a fall, showing a coccyx fracture. (*A, B*) Sagittal CT (*A*) and 18F-FDG PET/CT (*B*) reconstructions showing a coccygeal fracture with corresponding intense activity (*arrows*).

common in patients with cancer after chemotherapy and radiation therapy. Radiation can result in damage to osteoblasts, resulting in osteopenia. Combined with radiation-induced vascular injury, the ultimate result is structural weakness of the bone, which is susceptible to fracture following a normal or physiologic stress.[15] The typical pattern of bilateral fracture on bone scintigraphy is the Honda sign in the sacrum. As with bone scintigraphy, increased FDG uptake can be seen on PET-CT at the region corresponding to the Honda sign (**Fig. 6**). The SUVmax for this type of fracture has been reported to range from 2.2 to 8.9,[16–18] with the latter case (SUVmax of 8.9) being an acute fracture. However, the specific location and pattern of FDG uptake along with CT findings seems to be more helpful than the SUVmax value. These fractures are most easily visualized on the bone windows of unfused CT, in the coronal plane, as linear lucent lines in the sacral ala medial to the sacroiliac joints. Other characteristic pelvic insufficiency fractures can involve the pubic rami and supraacetabular iliac bones.[19] If MRI is available, fracture lines are detected as hypointense lines on T1 and T2, with areas of adjacent T2 hyperintensity representing edema adjacent to acute fractures.[20]

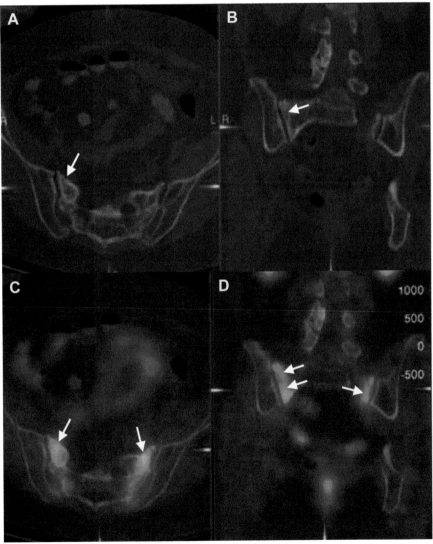

Fig. 6. An 81-year-old woman with monoclonal gammopathy demonstrating insufficiency fractures of the sacral alae. (*A, B*) Axial and coronal CT images show sclerosis and a subtle lucent fracture line (*arrows*). (*C, D*) Axial and coronal fused 18F-FDG PET/CT reconstructions show avidity (*arrows*) in these locations.

Shoulder dislocation

In the setting of shoulder dislocation, PET may show increased FDG uptake (**Fig. 7**) in the areas corresponding to bone marrow contusion on MRI because inflammation is often intensely FDG avid, which can be mistaken for malignancy.[21,22] For example, in posterior shoulder dislocation, anteromedial humeral head contusion with increased signal on fluid sensitive sequences on MRI and corresponding increased FDG uptake on PET can be seen. On the unfused CT images, a reverse Hill-Sachs impaction fracture and a reverse Bankart lesion can be seen. In the case of anterior shoulder dislocation, impaction and edema at the posterosuperior humeral head (Hill-Sachs lesions) and the anteroinferior glenoid (osseous Bankart lesions) may be noted. Findings on CT as well as clinical history of shoulder dislocation are helpful in avoiding misdiagnosis for a malignant process.

Benign Tumors and Tumorlike Processes of Bone

Enchondroma

It has been found that FDG uptake is generally higher in malignant primary bone tumors than benign ones. This is more reliable if tumors of the same histologic type are compared, for example, cartilaginous tumors.[23,24] This may not be true if tumors of different lineages are compared.

For example, benign giant cell tumors may show high FDG uptake and may demonstrate higher metabolic activity than malignant chondrosarcomas.[25]

In general for primary bone tumors, the morphologic characteristics of the tumor on radiographs and the CT portion of PET-CT are very important for deciding whether the tumor is benign or malignant, and the metabolic activity on PET should not be the only deciding factor. Some of the most metabolically active benign bone tumors and tumorlike conditions include giant cell tumor of bone, giant cell reparative granuloma, chondroblastoma, osteoblastoma, osteoid osteoma, Langerhans cell histiocytosis, chondromyxoid fibroma, brown tumor, fibrous dysplasia, nonossifying fibroma, desmoplastic fibroma, and aneurysmal bone cyst.[26] Containing a high number of multinucleated giant cells is associated with highly metabolically active bone tumors.[25]

Approximately less than 1% of enchondromas undergo malignant transformation into chondrosarcoma (**Fig. 8**). In a prospective study of 36 patients with long bone enchondromas and chondrosarcomas, the lesions with an SUVmax less than 2 were followed-up and those with SUVmax greater than 2 underwent surgery. Sixteen of the 17 lesions with SUVmax less than 2 were found to be enchondromas and 1 was found to be chondrosarcoma. On review, the 1 chondrosarcoma actually had an SUVmax of 2.18. Nineteen lesions

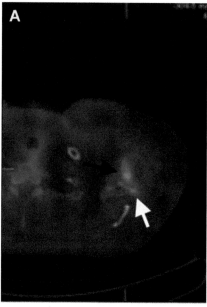
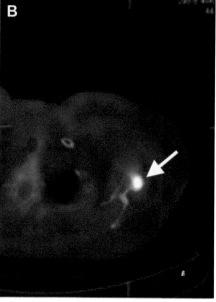

Fig. 7. A 41-year-old man with recent posterior dislocation of the glenohumeral joint status postreduction. Axial fused 18F-FDG PET/CT reconstructions at the level of the superior glenoid (*A*) and inferior glenoid (*B*) show a reverse Hill-Sachs defect (*black arrow*) as well as activity within the posterior glenoid (*white arrows*) areas, which correspond to bone marrow contusion (typically identified on MRI).

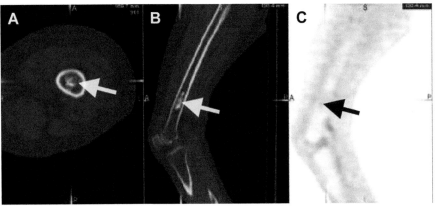

Fig. 8. 52-year-old woman referred for evaluation of a lesion in the distal femur, showing an enchondroma. (*A*) Axial and (*B*) sagittal CT, as well as (*C*) sagittal PET images show flocculant matrix mineralization (*white arrows*) within the central medullary region of the distal femur, with very low activity (*black arrow*) (SUVmax = 0.8). No endosteal scalloping or cortical destruction is present.

with SUVmax greater than 2 were found to be chondrosarcomas and only 1 was found to be an enchondroma.[27]

Pigmented villonodular synovitis

Pigmented villonodular synovitis (PVNS) is a benign intraarticular proliferative disease. As a tumor with abundant giant cells, PVNS as well as its extraarticular counterpart, the giant cell tumor of tendon sheath (tenosynovial giant cell tumor), demonstrate FDG avidity on PET[25] (**Fig. 9**) and hence can be mistaken for malignancy. Markedly elevated SUVmax values have been reported in the literature, up to values as high as 16.[28] The most commonly affected joint by PVNS is the knee. The involvement may range from a focal nodular mass to diffuse proliferation of the entire synovium. On MRI, a joint effusion with masslike lobulated synovial proliferation with lobulated margins can be seen, which may extend through

capsular defects along ligaments. In most cases, PVNS demonstrates low-signal intensity on T1 and T2 throughout the lesion due to the presence of hemosiderin. Gradient echo sequence may show blooming artifact. Postcontrast images demonstrate moderate to intense inhomogeneous enhancement.[29] On CT, the synovial proliferation seems as soft tissue mass and can be hyperdense to muscle if containing hemosiderin. Postcontrast behavior is similar to that of MRI. The intraarticular location of the lesion as well as the characteristic MRI appearance of PVNS helps in avoiding misinterpreting the lesion as a malignancy.

Heterotopic ossification

Previously referred to as myositis ossificans, heterotopic ossification is formation of bone outside of the skeletal system, which may include the skin, subcutaneous tissue, skeletal muscle,

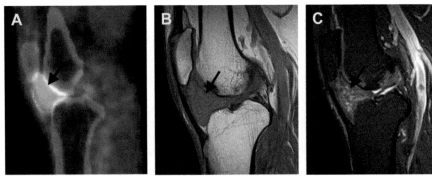

Fig. 9. A 59-year-old man with pathology-proven PVNS. (*A*) Sagittal fused 18F-FDG PET/CT reconstruction showing an intraarticular lesion in the region of the Hoffa fat pad (*arrows*) with intense FDG avidity (SUVmax = 16). (*B*) Sagittal proton density (PD) and (*C*) proton density-fat saturated (PD-FS) images showing the intraarticular lesion is isointense to muscle on PD and slightly hyperintense to muscle on PD FS.

fibrous tissue adjacent to joints, and intraabdominal mesentery.[30] The size is variable and can range from very minimal to massive. Intense metabolic activity may be detected on PET (**Fig. 10**). The best diagnostic clue for this entity is a zonal pattern of mineralization, meaning higher density in the periphery than centrally, in areas prone to trauma or prior surgery. Although any age can be affected, the most common demographic is young adults. The most commonly involved anatomic locations are the muscles of the thigh, buttocks, and the upper arm.[31]

In the early stages, CT may demonstrate soft tissue mass without any mineralization, which may be indistinguishable from sarcoma.[32] After 3 to 5 weeks, mineralization typically appears in the lesion. After 6 weeks, this mineralization typically becomes more organized with a peripheral rim of mineralization (the zonal pattern). As the lesion ages, it may blend with the cortex of an adjacent bone, and the zonal pattern may become less apparent and ultimately may evolve into mature cortical bone at the periphery with central fatty marrow component.[33] Close assessment of the CT portion of the PET-CT and knowledge of the common location and natural history can help avoid incorrect diagnosis and unnecessary biopsy because tissue biopsy can occasionally be confusing and may be misinterpreted by pathologists as a sarcoma.[34]

Desmoid tumor

Also known as aggressive fibromatosis, desmoid tumors are soft tissue masses with a firm consistency, composed of a monoclonal fibroblastic proliferation. They are benign with no potential for metastases, but can be locally aggressive. They are most common in adults 25 to 35 years of age, with 70% occurring in the extremities. Other common locations are the abdominal wall muscles and fascia (common in women 20–30 years of age) (**Fig. 11**) and intraabdominally, most commonly in the small bowel mesentery. They may present with moderate FDG uptake with reported median SUVmax of 3.1 and range of 2.0 to 7.3.[35] Desmoid tumors generally present as nonspecific ill-defined soft tissue masses with an infiltrative appearance, variable attenuation, and mild heterogeneous, or delayed enhancement due to fibrosis that may not be detected on typical venous phase of contrast on CT. On MRI, these lesions have similar signal to muscle on T1 images and iso- to hyperintense relative to muscle on T2-weighted images, with mildly heterogeneous postcontrast appearance.[36] Central areas of low T2 signal can be seen as a result of high collagen content.[37] Unfortunately, the imaging appearance may be similar to sarcoma. Desmoid tumors have a high recurrence rate and are usually managed by radical wide resection.

Elastofibroma dorsi

Elastofibroma dorsi is a benign soft tissue lesion, which is thought to represent a reactive process and not a true neoplasm. The location is characteristically in the subscapular region deep to the serratus anterior muscle.[38] It is thought to be secondary to friction between the scapula and chest wall. The shape is generally lenticular and may interdigitate with surrounding fat, which can be mistaken for invasion of surrounding fat or a fat-containing neoplasm, such as liposarcoma.

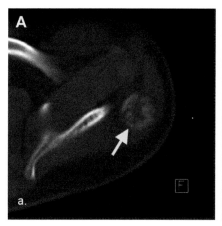
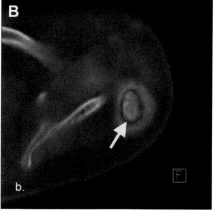

Fig. 10. A 51-year-old woman with L5 compression fracture and recent fall on the left shoulder referred for evaluation for possible malignancy, showing heterotopic ossification. (*A*) Axial CT and (*B*) axial fused 18F-FDG PET/CT show a zonal pattern of peripheral calcification within the posterior deltoid muscle with corresponding increased metabolism on the PET/CT fused image (*arrows*).

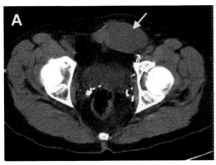
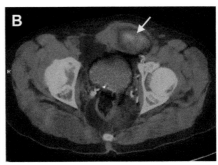

Fig. 11. A 39-year-old woman status postcolectomy showing a pathology-proven desmoid tumor of the anterior abdominal wall. (*A*) Axial CT and (*B*) axial fused 18F-FDG PET/CT images show a soft tissue mass (*arrows*) within the left rectus abdominis muscle with intense FDG avidity.

This lesion commonly enhances and demonstrates mild to moderate FDG avidity (**Fig. 12**). The SUVmax in a retrospective study of 75 cases of elastofibroma dorsi were reported as 2.0 ± 0.63.[39] SUVmax showed a weak positive correlation with lesion size, and no significant correlation was demonstrated between SUVmax and symptom severity in this study.[39] The mechanism of uptake is not clear but may be a combination of vascularity and increased metabolic activity within the mass.[40] Knowledge of the characteristic CT appearance (heterogeneous soft tissue mass with attenuation similar to skeletal muscle interlaced with strands of fat) of this lesion,[41] the typical location, and bilaterality (in up to 60% of cases) are very helpful features in distinguishing this lesion.

Intramuscular myxoma

Myxomas are rare benign well-circumscribed myxoid tumors that are intramuscular 82% of the time and have a predilection for the large muscles of the thigh, buttocks, and shoulder. They are characterized by a paucity of cells and diminished vascularity.[42] Mazabraud syndrome represents intramuscular myxomas in association with fibrous dysplasia (usually the polyostotic form). The few reported cases of intramuscular myxomas in the literature that have undergone PET-CT studies have demonstrated mild FDG uptake with SUVmax range of 1.7 to 1.8.[43] Mildly increased FDG uptake was noted in our case associated with an intramuscular myxoma in the vastus lateralis muscle (**Fig. 13**). The reason for increased uptake is uncertain. In a reported case of Mazabraud syndrome on PET-CT, the intramuscular myxomas again demonstrated mildly increased uptake with SUVmax of 2.6.[44] Intramuscular myxomas demonstrate low attenuation on CT. A small amount of peripheral fat is not uncommon. On MRI, the lesion is isointense to muscle on T1 with markedly increased signal on T2. Contrast enhancement is variable, and some lesions may demonstrate minimal enhancement and may be confused with cystic lesions.[45]

Fig. 12. A 70-year-old man referred for workup of adenocarcinoma of the right colon showing elastofibroma dorsi. (*A*) Axial CT and (*B*) axial fused 18F-FDG PET/CT reconstructions show bilateral soft tissue lesions (*arrows*) in the characteristic subscapular location deep to the serratus anterior muscles, with corresponding increased metabolic activity (SUVmax 3.7).

Osteonecrosis

Osteonecrosis can be caused by a variety of conditions, including sickle cell disease, alcohol abuse, trauma, long-term steroid use, systemic lupus erythematosus, or may be idiopathic. Although radiographs or MRI are more commonly

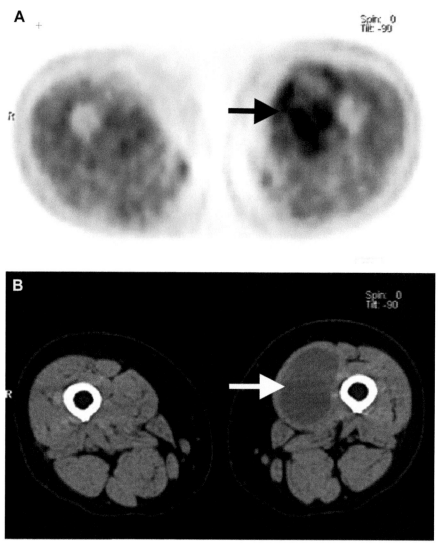

Fig. 13. A 59-year-old man with history of melanoma, with an incidental intramuscular myxoma. (*A*) Axial PET and (*B*) axial CT images show a well-circumscribed low attenuation lesion (*arrows*) in the left vastus medialis muscle with corresponding increased FDG uptake on PET. Biopsy showed paucicellular myxoid tissue consistent with myxoma.

performed when evaluating for osteonecrosis, this condition may be incidentally seen in patients undergoing routine surveillance PET studies, especially when steroids are part of the treatment regimen (**Fig. 14**). There have been reported cases in literature of osteonecrosis on PET, showing increased FDG uptake, for example, SUVmax of 2.9 was reported in a femoral head osteonecrosis case.[46] The increased FDG uptake may be due to associated inflammation and presence of inflammatory cells in the osteonecrotic lesions.[47] PET may have value in identifying early osteonecrosis when radiographs and MRI are initially negative, as noted on a study of 17 hip osteonecrosis, in which 9 hips demonstrated increased uptake on PET suspicious for early stage osteonecrosis but no evidence of osteonecrosis on MRI or bone scan.[48] MRI is more sensitive than radiographs and is commonly used in early diagnosis of osteonecrosis. MRI initially shows bone marrow edema (low T1 and high T2 signal), and the "double line" sign on T2 MR sequence is diagnostic. Serpentine or patchy sclerotic foci are characteristic findings on radiograph, and if the articular surface is involved, collapse and fragmentation may result. Most commonly involved locations for osteonecrosis are the hips, knees, shoulders, and ankles.

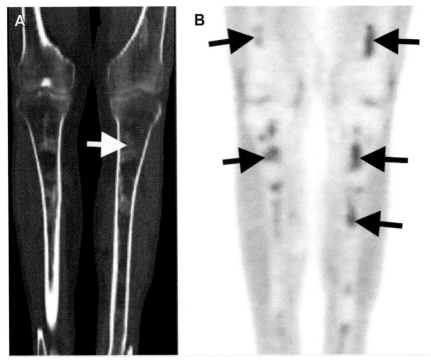

Fig. 14. A 42-year-old man with history of sickle cell anemia demonstrating multiple bone infarcts. (*A*) Coronal CT and (*B*) coronal PET show intramedullary areas of sclerosis, which is linear and serpentine (*arrows*) with an SUV-max of 1.9 (*arrows*).

Inflammation/Infection

Shingles (herpes zoster)

Herpes zoster infection occurs when cell-mediated immunity is compromised (such as in oncology patients undergoing chemotherapy and radiation), and the dormant virus replicates and is reactivated in the host, presenting as a vesicular rash in a dermatomal distribution. Herpes zoster infection is not a common finding on PET scans, but a few cases have been reported in the literature.[49] The acute infection typically displays moderately increased metabolic activity on PET (**Fig. 15**), thought to be secondary to inflammatory cells displaying increased metabolic activity. Clinical history of a painful erythematous pruritic rash in a dermatomal distribution and an imaging appearance of a superficial band of increased metabolic activity and mild skin thickening in a dermatomal distribution are suggestive of this diagnosis, and it is important to be aware of this entity so not to confuse it with cutaneous metastasis. The rash may appear on PET-CT as soft tissue nodules with increased FDG uptake instead of a superficial band of increased FDG uptake.[50]

Decubitus ulcer

Decubitus ulcers, also known as pressure sores, are open wounds involving the skin and

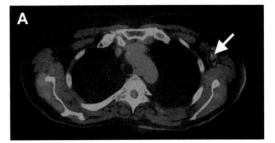

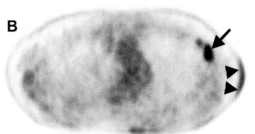

Fig. 15. A 60-year-old man with squamous cell carcinoma of the right temporal region with incidentally noted shingles (varicella zoster). (*A*) Axial fused 18F-FDG PET/CT reconstruction and (*B*) axial PET images show FDG uptake in a left axially lymph node (*arrow*) and a superficial band of increased metabolic activity in a dermatomal distribution in the adjacent skin (*arrowheads*). The patient had a new rash in a dermatomal distribution in this region.

subcutaneous tissues covering bony promi-
nences. Bed-bound and paralyzed individuals
are most prone to these lesions. Decubitus ulcers
may lead to sinus tract formation, abscesses, and
osteomyelitis.[51] PET is not typically used for evaluation of decubitus ulcers; however, they may
be incidentally seen on PET (**Fig. 16**), as areas
of increased FDG uptake. Hence awareness
of increased FDG avidity associated with these

lesions on PET is beneficial and essential. Physical examination and clinical history are extremely
helpful in this scenario. Also attention to the CT
portion of the PET-CT that usually shows skin or
soft tissue defect with inflammatory fat stranding
in the region is key in differentiating this condition
from metastasis. An associated fluid collection
may be seen on CT. Evaluation for underlying
bone osteomyelitis is best performed by MRI.
Osteomyelitis can also mimic malignancy due to
increased FDG uptake on PET. In osteomyelitis,
inflammatory cells cause increased FDG uptake.[52] MRI is the most sensitive and specific imaging modality for detection of early osteomyelitis
and for evaluation of extent of the infection and
better soft tissue evaluation. However, if encoun-
tered on PET-CT, CT can show osseous erosion,
sinus tracts, sequestra, cloacas, involucra, and
gas. Diagnosis of low-grade and chronic infection
is more easily performed with PET as FDG is
taken up by macrophages that predominate in
setting of chronic infection. The reported sensitivity and specificity for diagnosis of chronic osteomyelitis with FDG-PET have been 100% and
92%, respectively.[52] If the imaging appearance
and clinical picture are not definitive, MRI or biopsy may be considered to confirm diagnosis.
Confluent region of decreased signal intensity
on T1 and increased signal within bone and soft
tissues on fluid sensitive sequences are noted
on MRI.

Posttreatment and Postsurgical Hypermetabolism

Bisphosphonate-related osteonecrosis

Osteonecrosis of the maxillary and mandibular
bones is a discrete entity and is a known severe
complication of prolonged bisphosphonate treatment, which can be used for management of
bone metastases. In the setting of cancer, it may
be difficult to differentiate osteonecrosis in these
locations from tumor involvement. Even though
histology can confirm the diagnosis, biopsy can
cause further structural damage in cases of osteonecrosis. Bisphosphonate-related jaw osteonecrosis has been found to demonstrate increased
FDG uptake on PET, possibly secondary to inflammation, infection, or healing process at the site
(**Fig. 17**).

Technetium (^{99m}Tc)-sestamibi scintigraphy
combined with PET-CT has been reported to
aid in confirming the diagnosis, because
Tc99m sestamibi shows some oncotropic properties compared with the nontumor-specific
^{18}F-FDG. In a study of 4 patients with
multiple myeloma and oral osteonecrosis,

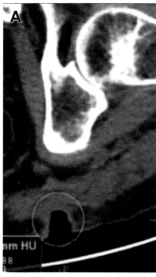

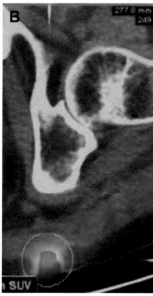

Fig. 16. A 47-year-old man referred for non-Hodgkin
lymphoma with a decubitus ulcer. (*A*) Axial CT and
(*B*) axial fused 18F-FDG PET/CT reconstructions show
a posterior soft tissue defect adjacent to the ischium
(*circled areas*) with associated focal increased FDG uptake in the skin and superficial soft tissues in this patient with a decubitus ulcer in this location.

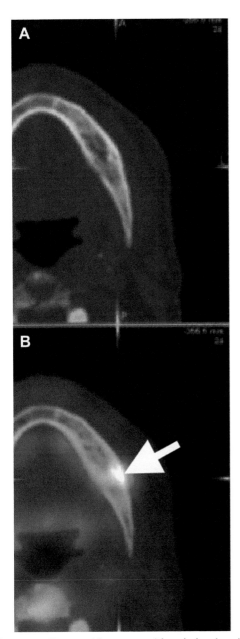

Fig. 17. A 60-year-old woman with zoledronic acid–related osteonecrosis referred for left breast infiltrating ductal carcinoma. (A) Axial CT and (B) axial fused 18F-FDG PET/CT images show a region of sclerosis within the left mandible with corresponding increased FDG activity (arrow). Follow-up images (not shown) after 3 months after discontinuing the medication showed interval improvement with a decrease in the SUVmax.

PET-CT showed focal uptake in all the cases, whereas Tc99m-sestamibi was not taken up by the areas of bone necrosis but was taken up by areas of osteolysis from multiple myeloma.[53] The CT appearance of bisphosphonate-related osteonecrosis is variable and can range from predominantly lytic, to mixed, to predominantly sclerotic. On MR, variable signal intensity is associated with the lesion likely related to disease stage.[54]

Subcutaneous injection sites

A variety of agents are administered via subcutaneous injection in patients. Interferon-alpha is a cytokine used in the treatment of patients with certain types of cancer and viral disease. It can be administered intramuscularly, subcutaneously, and intravenously. Subcutaneous injection sites can display FDG avidity. There have not been many reported cases of interferon injection as seen on PET-CT. A reported case in the literature demonstrated focal subcutaneous area of increased FDG uptake at the site of injection in the anterior thigh,[55] whereas the authors' case demonstrated a bandlike area of increased FDG uptake in the bilateral anterior thighs associated with interferon injections (Fig. 18). Similarly, enoxaparin sodium injection and other similar anticoagulation agents are injected subcutaneously for prophylactic or therapeutic purposes for deep vein thrombosis or pulmonary emboli. Patients with cancer are commonly under treatment with these anticoagulation agents. The granulomatous reaction in the subcutaneous tissues may present as soft tissue nodules with increased FDG uptake on PET-CT (Fig. 19) and may be mistaken for foci of metastases. Subcutaneous insulin injection in the diabetic population leads to similar appearance on PET-CT. There have been few cases reported in the literature of FDG-avid subcutaneous nodules of varying sizes in the anterior thighs and abdominal wall corresponding to sites of subcutaneous injection as confirmed clinically.[56] Metastases can involve the subcutaneous tissues and may have very similar appearance to these injection sites on PET-CT.[57,58] Cutaneous T-cell lymphoma can also have a similar appearance. However, the observation that these nodules are only found at the anterior aspect of the body where patients are most comfortable making injections and confirmation with clinical history of subcutaneous injections are helpful in establishing the correct diagnosis. Intramuscular gluteal injections have also been reported to display FDG avidity on PET-CT and found to be consistent with injection site granulomata on biopsy (macrophages within fibrous tissue).[59] The authors suspect that subcutaneous injection of recreational "street" drugs, which is commonly known as "skin popping," may also present as foci of increased activity subcutaneously through a similar

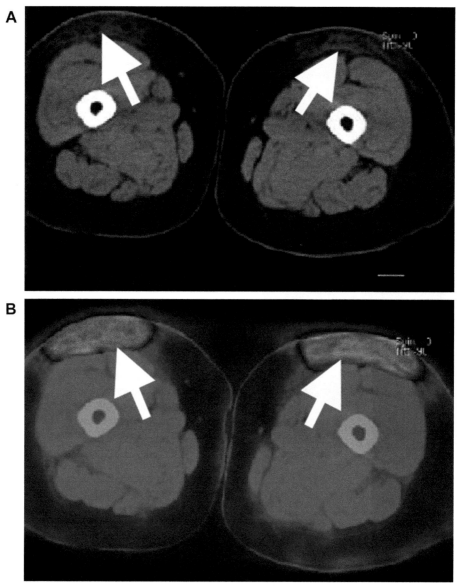

Fig. 18. A 61-year-old man receiving interferon immunotherapy injections in the anterior thigh soft tissues. (*A*) Axial CT and (*B*) axial fused 18F-FDG PET/CT images show bands of increased attenuation and metabolic activity in the anterior subcutaneous soft tissues of the thighs (*arrows*), a common location for interferon injection and uncommon location for presentation of malignancy.

process. Clinical correlation, however, can easily confirm the presence of these injection sites. Tattoos may also incite a foreign body reaction, which leads to FDG-avid lymph nodes that can be mistaken for malignancy.[60]

Hyperthermia therapy

Hyperthermia therapy, also known as thermal therapy or thermotherapy, is a type of cancer treatment in which body tissues are exposed to elevated temperatures up to 113°F. This treatment is commonly used with radiation therapy and

chemotherapy and is thought to make cancer cells more sensitive to the effects of radiation and chemotherapy.[61] Increased FDG uptake was noted in the skin and subcutaneous tissues on the PET in a patient who had undergone hyperthermia therapy for cancer (Fig. 20). The increased FDG uptake is suspected to be secondary to increased metabolic activity in the cells in the regions exposed to increased temperatures. To the authors' knowledge, other cases of this entity have not been reported in the literature. Being familiar with this entity and its potential to cause

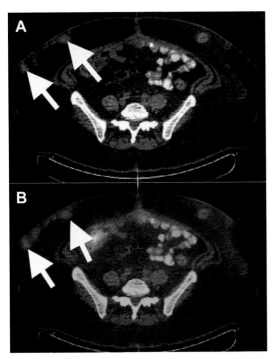

Fig. 19. A 49-year-old receiving enoxaparin injections (referred for diffuse large B-cell lymphoma). (*A*) Axial CT and (*B*) axial fused 18F-FDG PET/CT images show areas of soft tissue attenuation and increased metabolic activity within the anterior abdominal wall (*arrows*), a common location for subcutaneous injections and an uncommon location and presentation for malignancy.

a false-positive finding on PET scan can avoid confusion.

Aggressive granulomatosis (osteolysis)
Aggressive granulomatosis is a possible complication of hip arthroplasty placement. This is thought to be a consequence of inflammatory reaction to excessive wear, most commonly involving the polyethylene liner, and typically occurs 1 to 5 years after prosthesis surgery. Patients are asymptomatic in the beginning but with further bone loss, pain and loss of range of motion result. Normal lucency at the cement-bone interface is less than 2 mm. Granulomatous osteolysis usually causes multifocal lucencies, which may not conform to the shape of the prosthesis (**Fig. 21**). The particles from polyethylene wear lead to macrophage activation releasing bone-resorbing prostaglandins, resulting in progressive bone loss and granulomatous change, which may simulate infection.[62] However, the time course of bone resorption may be a helpful tool in differentiating this entity from infection.

Bone scintigraphy and FDG PET are generally not performed in the initial evaluation of prosthetic loosening and infection, whereas leukocyte (111In-labeled white blood cell) scan with bone marrow (^{99m}Tc-sulfur colloid) scintigraphy has a sensitivity, specificity, and accuracy of 100%, 91%, and 95%, respectively for periprosthetic infection.[63] Macrophage-specific PET probes currently being investigated, using radiolabeled macrophage surface peptide antagonists instead of FDG, have the potential to differentiate infection from loosening.[64] Of course, as explained in the attenuation artifacts section, both attenuation-corrected and uncorrected PET images should be reviewed because the prosthetic material itself may cause false-positive FDG uptake on attenuation-corrected PET images owing to its relatively high photon absorption. The time course of disease and clinical presentation including laboratory values are helpful differentiating tools. Serial radiographs are helpful in differentiation because changes occur more quickly in the presence of infection.[65] Ultimately, joint aspiration and culture may be required to exclude infection.

Physiologic Uptake and Artifacts

Diffuse muscular uptake
FDG uptake in normal muscle can be a common source of potential pitfall. The normal FDG uptake in skeletal muscles is mild, with SUVmax range of 0.5 to 2.2 and a mean of 1.0. During postprandial episodes, when insulin is quickly secreted in response to increased serum glucose, skeletal muscle glucose uptake increases.[66,67] Injection of FDG during postprandial episode or use of insulin by patients before FDG injection can cause diffusely increased muscle FDG uptake (**Fig. 22**). This is commonly symmetric and mild to moderate in intensity.[68] To avoid confusion and misdiagnosis, patients should fast for 4 to 6 hours before the PET-CT, and they should avoid insulin and oral hypoglycemic medications before the FDG injection. Vigorous exercise should also be avoided 24 hours before the examination because exercise also increases glucose uptake into skeletal muscles. Correlation with patient history for lack of appropriate fasting or recent use of insulin is helpful. In addition, this finding is expected to resolve on future examinations.

Asymmetric muscular activity
Prominent physiologic uptake can be seen in muscles depending on usage and activity immediately before or following FDG injection. For example,

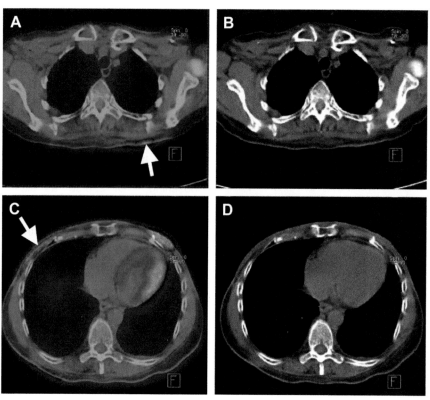

Fig. 20. A 45-year-old man receiving hyperthermia treatment for colon cancer with liver and peritoneal metastasis. (*A, B*) Axial fused 18F-FDG PET/CT and (*C, D*) corresponding axial CT images show increased FDG uptake in the skin and subcutaneous soft tissues (*arrows*).

increased uptake can be noted in the tongue and pterygoid muscles due to vocalization and chewing (**Fig. 23**), in the extraocular muscles due to eye movement, in the posterior cricoarytenoid muscles due to phonation, and in select skeletal muscles due to rigorous exercise.[69] FDG uptake related to muscle activity appears as linear or curvilinear tracer uptake that can be traced from muscle origin to insertion. To avoid false positives

regarding physiologic skeletal muscle uptake, patients are placed in a quiet room with limited stimulation for 60 to 90 minutes during the uptake phase before undergoing the examination. In addition, patients can display increased muscle contraction and FDG uptake in select muscles as a result of anxiety and stress, commonly in the neck, paravertebral muscles, and trapezius muscle.[70] Although rarely used in clinical practice,

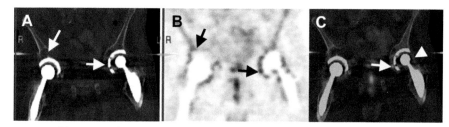

Fig. 21. A 77-year-old man with aggressive granulomatosis (referred for evaluation of lung cancer). (*A*) Coronal CT, (*B*) coronal PET, and (*C*) coronal fused 18F-FDG PET/CT reconstruction images show bilateral hip arthroplasties with loss of bone adjacent to the acetabular components bilaterally with corresponding increased FDG uptake (*arrows*). The left femoral head is asymmetrically positioned within the acetabular component (*arrowhead* in C) representing polyethylene liner wear, leading to particle disease (aggressive granulomatosis).

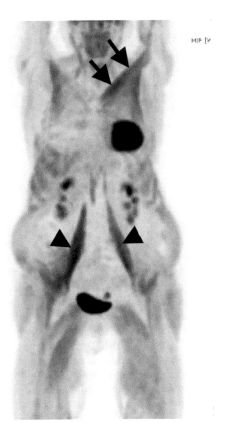

Fig. 22. A 60-year-old man who had received recent administration of insulin. Coronal PET image shows diffuse muscular increased FDG uptake, most prominently noted within the left pectoralis major muscle (*arrows*) and bilateral psoas muscles (*arrowheads*) in addition to the intense cardiac uptake.

benzodiazepines, such as diazepam, have been found to help reduce tracer uptake in these muscles when administered before tracer injection.[71] Knowledge of physiologic causes of increased skeletal muscle tracer uptake is useful in proper interpretation.

Brown fat

Brown adipose tissue is a thermogenic and metabolically active tissue. As such, it is not surprising that it is frequently FDG avid on PET. The incidence of FDG uptake in brown fat has been reported up to 2.3%.[72] This can be a source of confusion for foci of malignancy or metastases, especially in cases such as Hodgkin lymphoma, as brown fat is frequently found near areas of expected lymphadenopathy. Common locations for brown fat include the supraclavicular, neck, paratracheal, paraesophageal, and prevascular regions, along the pericardium and interatrial septum, paravertebral, perinephric, perihepatic, and subdiaphragmatic regions[73] (**Fig. 24**). In

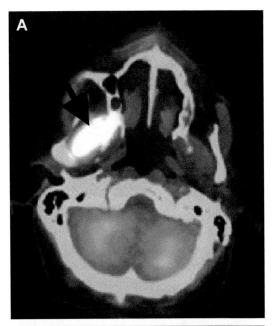

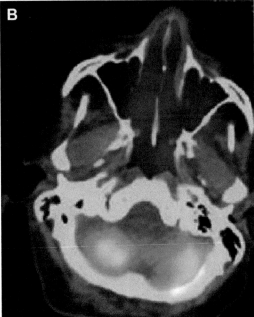

Fig. 23. A 61-year-old man with asymmetric muscle activity (referred for evaluation of melanoma). (*A*) Axial fused 18F-FDG PET/CT reconstruction show linear increased uptake corresponding to the right pterygoid muscle (*arrow*). This activity resolved on the follow-up images obtained 3 months later (*B*).

cases where these hypermetabolic foci occur in the expected locations of lymph nodes, comparison with CT images is very important in order to investigate for the presence of lymph nodes and for evaluation of lymph node size

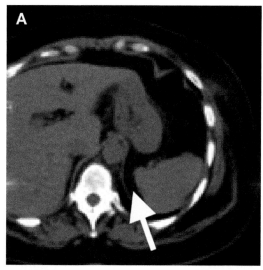

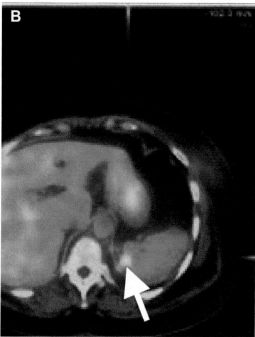

Fig. 24. A 66-year-old man with brown fat (referred for colon cancer). (*A*) Axial CT and (*B*) axial fused 18F-FDG PET/CT reconstruction images show increased FDG uptake in the left paraspinal region in an area with fat attenuation (*arrows*) consistent with brown fat.

and morphology. Presence of adipose tissue and absence of any pathologic lesion on CT is suggestive of brown fat as the cause of increased uptake on PET. Furthermore, it is helpful to remember that brown fat is more common in children than adults, women than men, in people with lower body mass index, and in colder temperatures.[72]

Knowledge of common areas for brown fat and the pattern of uptake, correlation with the CT portion of the study, and age and sex distribution are helpful tactics for differentiation of metastases from brown fat. In addition, warmer temperature at the injection room and waiting room decreases the likelihood of FDG uptake by brown fat and helps avoid confusion. It has also been found that a dose of oral propranolol may be helpful in reducing FDG uptake by brown fat because it is thought that sympathetic stimulation leads to glucose accumulation within brown fat.[74]

Attenuation artifacts

In PET-CT studies, the CT data are used for attenuation correction of the PET data to overcome the greater attenuation of photons arising in deep compared with superficial structures. After completion of the CT scan, the CT attenuation coefficients corresponding to various tissue types are mapped to their respective PET energies to generate a PET attenuation correction map.[75] The CT data are acquired with 120 to 140 kVp and is used to estimate the attenuation coefficients of the 511 keV PET photons. However, CT attenuation correction can cause artifacts in the PET images. Contrast media and metallic hardware and implants are important and common sources of artifact that can mimic focal tracer uptake. Vertebroplasty and infrequently sclerotic metastases can also cause artifacts (**Fig. 25**).[76] These artifacts occur because the CT scan is used instead of PET scan for attenuation correction of the PET data. High-density metallic implants have high Hounsfield units and generate streak artifact. These high numbers are mapped to high PET attenuation coefficients leading to overestimation of activity. This issue can be solved by correlation with nonattenuation-corrected PET images, which are not affected by this error.[77]

Similarly, high-density contrast media are associated with high density on CT leading to overcorrection of attenuation of PET data leading to appearance of increased FDG uptake on the attenuation-corrected PET images. Intravenous contrast media generally do not have significant effect because they are relatively dilute and clear quickly, whereas oral contrast media such as barium sulfate are dense and can stay in the colon for an extended time, lose water, become more concentrated, and cause more artifact.[78,79,80] Therefore, evaluation of the nonattenuated PET images is very helpful in avoiding misdiagnosis as increased metabolic activity.

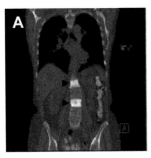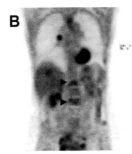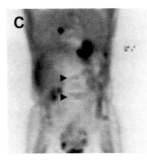

Fig. 25. (A, B) A 65-year-old man with prostate carcinoma and treated sclerotic vertebral body metastasis. Coronal CT reconstruction and corresponding attenuation-corrected PET images show apparent increased metabolic activity in the vertebral bodies (arrowheads). (C) The coronal nonattenuation-corrected images show that the apparent increased metabolic activity is an attenuation artifact related to the underlying sclerosis, in this patient with treated sclerotic metastasis, because the FDG uptake (arrowheads) is the same as the adjacent normal vertebral bodies.

SUMMARY

^{18}F-FDG PET-CT has revolutionized oncologic imaging by combining functional imaging with anatomic imaging and increasing sensitivity and specificity of diagnosis, staging, and response to therapy in patients with cancer. However, a major part of accurate interpretation entails knowledge of pitfalls and false positives on PET to avoid misdiagnosis. Many benign neoplastic, reactive, inflammatory, traumatic, degenerative, posttreatment, and physiologic entities can demonstrate increased FDG uptake on PET and can be mistaken for a malignant process. Awareness and prior knowledge of such entities as well as strategies to solve problem and further clarify are essential in clinical use of PET-CT in oncology.

ACKNOWLEDGMENTS

The authors would like to thank Dr John Seto and Dr Robert Henderson for providing cases for this article, and Marineh Asadoorian for her contribution and assistance with editing and drafting this article.

REFERENCES

1. Pauwels EK, Sturm EJ, Bombardieri E, et al. Positron-emission tomography with [18F]fluorodeoxyglucose. Part I. Biochemical uptake mechanism and its implication for clinical studies. J Cancer Res Clin Oncol 2000;126(10):549–59.

2. Gamelli RL, Liu H, He LK, et al. Augmentations of glucose uptake and glucose transporter-1 in macrophages following thermal injury and sepsis in mice. J Leukoc Biol 1996;59(5):639–47.

3. Kubota R, Yamada S, Kubota K, et al. Intratumoral distribution of fluorine-18-fluorodeoxyglucose in vivo: high accumulation in macrophages and granulation tissues studied by microautoradiography. J Nucl Med 1992;33(11):1972–80.

4. Beckers C, Ribbens C, Andre B, et al. Assessment of disease activity in rheumatoid arthritis with (18)F-FDG PET. J Nucl Med 2004;45(6): 956–64.

5. Palmer WE, Rosenthal DI, Schoenberg OI, et al. Quantification of inflammation in the wrist with gadolinium-enhanced MR imaging and PET with 2-[F-18]-fluoro-2-deoxy-D-glucose. Radiology 1995; 196(3):647–55.

6. Elzinga EH, van der Laken CJ, Comans EF, et al. 2-Deoxy-2-[F-18]fluoro-D-glucose joint uptake on positron emission tomography images: rheumatoid arthritis versus osteoarthritis. Mol Imaging Biol 2007;9(6):357–60.

7. Rosen RS, Fayad L, Wahl RL. Increased 18F-FDG uptake in degenerative disease of the spine: characterization with 18F-FDG PET/CT. J Nucl Med 2006;47(8):1274–80.

8. Bywaters EG, Evans S. The lumbar interspinous bursae and Baastrup's syndrome. An autopsy study. Rheumatol Int 1982;2(2):87–96.

9. Subramanyam P, Palaniswamy SS. Role of FDG PET/CT in Baastrup's disease. Indian J Nucl Med 2016; 31(3):235–7.

10. Lin E. Baastrup's disease (kissing spine) demonstrated by FDG PET/CT. Skeletal Radiol 2008; 37(2):173–5.

11. Shin DS, Shon OJ, Byun SJ, et al. Differentiation between malignant and benign pathologic fractures with F-18-fluoro-2-deoxy-D-glucose positron emission tomography/computed tomography. Skeletal Radiol 2008;37(5):415–21.

12. Zhuang H, Sam JW, Chacko TK, et al. Rapid normalization of osseous FDG uptake following traumatic or surgical fractures. Eur J Nucl Med Mol Imaging 2003;30(8):1096–103.

13. Bastawrous S, Bhargava P, Behnia F, et al. Newer PET application with an old tracer: role of 18F-NaF skeletal PET/CT in oncologic practice. Radiographics 2014;34(5):1295–316.

14. Drubach LA, Johnston PR, Newton AW, et al. Skeletal trauma in child abuse: detection with 18F-NaF PET. Radiology 2010;255(1):173–81.

15. Oh D, Huh SJ. Insufficiency fracture after radiation therapy. Radiat Oncol J 2014;32(4):213–20.

16. Fayad LM, Cohade C, Wahl RL, et al. Sacral fractures: a potential pitfall of FDG positron emission tomography. AJR Am J Roentgenol 2003;181(5):1239–43.

17. Tsuchida T, Kosaka N, Sugimoto K, et al. Sacral insufficiency fracture detected by FDG-PET/CT: report of 2 cases. Ann Nucl Med 2006;20(6):445–8.

18. Ravenel JG, Gordon LL, Pope TL, et al. FDG-PET uptake in occult acute pelvic fracture. Skeletal Radiol 2004;33(2):99–101.

19. Peh WC, Khong PL, Yin Y, et al. Imaging of pelvic insufficiency fractures. Radiographics 1996;16(2):335–48.

20. Kanberoglu K, Kantarci F, Cebi D, et al. Magnetic resonance imaging in osteomalacic insufficiency fractures of the pelvis. Clin Radiol 2005;60(1):105–11.

21. Cetik O, Uslu M, Ozsar BK. The relationship between Hill-Sachs lesion and recurrent anterior shoulder dislocation. Acta Orthop Belg 2007;73(2):175–8.

22. Ulaner G, Hwang S, Lefkowitz RA, et al. Musculoskeletal tumors and tumor-like conditions: common and avoidable pitfalls at imaging in patients with known or suspected cancer: part A: benign conditions that may mimic malignancy. Int Orthop 2013;37(5):871–6.

23. Dimitrakopoulou-Strauss A, Strauss LG, Heichel T, et al. The role of quantitative (18)F-FDG PET studies for the differentiation of malignant and benign bone lesions. J Nucl Med 2002;43(4):510–8.

24. Schulte M, Brecht-Krauss D, Heymer B, et al. Grading of tumors and tumorlike lesions of bone: evaluation by FDG PET. J Nucl Med 2000;41(10):1695–701.

25. Aoki J, Watanabe H, Shinozaki T, et al. FDG PET of primary benign and malignant bone tumors: standardized uptake value in 52 lesions. Radiology 2001;219(3):774–7.

26. Shin DS, Shon OJ, Han DS, et al. The clinical efficacy of (18)F-FDG-PET/CT in benign and malignant musculoskeletal tumors. Ann Nucl Med 2008;22(7):603–9.

27. Jesus-Garcia R, Osawa A, Filippi RZ, et al. Is PET-CT an accurate method for the differential diagnosis between chondroma and chondrosarcoma? SpringerPlus 2016;5:236.

28. Elumogo CO, Kochenderfer JN, Civelek AC, et al. Pigmented villonodular synovitis mimics metastases on fluorine 18 fluorodeoxyglucose position emission tomography-computed tomography. Quant Imaging Med Surg 2016;6(2):218–23.

29. Durr HR, Stabler A, Maier M, et al. Pigmented villonodular synovitis. Review of 20 cases. J Rheumatol 2001;28(7):1620–30.

30. Wilson JD, Montague CJ, Salcuni P, et al. Heterotopic mesenteric ossification ('intraabdominal myositis ossificans'): report of five cases. Am J Surg Pathol 1999;23(12):1464–70.

31. McCarthy EF, Sundaram M. Heterotopic ossification: a review. Skeletal Radiol 2005;34(10):609–19.

32. De Smet AA, Norris MA, Fisher DR. Magnetic resonance imaging of myositis ossificans: analysis of seven cases. Skeletal Radiol 1992;21(8):503–7.

33. Ehara S, Shiraishi H, Abe M, et al. Reactive heterotopic ossification. Its patterns on MRI. Clin Imaging 1998;22(4):292–6.

34. Lacout A, Jarraya M, Marcy PY, et al. Myositis ossificans imaging: keys to successful diagnosis. Indian J Radiol Imaging 2012;22(1):35–9.

35. Xu H, Koo HJ, Lim S, et al. Desmoid-type fibromatosis of the thorax: CT, MRI, and FDG PET characteristics in a large series from a tertiary referral center. Medicine 2015;94(38):e1547.

36. McDonald ES, Yi ES, Wenger DE. Best cases from the AFIP: extraabdominal desmoid-type fibromatosis. Radiographics 2008;28(3):901–6.

37. Tateishi U, Gladish GW, Kusumoto M, et al. Chest wall tumors: radiologic findings and pathologic correlation: part 1. Benign tumors. Radiographics 2003;23(6):1477–90.

38. Naylor MF, Nascimento AG, Sherrick AD, et al. Elastofibroma dorsi: radiologic findings in 12 patients. AJR Am J Roentgenol 1996;167(3):683–7.

39. Onishi Y, Kitajima K, Senda M, et al. FDG-PET/CT imaging of elastofibroma dorsi. Skeletal Radiol 2011;40(7):849–53.

40. Patrikeos A, Breidahl W, Robins P. F-18 FDG uptake associated with Elastofibroma dorsi. Clin Nucl Med 2005;30(9):617–8.

41. Battaglia M, Vanel D, Pollastri P, et al. Imaging patterns in elastofibroma dorsi. Eur J Radiol 2009;72(1):16–21.

42. Charron P, Smith J. Intramuscular myxomas: a clinicopathologic study with emphasis on surgical management. Am Surg 2004;70(12):1073–7.

43. Nishio J, Naito M. FDG PET/CT and MR imaging of intramuscular myxoma in the gluteus maximus. World J Surg Oncol 2012;10:132.

44. Singnurkar A, Phancao JP, Chatha DS, et al. The appearance of Mazabraud's syndrome on 18F-FDG PET/CT. Skeletal Radiol 2007;36(11):1085–9.

45. Murphey MD, McRae GA, Fanburg-Smith JC, et al. Imaging of soft-tissue myxoma with emphasis on CT and MR and comparison of radiologic and pathologic findings. Radiology 2002;225(1):215–24.

46. Choi KH, Oh JK, Kim SH, et al. Osteonecrosis mimicking bone metastasis in femoral head on (18)F-FDG PET/CT: a case report. Nucl Med Mol Imaging 2011;45(1):68–71.

47. Grigolon MV, Delbeke D. F-18 FDG uptake in a bone infarct: a case report. Clin Nucl Med 2001;26(7):613–4.

48. Dasa V, Adbel-Nabi H, Anders MJ, et al. F-18 fluoride positron emission tomography of the hip for osteonecrosis. Clin Orthop Relat Res 2008;466(5):1081–6.

49. Muzaffar R, Fesler M, Osman MM. Active shingles infection as detected on (18)F-FDG PET/CT. Front Oncol 2013;3:103.

50. Joyce JM, Carlos T. Herpes Zoster mimicking recurrence of lymphoma on PET/CT. Clin Nucl Med 2006; 31(2):104–5.

51. Hendrix RW, Calenoff L, Lederman RB, et al. Radiology of pressure sores. Radiology 1981;138(2):351–6.

52. Guhlmann A, Brecht-Krauss D, Suger G, et al. Chronic osteomyelitis: detection with FDG PET and correlation with histopathologic findings. Radiology 1998;206(3):749–54.

53. Catalano L, Del Vecchio S, Petruzziello F, et al. Sestamibi and FDG-PET scans to support diagnosis of jaw osteonecrosis. Ann Hematol 2007;86(6):415–23.

54. Morag Y, Morag-Hezroni M, Jamadar DA, et al. Bisphosphonate-related osteonecrosis of the jaw: a pictorial review. Radiographics 2009;29(7):1971–84.

55. Bombardieri E, Buscombe J, Lucignani G, et al. Advances in nuclear oncology: diagnosis and therapy. CRC Press; 2007.

56. Liu B, Chan S, Servaes S, et al. Multiple FDG-avid injection site granulomas due to lovenox injection. Clin Nucl Med 2014;39(3):308–11.

57. Ravizzini G, Meirelles GS, Horwitz SM, et al. F-18 FDG uptake in subcutaneous panniculitis-like T-cell lymphoma. Clin Nucl Med 2008;33(12):903–5.

58. Nguyen VX, Nguyen BD, Ram PC. Occult colon cancer with initial cutaneous metastatic manifestation: PET/CT detection. Clin Nucl Med 2012;37(5):506–8.

59. Prosch H, Mirzaei S, Oschatz E, et al. Case report: gluteal injection site granulomas: false positive finding on FDG-PET in patients with non-small cell lung cancer. Br J Radiol 2005;78(932):758–61.

60. Grove N, Zheng M, Bristow RE, et al. Extensive tattoos mimicking lymphatic metastasis on positron emission tomography scan in a patient with cervical cancer. Obstet Gynecol 2015;126(1):182–5.

61. Wust P, Hildebrandt B, Sreenivasa G, et al. Hyperthermia in combined treatment of cancer. Lancet Oncol 2002;3(8):487–97.

62. Spector M, Shortkroff S, Hsu HP, et al. Tissue changes around loose prostheses. A canine model to investigate the effects of an antiinflammatory agent. Clin Orthop Relat Res 1990;(261):140–52.

63. Love C, Marwin SE, Tomas MB, et al. Diagnosing infection in the failed joint replacement: a comparison of coincidence detection 18F-FDG and 111In-labeled leukocyte/99mTc-sulfur colloid marrow imaging. J Nucl Med 2004;45(11):1864–71.

64. Zhang Y, Kundu B, Zhong M, et al. PET imaging detection of macrophages with a formyl peptide receptor antagonist. Nucl Med Biol 2015;42(4):381–6.

65. Spangehl MJ, Younger AS, Masri BA, et al. Diagnosis of infection following total hip arthroplasty. Instr Course Lect 1998;47:285–95.

66. Abouzied MM, Crawford ES, Nabi HA. 18F-FDG imaging: pitfalls and artifacts. J Nucl Med Technol 2005;33(3):145–55 [quiz: 162–3].

67. Turcotte E, Leblanc M, Carpentier A, et al. Optimization of whole-body positron emission tomography imaging by using delayed 2-deoxy-2-[F-18]fluoro-D: -glucose injection following I.V. Insulin in diabetic patients. Mol Imaging Biol 2006;8(6):348–54.

68. Liu Y, Ghesani NV, Zuckier LS. Physiology and pathophysiology of incidental findings detected on FDG-PET scintigraphy. Semin Nucl Med 2010; 40(4):294–315.

69. Reinking MF, Osman MM. Prospective evaluation of physiologic uptake detected with true whole-body 18F-FDG PET/CT in healthy subjects. J Nucl Med Technol 2009;37(1):31–7.

70. Shreve PD, Anzai Y, Wahl RL. Pitfalls in oncologic diagnosis with FDG PET imaging: physiologic and benign variants. Radiographics 1999;19(1):61–77 [quiz: 150–1].

71. Barrington SF, Maisey MN. Skeletal muscle uptake of fluorine-18-FDG: effect of oral diazepam. J Nucl Med 1996;37(7):1127–9.

72. Yeung HW, Grewal RK, Gonen M, et al. Patterns of (18)F-FDG uptake in adipose tissue and muscle: a potential source of false-positives for PET. J Nucl Med 2003;44(11):1789–96.

73. Truong MT, Erasmus JJ, Munden RF, et al. Focal FDG uptake in mediastinal brown fat mimicking malignancy: a potential pitfall resolved on PET/CT. AJR Am J Roentgenol 2004;183(4):1127–32.

74. Soderlund V, Larsson SA, Jacobsson H. Reduction of FDG uptake in brown adipose tissue in clinical patients by a single dose of propranolol. Eur J Nucl Med Mol Imaging 2007;34(7):1018–22.

75. Sureshbabu W, Mawlawi O. PET/CT imaging artifacts. J Nucl Med Technol 2005;33(3):156–61 [quiz: 163–4].

76. Kuo PH, Cheng DW. Artifactual spinal metastases imaged by PET/CT: a case report. J Nucl Med Technol 2005;33(4):230–1.

77. Beyer T, Antoch G, Muller S, et al. Acquisition protocol considerations for combined PET/CT imaging. J Nucl Med 2004;45(Suppl 1):25S–35S.

78. Dizendorf E, Hany TF, Buck A, et al. Cause and magnitude of the error induced by oral CT contrast agent in CT-based attenuation correction of PET emission studies. J Nucl Med 2003;44(5):732–8.

79. Cohade C, Osman M, Nakamoto Y, et al. Initial experience with oral contrast in PET/CT: phantom and clinical studies. J Nucl Med 2003;44(3):412–6.

80. Gholamrezanezhad A, Basques K, Batouli A, et al. Clinical Nononcologic Applications of PET/CT and PET/MRI in Musculoskeletal, Orthopedic, and Rheumatologic Imaging. AJR Am J Roentgenol 2018; 210(6):W245–63.

PET in the Diagnostic Management of Soft Tissue Sarcomas of Musculoskeletal Origin

Sanaz Katal, MD, MPH[a], Ali Gholamrezanezhad, MD[b],*,
Michael Kessler, MD[c], Mojtaba Olyaei, MD[a],
Hossein Jadvar, MD, PhD, MPH, MBA[b]

KEYWORDS

- Positron emission tomography • Liposarcoma • Malignant fibrous histiocytoma
- Pleomorphic undifferentiated sarcoma • Malignant nerve sheath tumor • Rhabdomyosarcoma
- Synovial cell sarcoma • Angiosarcoma

KEY POINTS

- A soft tissue sarcoma (STS) is relatively rare. (18) Fluorine-2-fluoro-2-deoxy-D-glucose (FDG) PET–computed tomography (CT) offers complementary information in the management of an STS.
- Additional research is needed to strengthen the current evidence and to elaborate on the application of FDG PET-CT, particularly for rare subtypes of STS.
- Though FDG PET-CT cannot replace direct tissue sampling, it can significantly enhance the biopsy diagnostic yield by targeting the hypermetabolic part of lesion.
- FDG PET-CT can be used to detect malignant transformation of a benign lesion into an aggressive lesion.
- Because classic size-based assessment of treatment response is inadequate, metabolic FDG PET data is valuable in posttreatment evaluation of cancer, including STS.

INTRODUCTION

Soft tissue sarcomas (STSs) are a relatively rare group of heterogeneous tumors derived from mesenchymal tissue elements. An STS can occur at any age, accounting for less than 1% of all adult solid tumors and about 7% of pediatric malignancies. As a result, STSs are the cause of 2% of all cancer-related deaths.[1,2]

Typically, the clinical manifestation of an STS is of a heterogeneous soft tissue mass that grows over time. Symptoms usually develop due to the mass effect on nerves, vessels, and other adjacent structures. The anatomic locations at which STSs of musculoskeletal origin most often occur are the extremities (70%), followed by the thoracic wall.[3] Within these locations, the muscular compartments are the most common spaces. Distinguishing between the more than 50 discrete histologic subtypes of STSs is possible through tissue biopsy. In adults, the most common histologic subtypes are liposarcoma, malignant fibrous histiocytoma (MFH), and leiomyosarcoma. In children, almost all STSs are rhabdomyosarcomas at 40%.[4,5] Prognosis of disease is subsequently determined

[a] Tehran University of Medical Sciences (TUMS), Tehran, Iran; [b] Keck School of Medicine, University of Southern California (USC), 1520 San Pablo Street, Suite L1600, Los Angeles, CA 90033; [c] Case Medical Center, University Hospitals of Cleveland, Case Western Reserve University, Cleveland, OH, USA
* Corresponding author.
E-mail address: A.gholamrezanezhad@yahoo.com

PET Clin 13 (2018) 609–621
https://doi.org/10.1016/j.cpet.2018.05.011
1556-8598/18/© 2018 Elsevier Inc. All rights reserved.

through the combination of the histologic subtype, the tumor's grade, the size and depth of the primary tumor, the stage of the disease at its initial presentation, and the patient's age. Following treatment, additional indicators of prognosis are incorporated, including the presence of disease at the margins of the resected specimen and the recurrence of disease on successive follow-up imaging studies. Treatment protocols often focus on surgical resection with the addition of adjuvant chemotherapy and radiotherapy. With current management strategies, the resulting 5-year survival for patients with an STS is 50% for adults and 71% for pediatric patients.[3]

With the advent of PET–computed tomography (CT), many clinicians and researchers have explored the use of (18) fluorine-2-fluoro-2-deoxy-D-glucose (FDG) PET imaging to improve the management of STSs. This article reviews the current evidence for use of FDG PET-CT in the general diagnosis, staging or prognosis, and treatment monitoring of STSs. Additionally, a brief overview of several of the most common histologic subtypes of STS are discussed with more specific information regarding the use of FDG PET-CT in the management of each subtype.

VALUE OF PET IN THE DIFFERENTIAL DIAGNOSIS OF PRIMARY SOFT TISSUE MASSES

FDG PET-CT is rarely the modality of discovery for a mass concerning for a STS. However, FDG PET-CT may be used for specific patient populations as a method for detecting malignant transformation of benign lesions into biologically aggressive lesions. One example of this is the case of plexiform neurofibroma transformation into a malignant peripheral nerve sheath tumor (MPNST).[6,7] On finding a suspected malignancy, evaluation proceeds with tissue sampling and histologic grading. Though FDG PET-CT cannot replace a direct tissue sampling, it can significantly increase the diagnostic yield of the biopsy by targeting the hypermetabolic part of a heterogeneous lesion.[3]

Grading a tumor is the most reliable predictor of a tumor's biological behavior and the patient's ultimate clinical outcome. The most commonly used grading system for STSs is the French Federation of Cancer Centers Sarcoma Group (Fédération Nationale des Centers de Lutte Contre le Cancer [FFNLCC]) grading system. The FFNLCC system categorizes tumors based on the mitotic rate, cellularity, and degree of differentiation. Recently, many studies have explored the complementary role of FDG PET-CT in the grading of STSs.[8–11] Benz and colleagues[12] analyzed 120 subjects with 12

different STS subtypes. Their study revealed a significant relationship between the standard uptake value (SUV) at maximum SUV (SUV_{max}) of a lesion and the histologic grade given by the 3-tiered FFNLCC system when using a cutoff of 6.6 g/mL. On a meta-analysis examining a total 441 tumoral lesions that attempted to distinguish malignant STSs from benign lesions with FDG PET, Ioannidis and Lau[13] reported a sensitivity and specificity of 87% and 79% using an SUV_{max} threshold of 2.0, and 70% and 87% using an SUV_{max} threshold of 3.0, respectively. In their study, 100% of the intermediate and high-grade sarcomas were detected, whereas 74% of lower grade sarcomas and 39% of benign lesions were correctly characterized. Furthermore, several additional studies have shown similarly high sensitivities in distinguishing high-grade sarcomas from lower grade tumors.[14,15] Another meta-analysis, which included 341 subjects with STSs, revealed a sensitivity and specificity of 88% and 86%, respectively, when using the mean SUV to discriminate between low-grade sarcomas and high-grade sarcomas.[16]

Several recent studies have attempted to achieve better performance in STS and benign tumor differentiation by examining the lesion FDG kinetics. Lodge and colleagues[17] reported that malignant STSs achieve the maximal FDG uptake 4 hours following the radiotracer injection, whereas benign lesions reached peak uptake after only 30 minutes. They found that these indices had a sensitivity and specificity of 100% and 76%, respectively. In another approach, Dancheva and colleagues[18] studied the method of dual time point imaging for the detection of recurrent tumor in restaging FDG PET-CT studies. They reported that an increase in SUV greater than 10% on delayed imaging could detect high-grade sarcomas with a sensitivity and specificity of 100% and 80%, respectively.

With the many potential benefits of evaluating a primary tumor with FDG PET-CT, it is important to know its limitations. Though FDG PET-CT has shown the ability to differentiate between high-grade and benign tumors on multiple studies, there is lack of evidence of its ability to differentiate between low-grade and benign soft tissue lesions.[3] One study found that false-negative interpretations of low-grade sarcomas was found to be primarily related to their low metabolic rate, whereas false-positive results of benign lesions were often the result of associated inflammation.[16]

PET IN INITIAL STAGING OF SOFT TISSUE SARCOMAS

Staging a patient's STS is among the most important prognostic indicators for a patient's clinical outcome. The most common site for STS metastasis is the lung (75%), whereas metastasis to lymph nodes and bones occur less frequently or more often with specific subtypes. The American Joint Committee on Cancer (AJCC) system of staging, based on the evaluation of the primary tumor, lymph node involvement, and distal metastasis, is the most commonly used staging system for STSs. Typically, the AJCC system uses CT scan and MR imaging to evaluate the primary tumor and assess for spread. More recently, the use of whole-body FDG PET-CT has been shown to play a complementary role in the staging and restaging of many cancers, including STSs. Lucas and colleagues[19] reported a sensitivity and specificity of 86.7% and 100%, respectively, for detecting pulmonary metastases with FDG PET compared with 100% and 96.4%, respectively, for CT scan alone. Furthermore, FDG PET-CT found 13 additional, unexpected sites of metastases. Researchers, Volker and colleagues,[20] and Ricard and colleagues,[21] showed that PET-CT can detect a greater number of lymph nodes and bone lesions in the initial staging of an STS than conventional imaging alone; however, it had a lower sensitivity and specificity for detecting pulmonary metastases. A similar limitation was found by Fortes and colleagues[22] in a study of 154 subjects with pulmonary nodules, 18 of which were STSs. They concluded that lack of high FDG uptake in a suspicious pulmonary nodule on a CT scan cannot exclude malignancy. Therefore, use of dedicated chest CT scan on full inspiration has been advocated.[20,21]

As mentioned previously, FDG PET-CT has been shown to be effective at detecting malignancy deposited in lymph nodes.[23] This has proven useful for excluding distant metastases in patients who may otherwise be surgical candidates.[3] In the evaluation of osseous metastases, a meta-analysis reported a greater sensitivity and specificity for detecting bone metastases with FDG PET-CT than with CT scan alone but with equal sensitivity and specificity to that of MR imaging.[24–26] In either case, it is important to analyze both the PET and CT components to avoid missing lesions that demonstrate minimal metabolic activity, such as in densely sclerotic lesions.

RESTAGING AND TREATMENT RESPONSE ASSESSMENT

FDG PET imaging has also been found to be useful in both restaging the disease and assessing response to treatment. Kole and colleagues[27] performed an analysis of 14 subjects involving the detection of recurrence of an STS using FDG PET-CT and reported 93% sensitivity. Al-Ibraheem and colleagues[28] found that FDG PET-CT offered a higher accuracy of detection for recurrent bone or soft tissue tumors compared with conventional CT scan. This superiority is mainly due to its ability to discriminate local tumor recurrence from scar tissue in a treated area.[28,29] However, an important finding to note when comparing FDG PET-CT in restaging versus the initial staging of a tumor is that calculated SUV cannot reliably predict a tumor's grade at recurrence.[30]

Furthermore, it is becoming common knowledge that observing for a decrease in tumor size is a poor anatomic metric for the evaluation of treatment response. In particular, heterogeneous tumors can contain various tissue types with differential sensitivity to chemoradiation and may demonstrate no significant change in size even with effective treatment. Often, a tumor may even appear to grow in size due to changes such as increased edema or internal hemorrhage. Additionally, with the advent of new targeted therapies and cytostatic versus cytotoxic agents, classic treatment assessment based only on size is even less accurate. In a study by Evilevitch and colleagues,[31] the reduction of metabolic activity, as measured by FDG PET-CT, was shown to be a more accurate predictor of tumor response to chemotherapy than the change in size as evaluated by the Response Evaluation Criteria In Solid Tumors (RECIST) criteria. Schuetze and colleagues[32] found that a 40% decline in the SUV_{max} of a tumor in which the baseline SUV_{max} was greater than or equal to 6 g/mL could discriminate responders from nonresponders and help predict patient outcome. Similarly, another study stated that a 35% reduction in SUV_{max} is capable of predicting a histopathologic response in high-grade sarcomas even after only 1 cycle of chemotherapy.[33] Moreover, Eary and colleagues[34] showed that the percentage reduction of FDG uptake after 2 cycles of chemotherapy was also a good prognostic indicator. Though current evidence for FDG PET-CT is promising for use in evaluation of treatment response, additional studies with larger subject groups are needed.

HISTOLOGIC SUBTYPES

The following sections briefly review some of the most common STSs and the subtype-specific use of FDG PET-CT in their management.

Liposarcoma

Liposarcoma is among the most common STSs. They arise most often from the deep soft tissues of the extremities and retroperitoneum, and can demonstrate multiple histologic subtypes, including myxoid, pleomorphic, and dedifferentiated tumor cells.[35-39] Considered a low-grade to intermediate-grade sarcoma, pleomorphic type accounts for 20% to 50% of all liposarcomas (Fig. 1) with a 5-year survival of about 90%.[38,40,41] The standard treatment is complete tumor resection with negative surgical margins. The myxoid subtype demonstrates chemoradiotherapy sensitivity and often receives neoadjuvant therapy. Additionally, novel methods, such as photodynamic therapy with acridin, have been proposed as alternative therapy.[42]

CT and MR imaging are often sufficiently able to visualize the fat and nonfat tissue components (see Fig. 1A–F) of a liposarcoma and predict a subtype; however, anatomic imaging is unable to distinguish the well-differentiated liposarcomas from benign lesions.[43] Suzuki and colleagues[44] found that both visual and quantitative analysis of FDG PET images could allow for differentiation of liposarcomas from lipomas. They stated that the mean SUV of the myxoid-type lipomas, as well as other types of liposarcoma, were significantly higher than that of well-differentiated liposarcoma by 2-fold and 3-fold, respectively.[45]

Another study by Schwarzbach and colleagues[46] showed that more well-differentiated myxoid liposarcoma present with a lower FDG uptake than a dedifferentiated or pleomorphic tumor. They also demonstrated that an SUV_{max} greater than or equal to 3.6 was associated with a significantly reduced progression-free survival. Suzuki and colleagues[46] offered a cutoff SUV of 0.81 to discern benign lipomatous lesions from sarcomas with a high level of accuracy. Lucas and colleagues,[19] and Tateishi and colleagues,[47] further reported that FDG uptake in liposarcoma depends on specific tumoral histologic features. Conill and colleagues[48] proposed that the pleomorphic, mixed, and/or higher grade liposarcomas should be selected preferentially for FDG PET evaluation, whereas the The National Comprehensive Cancer Network (NCCN) guidelines have recommended that FDG PET-CT be used only for high-grade tumors larger than 3 cm.[49] FDG PET-CT has a lower sensitivity of pulmonary metastasis detection and often underestimates the extent of osseous metastatic disease. The combination of FDG-PET-CT and MR imaging for the staging of myxoid-type liposarcomas may be helpful in this clinical setting.[48]

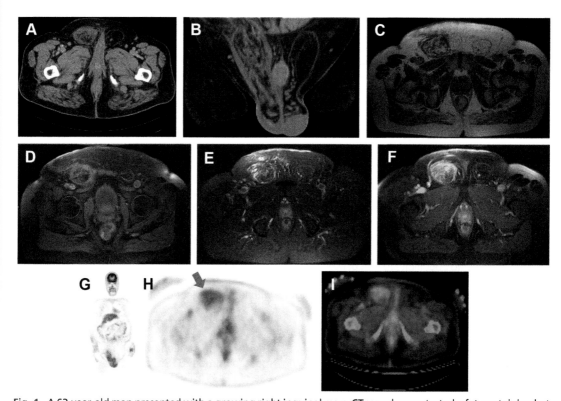

Fig. 1. A 63-year-old man presented with a growing right inguinal mass. CT scan demonstrated a fat-containing heterogeneous soft tissue mass (A, B). The lesion is heterogeneous with both fat and nonfat components on T1-weighted image (C), fat-saturated T1 (D) weighted image, heterogeneous short tau inversion recovery (STIR) hypersignal intensity (E), and postcontrast enhancement (F). The lesions is mildly hypermetabolic on PET-CT with an SUV_{max} of 3.6 (G–I). STIR, short t1 inversion recovery. The pathologic assessment of the lesion confirmed pleomorphic liposarcoma.

Malignant Fibrous Histiocytoma

MFH, also known as pleomorphic undifferentiated sarcoma or fibrosarcoma, is the most common STS in adults. This STS arises from histiocytic and fibroblastic cells or directly from more primitive mesenchymal cells.[50,51] This aggressive tumor typically occurs in the deep fascia and skeletal muscles of the extremities, most commonly occurring in the thigh or retroperitoneum. Of the 5 histologic types of MFH, storiform-pleomorphic type is the most common subtype (50%–60%). It is composed of spindle cells (fibroblastic-like) and round cells (histiocytic-like) arranged in a storiform pattern with intervening inflammatory cells.[52] Similar to liposarcomas, MFH is treated with surgical resection with or without adjuvant treatment.[53–59] However, MFH is considered a higher grade sarcoma and frequently metastasizes, leading to a poorer prognosis with an overall 5-year survival of about 14%.[52]

Diagnosing MFH can be difficult because neither the clinical features nor its gross appearance distinguishes this tumor from the other subtypes of STS. With 25% of MFH tumors demonstrating a highly myxoid composition, the tumor may mimic myxoid liposarcoma.[52] Though few studies describe MFH explicitly, this subtype has been included in other studies of malignant STS, demonstrating that it is also hypermetabolic.[60,61] Unlike MFH of the torso, only few reports exist describing MFH in extremities; the limited available publications describe MFH and other STSs as hypermetabolic masses.[60,61] The study of Kern and colleagues,[8] among the first studies showing the value of FDG-PET in STSs,

established that FDG-PET is among the most useful tools for STS metabolic evaluation. Since then, studies have been done that applied FDG-PET for grading,[13,17,19,62–67] staging, assessment of response to treatment,[31–33,60,68–72] and surgical planning of STSs. Hoshi and colleagues,[60] in an analysis of 113 subjects with STSs, including MFH, demonstrated that an SUV_{max} greater than or equal to 2 (**Fig. 2**) and a tumor size greater than or equal to 5 cm (**Fig. 3**) would infer a worse prognosis and would likely benefit from more aggressive therapy. Again, this generalized knowledge can be helpful in the management of MFH; however, more research specifically directed toward MFH and FDG PET-CT use is necessary.

Rhabdomyosarcoma

Rhabdomyosarcoma is the most common STS in children and adolescents. It arises from mesenchymal cells during skeletal muscle differentiation.[73–75] The most common anatomic locations for rhabdomyosarcoma are the head and neck, genitourinary tract, and limbs. Histologically, the embryonal form is the most common subtype. The embryonal form accounts for about 57% of all childhood rhabdomyosarcoma versus about 23% and 20% for the alveolar form and all other types of this sarcoma, respectively. The treatment most often includes surgical removal of the tumor with accompanying systemic chemotherapy followed by local radiotherapy.[73] The therapeutic management almost completely depends on initial staging, highlighting the need for a reliable tool for accurate evaluation of the tumor.

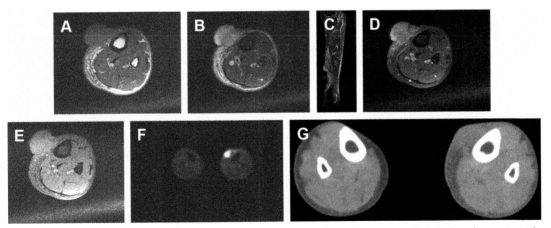

Fig. 2. A 72-year-old woman presented with a growing left leg fungating mass. MR imaging demonstrated a 2.3 cm heterogeneous T1 hyposignal (*A*), Proton Density (PD) intermediate (*B*), and STIR hypersignal (*C*) intensity lesion with heterogeneous postcontrast enhancement (*D*) compared with precontrast imaging (*E*). The lesion was highly hypermetabolic on PET (*F*) with an SUV_{max} of 12.7. The CT component of PET demonstrates a nonspecific fungating soft tissue density mass (*G*). The lesion was pathologically diagnosed as MFH or pleomorphic undifferentiated sarcoma (PUS).

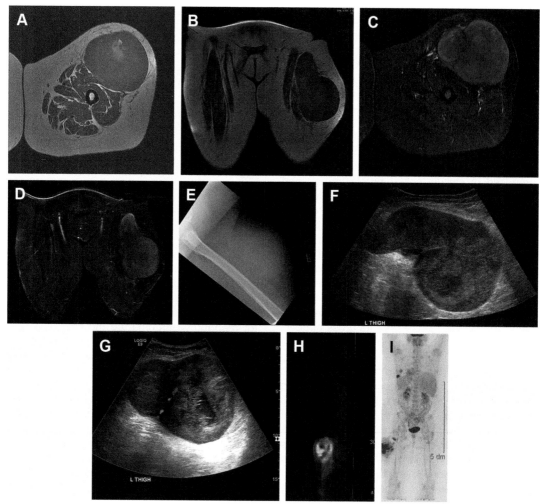

Fig. 3. MFH or PUS: multilobulated T1 intermediate signal intensity mass with areas of hyperintensity suggestive of internal hemorrhage (*A, B*), centered in the subcutaneous adipose tissues of the left anterolateral thigh, measuring approximately 18.1 by 9.9 by 11.4 cm, with areas of central T1 hyperintensity, which do not suppress on the fat-saturated sequences, likely representing areas of necrosis and hemorrhage. The mass abuts a short segment of the rectus femoris muscle and anterior aspect of the vastus lateralis muscle with no evidence of neurovascular involvement. The lesion demonstrates heterogeneous postcontrast enhancement (*C, D*). There is no evidence of bone invasion to the underlying osseous structures on radiograph (*E*). On ultrasound, the lesion is heterogeneous in echogenicity with mild internal vascularity (*F, G*). On PET-CT, the lesion is heterogeneously hypermetabolic with an SUV$_{max}$ of 14.3 (*H, I*).

Ricard and colleagues[21] concluded that FDG PET-CT is a useful method for staging and restaging of pediatric rhabdomyosarcoma with particular emphasis on the detection of lymph node and bone involvement.[21] Multiple studies have also demonstrated the utility of FDG PET-CT in the detection and evaluation of primary lesions with a higher sensitivity (95%–100%) and specificity (80%–100%) than that achieved by conventional imaging (17%–83% and 43%–100%, respectively).[20,21,76–80] For nonpulmonary and distal lymph node involvement, FDG PET-CT has shown a higher sensitivity with the same specificity compared with conventional imaging tools. In many of these studies, a greater total number of lymph nodes were detected using FDG PET-CT. In their 41 subject study of rhabdomyosarcoma, Baum and colleagues[21,77–83] noted that nodal involvement, primary tumoral metabolic activity, and other metastatic site involvements are the major determinants of patient survival in rhabdomyosarcoma. Concerning treatment response, Eugene and colleagues[26,77–80,82] demonstrated FDG PET-CT has a greater ability to detect complete response compared with conventional imaging. However, similar to other STSs, the major limitation of FDG

PET-CT in rhabdomyosarcoma is related to the evaluation of pulmonary metastases.[77,79]

Angiosarcoma

Angiosarcoma is an uncommon malignant tumor of vascular and lymphatic endothelial origin, accounting for less than 5% of all STSs.[84] Most often appearing in thighs and retroperitoneum, angiosarcomas can occur anywhere in the extremities, trunk, and head and neck regions.[85] Clinically, an angiosarcoma often presents as an enlarging, painful mass frequently associated with a vascular disorder such as anemia or a coagulopathy. They are aggressive tumors that tend to reoccur and metastasize widely. Prognosis is poor, as demonstrated in a case series study of 49 subjects that showed a 53% median survival at 11 months.[84] Epithelioid angiosarcoma is the most common subtype of angiosarcoma. Similar to other STSs, wide excisional resection remains the treatment of choice, with the addition of chemotherapy and radiotherapy if complete resection is not possible. Early diagnosis is of great importance in providing the greatest chance of total tumor resection.

There are only a few case reports in literature regarding the usefulness of FDG PET-CT in the management of angiosarcoma, primarily due to its low incidence; however, FDG PET-CT has provided some reliability in the early detection of distant metastases, staging, and its prognostication of disease.[86–92] Benign vascular lesions, such as hemangiomas and hemangioendotheliomas, demonstrate significantly lower FDG avidity compared with angiosarcoma, allowing distinguishability.[93–95] In a study by Lee and colleagues,[93] FDG uptake levels, as expressed by SUV_{max}, were able to effectively predict the prognosis of subjects with vascular tumors. Their study showed a significant reduction in survival with an SUV_{max} greater than or equal to 3 g/mL.[93] Clearly, much more research is needed to examine the value of FDG PET-CT in this setting.

Synovial Cell Sarcoma

Synovial cell sarcoma is the third most common STS, accounting for 6% to 10% of STSs. Synovial cell sarcoma occurs primarily in the extremities of young adults with a predilection for the periarticular regions, with the popliteal area being most common. However, rarely, synovial cell sarcoma may involve the trunk, near the joints (**Fig. 4**). Clinically, they present as slow growing and often painless masses. Like most STSs, synovial cell sarcoma metastasizes to the lungs.[96,97] Although, local surgical excision and radiotherapy give excellent local control of the tumor, it is a metastatic disease that is more difficult to treat.

MR imaging is the primary imaging modality for diagnosis and initial tumor staging, with CT scan useful for detection of distant disease.[98] There are very few studies that have evaluated FDG PET-CT in synovial cell sarcomas. Rayamajhi and colleagues[99] demonstrated that FDG PET-CT is a useful method for staging and restaging of patients with synovial cell sarcoma. Other studies suggested that a pretherapy SUV_{max} could be used for prediction of survival and pathologic response to neoadjuvant therapy.[100] It was shown that an SUV greater than 4.35 g/mL is associated with shorter progression-free survival and increased risk for developing recurrence or metastases of synovial sarcoma.[100] General STS studies that included synovial cell sarcoma have demonstrated

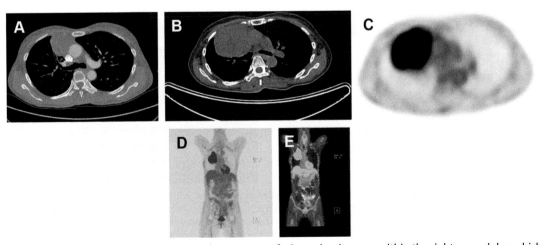

Fig. 4. A 61-year-old woman presented with a 10.4 cm soft tissue density mass within the right upper lobe, which abuts the pleural, pericardial, and mediastinal surfaces (*A, B*). The lesion is hypermetabolic on PET-CT with an SUV_{max} of 17.7 (*C–E*), the biopsy of which confirmed synovial cell carcinoma of the chest wall.

an ability to distinguish low-grade from high-grade sarcomas with 80% sensitivity.[101,102]

Malignant Peripheral Nerve Sheath Tumors

MPNSTs are a rare group of STSs that account for 5% to 10% of all STSs with an expected incidence of 0.1 out of 100,000 per year in the general population.[103] MPNSTs are of ectomesenchymal origin, deriving from Schwann cells or pluripotent cells of the neural crest and they arise along peripheral nerve branches or their sheaths.

About 25% to 50% of observed MPNSTs present in patients with neurofibromatosis (NF)-1, and 2% to 29% of patients with plexiform NF will develop MPNST,[6,7] whereas the total lifetime prevalence of MPNST in NF1 is only 10%.[104,105] These high numbers, along with the poor prognosis associated with MPNST, stress the need for early detection.

Detection of the malignant transformation of plexiform NF to MPNST is difficult using clinical history and conventional CT and MR imaging alone. Clinical symptoms, such as an enlarging, painful mass, are nonspecific and unreliable. Similar to other STSs, the blind tissue sampling of a small portion of the heterogeneous tumor cannot reliably determine an entire tumor's biological behavior because a higher grade component may have been missed. Additionally, excisional biopsies may not be feasible due to the high resultant morbidity from the involvement of the adjacent structures. Luckily, FDG PET-CT has shown the ability to detect malignant transformation in the patients with NF1, offering a promising tool for surveillance.[3,105–108] Ferner and colleagues[108] reported a significant difference between the SUV_{max} of malignant and benign lesions using an SUV_{max} cutoff of 2.5 g/mL for NF1 subjects 200 minutes following FDG injection (**Fig. 5**).

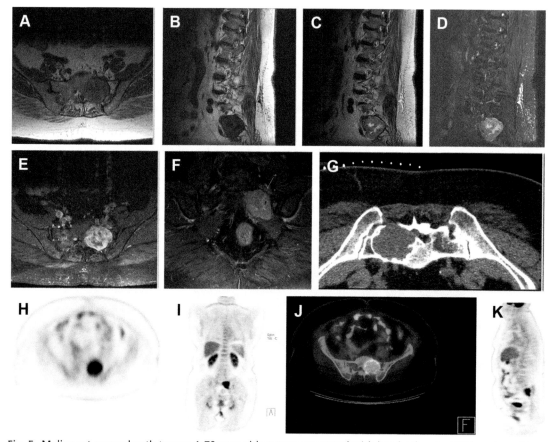

Fig. 5. Malignant nerve sheath tumor: A 70-year-old woman presented with low back pain. MR imaging of lumbar spine incidentally found a 4.7 by 4.4 by 4.8 cm lobular, well-defined heterogeneous T1 hyposignal (*A, B*), T2 intermediate to hypersignal (*C*), and STIR hypersignal intensity (*D*) mass centered at the left sacrum vertebra (S1) foramen, containing foci of central necrosis. On further postcontrast imaging, the lesion shows heterogeneous enhancement (*E, F*). The lesion underwent CT-guided biopsy with which osseous erosion with extension of the mass into the left S1 vertebral body and the left aspect of the sacral spinal canal was identified (*G*). PET-CT showed an intensely FDG avid lesion centered at left S1 foramen with an SUV_{max} of 8.9 (*H–K*).

Additional potential metrics for the assessment of malignant transformation to MPNST and tumor burden are total lesion glycolysis and total metabolic tumor volume.[101] One study even used a combination of FDG PET-CT and 11C-Methionine to demonstrate an even greater sensitivity and specificity.[109]

Despite its ability to detect malignant transformation from NF to MPNST, FDG PET-CT is unable to differentiate schwannomas from malignant sarcomas. Schwannomas are benign and often solitary peripheral nerve sheath tumors unassociated with NF1 and can present with a wide range of FDG uptake values. It is for these reasons that FDG PET-CT must be used with caution in distinguishing MPNSTs and other tumors from schwannomas.[110,111]

SUMMARY

FDG-PET-CT offers important complementary information that can be used in the diagnosis, staging, restaging, treatment response monitoring, and prognostication of STSs. Additional research is needed to strengthen the current evidence and to further elaborate on the application of FDG PET-CT, particularly for rare subtypes of STS.

REFERENCES

1. Burningham Z, Hashibe M, Spector L, et al. The epidemiology of sarcoma. Clin Sarcoma Res 2012;2:14.
2. Weitz J, Antonescu CR, Brennan MF. Localized extremity soft tissue sarcoma: improved knowledge with unchanged survival over time. J Clin Oncol 2003;21:2719–25.
3. Rodrigues-Alfonso B, Mucientes Rasilla J, Casanovas M, et al. 18F-FDG PET in STS; when to image? Rev Esp Med Nucl Imagen Mol 2014; 33(1):43–9.
4. American Cancer Society. Cancer facts and figures 2015. Available at: http://www.cancer.org/cancer/sarcoma-adultsofttissuecancer/detailed guide/sarcoma-adult-soft-tissue-cancer-key-statistics. Accessed June 2, 2015.
5. Early JF, Conrad EU. Imaging in sarcoma. J Nucl Med 2011;52:1903–13.
6. Sorensen SA, Mulvihill JJ, Nielsen A. Long-term follow up of von Recklinghausen neurofibromatosis. N Engl J Med 1986;314:1010–5.
7. D'Agostino AN, Soule EH, Miller RH. Sarcomas of the peripheral nerves and somatic soft tissue associated with multiple neurofibromatosis (von Recklinghausen's disease). Cancer 1963;16: 1015–27.
8. Kern KA, Brunetti A, Norton JA, et al. Metabolic imaging of human extremity musculoskeletal tumors by PET. J Nucl Med 1988;29:181–6.
9. Schulte M, Brecht-Krauss D, Heymer B, et al. Grading of tumors and tumorlike lesions of bone: evaluation by FDG PET. J Nucl Med 2000;41: 1695–701.
10. Schulte M, Brecht-Krauss D, Heymer B, et al. Fluorodeoxyglucose positron emission tomography of soft tissue tumours: is a non-invasive determination of biological activity possible? Eur J Nucl Med 1999;26:599–605.
11. Cobben DC, Elsinga PH, Suurmeijer AJ, et al. Detection and grading of soft tissue sarcomas of the extremities with (18) F-30 -fluoro-30 -deoxy-L-thymidine. Clin Cancer Res 2004;10:1685–90.
12. Benz MR, Dry SM, Eilber FC, et al. Correlation between glycolytic phenotype and tumor grade in soft-tissue sarcomas by 18F-FDG PET. J Nucl Med 2010;51:1174–81.
13. Ioannidis JP, Lau J. 18F-FDG PET for diagnosis and grading of soft tissue sarcoma: a meta-analysis. J Nucl Med 2003;37(2):257–61.
14. Shwarzbach MH, Dimirakopoulou-Strauss A, Willeke F, et al. Clinical value of [18-F] Fluorodeoxyglucose positron emission tomography imaging in soft tissue sarcoma. Ann Surg 2000;231(3):380–6.
15. Nieweg OE, Pruim J, Van Ginkel RJ, et al. Fluorodeoxyglucose PET imaging of soft tissue sarcoma. J Nucl Med 1996;37(2):2257–61.
16. Bastiannet E, Groen H, Jager PL, et al. The value of FDG-PET in the detection, grading and response to therapy of soft tissue sarcoma and bone sarcomas; a systematic review and meta-analysis. Cancer Treat Rev 2004;30(1):83–101.
17. Lodge MA, Lucas JD, Marsden MPK, et al. A PET study of 18FDG uptake in soft tissue masses. Eur J Nucl Med 1999;26(1):22–30.
18. Dancheva Z, Bochev P, Chaushev B, et al. Dual-time point imaging 18FDG-PET/CT imaging may be useful in assessing local recurrent disease in high grade bone and soft tissue sarcoma. Nucl Med Rev Cent East Eur 2016;19(1):22–7.
19. Lucas JD, O'Dohetry MJ, Wong JC, et al. Evaluation of Fluorodeoxyglucose positron emission tomography in the management of soft tissue sarcomas. J Bone Joint Surg Br 1998;80(3):441–7.
20. Volker T, Denecke T, Steffen I, et al. Positron emission tomography for staging of pediatric sarcoma patients: results of a prospective multicenter trial. J Clin Oncol 2007;25:5435–41.
21. Ricard F, Cimarelli S, Deshayes E, et al. Additional benefit of F-18 FDG PET/CT in the staging and follow-up of pediatric rhabdomyosarcoma. Clin Nucl Med 2011;36:672–7.
22. Fortes DL, Allen MS, Lowe VJ, et al. The sensitivity of 18F-fluorodeoxyglucose positron emission

tomography in the evaluation of metastatic pulmonary nodules. Eur J Cardiothorac Surg 2008;34:1223–7.

23. Fuglo HM, Jorgensen SM, Loft A, et al. The diagnostic and prognostic value of 18F-FDG PET/CT in the initial assessment of high-grade bone and soft tissue sarcoma. A retrospective study of 89 patients. Eur J Nucl Med Mol Imaging 2012;39:1416–24.

24. Yang HL, Liu T, Wang XM, et al. Diagnosis of bone metastases: a meta-analysis comparing 18FDG PET, CT, MRI and bone scintigraphy. Eur Radiol 2011;21:2604–17.

25. Roberge D, Vakilian S, Alabed YZ, et al. FDG PET/CT in initial staging of adult soft-tissue sarcoma. Sarcoma 2012;2012:960194.

26. Eugene T, Corradini N, Carlier T, et al. 18F-FDG–PET/CT in initial staging and assessment of early response to chemotherapy of pediatric rhabdomyosarcomas. Nucl Med Commun 2012;33:1089–95.

27. Kole AC, Nieweg OE, van Ginkel RJ, et al. Detection of local recurrence of soft-tissue sarcoma with positron emission tomography using [18F] fluorodeoxyglucose. Ann Surg Oncol 1997;4(1):57–63.

28. Al-Ibraheem A, Buck AK, Benz MR, et al. (18) F-fluorodeoxyglucose positron emission tomography/computed tomography for the detection of recurrent bone and soft tissue sarcoma. Cancer 2013; 119:1227–34.

29. Franzius C, Daldrup-Link HE, Wagner-Bohn A, et al. FDG-PET for detection of recurrences from malignant primary bone tumors: comparison with conventional imaging. Ann Oncol 2002;13:157–60.

30. Fendler WP, Chalkidis RP, Ilhan H, et al. Evaluation of several FDG PET parameters for prediction of soft tissue tumour grade at primary diagnosis and recurrence. Eur Radiol 2015;25:2214–21.

31. Evilevitch V, Weber WA, Tap WD, et al. Reduction of glucose metabolic activity is more accurate than change in size at predicting histopathologic response to neoadjuvant therapy in high-grade soft tissue sarcomas. Clin Cancer Res 2008;14(3): 715–8.

32. Schuetze SM, Rubin BP, Vernon C, et al. Use of positron emission tomography in localized extremity soft tissue sarcoma treated with neoadjuvant chemotherapy. Cancer 2005;103:339–48.

33. Benz MR, Czernin J, Allen-Auerbach MS, et al. FDG-PET/CT imaging predicts histopathologic treatment responses after the initial cycle of neoadjuvant chemotherapy in high-grade soft-tissue sarcomas. Clin Cancer Res 2009;15:2856–63.

34. Eary JF, Conrad EU, O'Sullivan J, et al. Sarcoma mid-therapy [F-18] fluorodeoxyglucose positron emission tomography (FDG PET) and patient outcome. J Bone Joint Surg Am 2014;96:152–8.

35. Baffle A, Zugaro L, Catalucci A, et al. Soft tissue liposarcoma: histological subtypes, MRI and CT findings. Radiol Med 2002;104:140–9.

36. Kudo H, Inaoka T, Tokuyama W, et al. Round cell liposarcoma arising left foot. Jpn J Radiol 2012; 30(10):852–7.

37. Enzinger FM, Weiss SW. Liposarcoma. In: Glodblum JR, Weiss SW, Folpe AL, editors. Soft tissue tumors. 5th edition. St Louis (MO): Mosby; 2008. p. 477–516.

38. Murphey MD, Arcara LK, Fanburg-Smith J. Imaging of musculoskeletal liposarcoma with radiologic–pathologic correlation. Radiographics 2005;25:1371–95.

39. Haniball J, Sumathi VP, Kindblom LG, et al. Prognostic factors and metastatic patterns in primary myxoid/round-cell liposarcoma. Sarcoma 2011; 2011:538085.

40. Antonescu CR, Tschernyavsky SJ, Decuseara R, et al. Prognostic impact of P53 status, TLS-CHOP fusion transcript structure, and histological grade in myxoid liposarcoma: a molecular and clinicopathologic study of 82 cases. Clin Cancer Res 2001;7(12):3977–87.

41. Nishida Y, Tsukushi S, Nakashima H, et al. Clinicopathologic prognostic factors of pure myxoid liposarcoma of the extremities and trunk wall. Clin Orthop Relat Res 2010;468(11):3041–6.

42. Matsubara T, Kusuzaki K, Matsumine A, et al. Can a less radical surgery using photodynamic therapy with acridine orange be equal to a wide-margin resection? Clin Orthop Relat Res 2013;471(3):792–802.

43. Kransdorf MJ, Bancroft LW, Peterson JJ, et al. Imaging of fatty tumors: distinction of lipoma and well-differentiated liposarcoma. Radiology 2002; 224:99–104.

44. Suzuki R, Watanabe H, Yanagava T, et al. PET evaluation of fatty tumors in the extremity: possibility of using the standardized uptake value (SUV) to differentiate benign tumors from liposarcoma. Ann Nucl Med 2005;19(8):661–70.

45. Brenner W, Eary JF, Hwang W, et al. Risk assessment in liposarcoma patients based on FDG PET imaging. Eur J Nucl Med Mol Imaging 2006;33:1290–5.

46. Schwarzbach MH, Dimitrakopoulou-Strauss A, Mechtersheimer G, et al. Assessment of soft tissue lesions suspicious for liposarcoma by F18-deoxyglucose (FDG) positron emission tomography (PET). Anticancer Res 2001;21(5):3609–14.

47. Tateishi U, Yamaguchi U, Seki K, et al. Bone and soft-tissue sarcoma: preoperative staging with fluorine 18 fluorodeoxyglucose PET/CT and conventional imaging. Radiology 2007;245:839–47.

48. Conill C, Setoain X, Colomo L, et al. Diagnostic efficacy of bone scintigraphy, magnetic resonance imaging, and positron emission tomography in bone metastases of myxoid liposarcoma. J Magn Reson Imaging 2008;27(3):625–8.

49. NCCN clinical practice guidelines in oncology. Soft tissue sarcoma. Version 3. 2012. Available at:

http://www.nccn.org/professionals/physician_gls/pdf/sarcoma.pdf. Accessed October 1, 2012.

50. Dei Tos AP. Classification of pleomorphic sarcomas: where are we now? Histopathology 2006; 48:51–62.

51. Al-Agha OM, Igbokwe AA. Malignant fibrous histiocytoma: between the past and the present. Arch Pathol Lab Med 2008;132:1030–5.

52. Weiss SW, Enzinger FM. Malignant fibrous histiocytoma: an analysis of 200 cases. Cancer 1978;41:2250–66.

53. Leite C, Goodwin JW, Sinkovics JG, et al. Chemotherapy of malignant fibrous histiocytoma: a southwest oncology group report. Cancer 1977;40:2010–4.

54. Kobayashi E, Kawai A, Seki K, et al. Bilateral adrenal gland metastasis from malignant fibrous histiocytoma: value of [F-18] FDG PET-CT for diagnosis of occult metastases. Ann Nucl Med 2006;20:695–8.

55. Murakawa T, Nakajima J, Fukami T, et al. Malignant fibrous histiocytoma in the anterior mediastinum. Jpn J Thorac Cardiovasc Surg 2001;49:722–7.

56. Noh HW, Park KJ, Sun JS, et al. Primary pulmonary malignant fibrous histiocytoma mimics pulmonary artery aneurysm with partial thrombosis: various radiologic evaluations. Eur Radiol 2008;18:1653–7.

57. Hwang SS, Park SY, Park YH. The CT and 18-F FDG PET/CT appearance of primary renal malignant fibrous histiocytoma. J Med Imaging Radiat Oncol 2010;54:365–7.

58. Ho L, Meka M, Gamble BK, et al. Left maxillary sinus malignant fibrous histiocytoma on FDG PET-CT. Clin Nucl Med 2009;34:967–8.

59. Yoo RE, Choi SH, Park SH, et al. Primary intracerebral malignant fibrous histiocytoma: CT, MRI and PET-CT findings. J Neuroimaging 2013;23(1):141–4.

60. Hoshi M, Oebisu N, Takada J, et al. Role of FDG-PET/CT for monitoring soft tissue tumors. Oncol Lett 2014;7(4):1243–8.

61. Jadvar H, Fishman AJ. Evaluation of rare tumors with [F-18] fludeoxyglucose positron emission tomography. Clin Positron Imaging 1999;2(3):153–8.

62. Adler LP, Blair HF, Williams RP, et al. Grading liposarcoma with PET using [18F] FDG. J Comput Assist Tomogr 1990;14(6):960–2.

63. Eary JF, Conrad EU, Bruckner JD, et al. Quantitative [F-18] fluorodeoxyglucose positron emission tomography in pretreatment and grading of sarcoma. Clin Cancer Res 1998;4:1215–20.

64. Warbey VS, Ferner RE, Dunn JT, et al. [(18) F] FDG PET/CT in the diagnosis of malignant peripheral nerve sheath tumours in neurofibromatosis type-1. Eur J Nucl Med Mol Imaging 2009;36:751–7.

65. Griffeth LK, Dehdashti F, McGuire AH, et al. PET evaluation of soft-tissue masses with fluorine-18 fluoro-2-deoxy-D-gtucose. Radiology 1992;182:185–94.

66. Watanabe H, Shinozaki T, Yanagawa T, et al. Glucose metabolic analysis of musculoskeletal tumors using fluorine-I 8-FDG PET as an aid to preoperative planning. J Bone Joint Surg Br 2000;82-B:760–7.

67. Kole AC, Nieweg OE, Hoekstra HJ, et al. Fluorine-18-fluorodeoxyglucose assessment of glucose metabolism in bone tumors. J Nucl Med 1998;39(5):810–5.

68. Tewfik JN, Greene GS. Fluorine-18-deoxyglucose–positron emission tomography imaging with magnetic resonance and computed tomographic correlation in the evaluation of bone and soft-tissue sarcomas: a pictorial essay. Curr Probl Diagn Radiol 2008;37(4):178–88.

69. Tateishi U, Kawai A, Chuman H, et al. PET/CT allows stratification of responders to neoadjuvant chemotherapy for high-grade sarcoma: a prospective study. Clin Nucl Med 2011;36:526–32.

70. Aoki J, Endo K, Watanabe H, et al. FDG-PET for evaluating musculoskeletal tumors: a review. J Orthop Sci 2003;8:435–41.

71. Jones DN, McCowage GB, Sostman HD, et al. Monitoring of neoadjuvant therapy response of soft-tissue and musculoskeletal sarcoma using fluorine- 18-FDG PET. J Nucl Med 1996;37(9):1438–44.

72. Charest M, Hickeson M, Lisbona R, et al. FDG PET/CT imaging in primary osseous and soft tissue sarcomas: a retrospective review of 212 cases. Eur J Nucl Med Mol Imaging 2009;36(12):1944–51.

73. Dagher R, Helman L. Rhabdomyosarcoma: an overview. Oncologist 1999;4:34–44.

74. Ries LAG, Smith MA, Gurney JG, et al, editors. Cancer incidence and survival among children and adolescents: United States SEER Program 1975–1995. NIH Pub. No. 99-4649. Bethesda (MD): National Cancer Institute; 1999.

75. Hayes-Jordan A, Andrassy R. Rhabdomyosarcoma in children. Curr Opin Pediatr 2009;21:373–8.

76. Klem ML, Grewal RK, Wexler LH, et al. PET for staging in rhabdomyosarcoma: an evaluation of PET as an adjunct to current staging tools. J Pediatr Hematol Oncol 2007;29:9–14.

77. Dharmarajan KV, Wexler LH, Gavane S, et al. Positron emission tomography (PET) evaluation after initial chemotherapy and radiation therapy predicts local control in rhabdomyosarcoma. Int J Radiat Oncol Biol Phys 2012;84:996–1002.

78. Federico SM, Wu J, Spunt SL, et al. Comparison of PET–CT and conventional imaging in staging pediatric rhabdomyosarcoma. Pediatr Blood Cancer 2012;60:1128–34.

79. Tateishi U, Hosono A, Makimoto A, et al. Comparative study of FDG PET/CT and conventional

imaging in the staging of rhabdomyosarcoma. Ann Nucl Med 2009;23:155–61.

80. Baum SH, Fruhwald M, Rahbar K, et al. Contribution of PET/CT to prediction of outcome in children and young adults with rhabdomyosarcoma. J Nucl Med 2011;52:1535–40.

81. Krasin M, Hua C, Spunt SL, et al. FDG-PET/CT prior or subsequent to radiation is a poor predictor of local outcome in patients with group III rhabdomyosarcoma. Int J Radiat Oncol Biol Phys 2011; 1:S116.

82. Quartuccio N, Treglia G, Salsano M, et al. The role of fluorine-18- fluorodeoxyglucose positron emission tomography in staging and restaging of patients with osteosarcoma. Radiol Oncol 2013;47: 97–102.

83. Barger RL, Nandalur KR. Diagnostic performance of dual-time 18F-FDG PET in the diagnosis of pulmonary nodules: a meta-analysis. Acad Radiol 2012;19:153–8.

84. Meis-Kindblom JM, Kindblom LG. Angiosarcoma of soft tissue: a study of 80 cases. Am J Surg Pathol 1998;22(6):683–97.

85. Fedok FG, Levin RJ, Maloney ME, et al. Angiosarcoma: current review. Am J Otolaryngol 1999; 20(4):223–31.

86. Hori Y, Funabashi N, Miyauchi H, et al. Angiosarcoma in the right atria demonstrated by fusion images of multislice computed tomography and positron emission tomography using F-18 fluoro-deoxyglucose. Int J Cardiol 2007;123(1): 15–7.

87. Watanabe S, Yano F, Kita T, et al. 18F-FDG-PET/CT as an indicator for resection of pulmonary epithelioid hemangioendothelioma. Ann Nucl Med 2008; 22:521–4.

88. Freudenberg LS, Rosenbaum SJ, Schulte-Herbrüggen J, et al. Diagnosis of a cardiac angiosarcoma by fluorine-18 fluorodeoxyglucose positron emission tomography. Eur Radiol 2002;12(3): 158–61.

89. Oe A, Habu D, Kawabe J, et al. A case of diffuse hepatic angiosarcoma diagnosed by FDG-PET. Ann Nucl Med 2005;19(6):519–21.

90. Lin E. Diagnosis of venous angiosarcoma by FDG PET/CT. Clin Nucl Med 2008;33(1):66–7.

91. Tokmak E, Özkan E, Yağcı S, et al. F18-FDG PET/CT scanning in angiosarcoma: report of two cases. Mol Imaging Radionucl Ther 2011;20(2): 63–6.

92. Vasanawala MS, Wang Y, Quon A, et al. F-18 fluorodeoxyglucose PET/CT as an imaging tool for staging and restaging cutaneous angiosarcoma of the scalp. Clin Nucl Med 2006;31(9): 534–7.

93. Lee WW, So Y, Kang SY, et al. F-18 fluorodeoxyglucose positron emission tomography for differential diagnosis and prognosis prediction of vascular tumors. Oncol Lett 2017;14(1):665–72.

94. Rest CC, Botton E, Robinet G, et al. FDG PET in epithelioid hemangioendothelioma. Clin Nucl Med 2004;29:789–92.

95. Jadhav R, Gupta K, Prasad R, et al. Case based pictorial review of FDG PET CT imaging in angiosarcoma. J Nucl Med 2017;58(Suppl 1):1000.

96. Chang KJ, Lim I, Park JY, et al. The role of 18F-FDG PET/CT as a prognostic factor in patients with synovial sarcoma. Nucl Med Mol Imaging 2015;49(1): 33–41.

97. Bakri A, Shinagare AB, Krajewski KM, et al. Synovial sarcoma: imaging features of common and uncommon primary sites, metastatic patterns, and treatment response. AJR Am J Roentgenol 2012; 199(2):208–15.

98. Kransdorf MJ, Murrphy MD. Radiologic evaluation of soft-tissue masses: a current perspective. AJR Am J Roentgenol 2000;175(3):575–87.

99. Rayamajhi S, Reddy A, Agrawl K, et al. Utility of F-18 FDG PET/CT in synovial cell sarcoma. J Nucl Med 2015;56(Suppl 3):37.

100. Lisle JW, Early JF, O'Sullivan J, et al. Risk assessment based on FDG-PET imaging in patients with synovial sarcoma. Clin Orthop Relat Res 2009; 467(6):1605–11.

101. Van Der Guucht A, Zehou O, Djelbani-Ahmad S, et al. Metabolic tumor burden measured by FDG PET/CT predicts malignant transformation in patients with neurofibromatosis typer-1. PLoS One 2016;11(3):e0151809.

102. Cardona S, Schwarzbach M, Hinz U, et al. Evaluation of FDG to assess the nature of neurogenic tumors. Eur J Surg Oncol 2003;29:536–41.

103. Enzinger FM, Weiss SW. Malignant tumours of peripheral nerves. In: Enzinger FM, Weiss SW, editors. Soft tissue tumors. Elsevier Health Sciences :2001; 31: p. 1209–63.

104. Anghileri M, Miceli R, Fiore M, et al. Malignant peripheral nerve sheath tumors: prognostic factors and survival in a series of patients treated at a single institution. Cancer 2006;107:1065–74.

105. Brenner W, Friedrich RE, Gawad KA, et al. Prognostic relevance of FDG PET in patients with neurofibromatosis type-1 and malignant peripheral nerve sheath tumours. Eur J Nucl Med Mol Imaging 2006; 33:428–32.

106. Khiewvan B, Macapinlac HA, Lev D, et al. The value of 18F-FDG PET/CT in the management of malignant peripheral nerve sheath tumors. Eur J Nucl Med Mol Imaging 2014;41:1756–66.

107. Benz MR, Czernin J, Dry SM, et al. Quantitative F18-fluorodeoxyglucose positron emission tomography accurately characterizes peripheral nerve sheath tumors as malignant or benign. Cancer 2010;116:451–8.

108. Ferner RE, Golding JF, Smith M, et al. [18F]2-flu-oro-2-deoxy-D-glucose positron emission tomography (FDG PET) as a diagnostic tool for neurofibromatosis 1 (NF1) associated malignant peripheral nerve sheath tumours (MPNSTs): a long-term clinical study. Ann Oncol 2008;19: 390–4.

109. Bredella MA, Torriani M, Hornicek F, et al. Value of PET in the assessment of patients with neurofibromatosis type 1. AJR Am J Roentgenol 2007;189(4):928–35.

110. Ahmed AR, Watanabe H, Aoki J, et al. Schwannoma of the extremities. Eur J Nucl Med 2001; 28(10):1541–51.

111. Beaulieu S, Rubin B, Djang D, et al. Positron emission tomography of schwannoma: emphasizing its potential in preoperative planning. AJR Am J Roentgenol 2004;182(4):971–4.

Applications of PET/CT and PET/MR Imaging in Primary Bone Malignancies

Ashkan Heshmatzadeh Behzadi, MD[a],*,
Syed Imran Raza, MBBS[a], John A. Carrino, MD, MPH[b],
Christos Kosmas, MD[c], Ali Gholamrezanezhad, MD[d],
Kyle Basques, MD[c], George R. Matcuk Jr, MD[d],
Jay Patel, MD[a], Hossein Jadvar, MD, PhD, MPH, MBA[e]

KEYWORDS

• PET/CT • PET/MRI • Primary bone malignancies

KEY POINTS

- The hybrid modalities of FDG PET/CT and PET/MRI have improved oncologic imaging that combine the sensitivity of metabolic imaging with the specificity of anatomic imaging.
- PET/CT is a valuable modality in the diagnosis, staging, and assessment of therapeutic response to treatment of several primary musculoskeletal malignancies.
- PET/MRI is promising modality, which allowed detailed local staging and tissue characterization, all while reducing patient's exposure to radiation.

INTRODUCTION

Diagnostic imaging plays a central role in the evaluation and management of oncologic disease involving the musculoskeletal system (Figs. 1–5). Standard imaging modalities used in current practice include conventional radiography, computed tomography (CT) scanning, Magnetic resonance imaging (MRI), and skeletal scintigraphy.[1,2] In recent years, PET imaging has also emerged as a complementary modality in musculoskeletal imaging, using various radiopharmaceutical agents to improve detection and characterization of the pathophysiology of disease.[3] Fusion of PET-acquired images with CT scans or MRI has significantly improved the overall diagnostic accuracy.[4] The objective of this article is to review the current role of PET/CT scans and PET/MRI hybrid imaging in the evaluation of primary malignancies of the skeletal system, with an emphasis on clinical usefulness, imaging findings, and current limitations.

ROLE OF HYBRID IMAGING IN BONE MALIGNANCY

Viable malignant primary bone tumors are usually 18F-fluorodeoxyglucose (FDG) avid.[4,5] PET

[a] Department of Radiology, Weill Cornell Medical Center, 525 East 68th Street, New York, NY 10065, USA; [b] Department of Radiology and Imaging, 535 East 70th Street, Hospital for Special Surgery, New York, NY 10021, USA; [c] Department of Radiology and Imaging, University Hospitals of Cleveland, Case Western Reserve University, 10900 Euclid Avenue, Cleveland, OH 44106, USA; [d] Division of Musculoskeletal Radiology, Department of Radiology, Keck School of Medicine, University of Southern California (USC), Los Angeles, CA 90007, USA; [e] Division of Nuclear Medicine, Department of Radiology, Keck School of Medicine, University of Southern California, Los Angeles, CA 90007, USA
* Corresponding author. Department of Radiology, Weill Cornell Medical College, 416 East 55th Street, New York, NY 10022.
E-mail address: ashkan.hbehzadi@gmail.com

PET Clin 13 (2018) 623–634
https://doi.org/10.1016/j.cpet.2018.05.012
1556-8598/18/Published by Elsevier Inc.

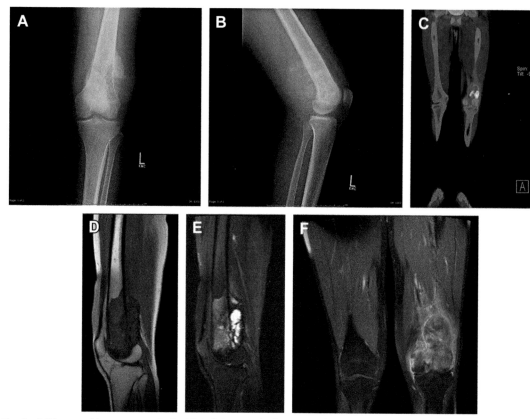

Fig. 1. A 19-year-old man presented with left knee pain for 1 month. The radiograph (*A*, *B*) shows aggressive osteolytic lesion of the distal left femur with sunburst periosteal reaction. The lesion demonstrates heterogeneous increased metabolic activity on PET/CT with fludeoxyglucose F 18 (FDG) with a maximum standardized uptake value of 8.8 (*C*). On MRI, the lesion demonstrates heterogeneous intermediate signal intensity on T1-weighted imaging (*D*), hypersignal on short tau inversion recovery imaging (*E*), and heterogeneous postcontrast enhancement (*F*) with cortical breakthrough, aggressive periosteal reaction, and associated soft tissue mass. Histopathologic evaluation confirmed osteosarcoma.

imaging using FDG produces images that allow for the diagnosis of these neoplasms, initial staging, selection of biopsy sites, evaluation of treatment response, and assessment for tumor recurrence.[3,4,6,7] When CT images are contemporaneously acquired, the PET and CT data are spatially co-registered, allowing for significantly improved localization of metabolic abnormalities. Integrated PET/CT devices allow for reduced scanning time and improved PET image quality and quantitation using CT attenuation correction reconstruction techniques.[6]

In the FDG PET component of these studies, lesions are assessed primarily based on their maximum standardized uptake value (SUV_{max}) and graded accordingly.[8] As methods evolve, metabolic activity will become a useful marker for differentiating between benign and malignant lesions. Moreover, dual time point imaging, which involves measuring the SUV_{max} at multiple sequential intervals after radiotracer injection, may also be beneficial in differentiating benign lesions from malignant processes.[9–11]

Recently, interest in hybrid PET/MRI has grown, particularly in evaluation of the musculoskeletal system. This new modality couples the physiologic information acquired from PET with the unparalleled soft tissue resolution and contrast of MRI to provide more accurate diagnoses.[12] In addition, MRI can be used to provide additional functional information using perfusion techniques and diffusion-weighted imaging.[13–15] With hybrid PET/MRI, a patient's oncologic disease can potentially be fully characterized and staged in a single imaging session.[14]

The morphologic characteristics of tumors are critical in making the correct diagnosis.[2,7,16] The MRI and CT components of hybrid imaging provide important morphologic information that PET scans alone cannot provide and, therefore, it is

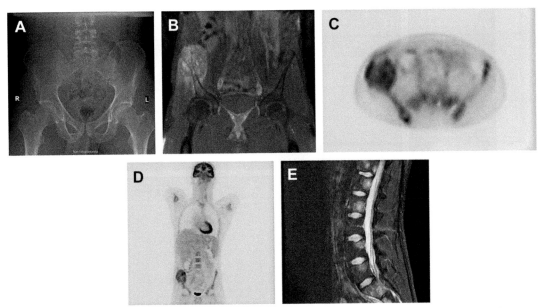

Fig. 2. A 21-year-old man presented with right hemipelvic pain. Initial radiographs were interpreted as unremarkable, but retrospectively demonstrated asymmetric thinning of the right iliac and suspect rarefaction of the right iliac bone compared with the contralateral side (A). On MRI (B), a large enhancing destructive lesion involving the anterior right iliac crest was identified, the biopsy of which showed Ewing's sarcoma. PET/CT with fludeoxyglucose F 18 for initial staging demonstrated a heterogeneously hypermetabolic lesion centered at the right iliac crest with maximum standardized uptake value of 8.2 and several metastatic foci involving the posterior right iliac crest, left hemisacrum, and thoracolumbar spine (C, D). MRI of the spine confirmed metastatic disease to the vertebrae (E).

essential that the interpreting radiologist be familiar with the conventional imaging appearance of bone tumors.[9,10] The morphologic characteristics of lesions can be preliminarily evaluated on the whole-body CT or MRI portion of the examination, which is obtained contemporaneously with the PET dataset, and then further correlated with dedicated small field-of-view MRI sequences or other anatomic imaging as necessary.[2,4,17]

CLINICAL APPLICATIONS
Osteosarcoma

Osteosarcoma is the most common primary malignant bone tumor.[18,19] Accurate initial staging and restaging after treatment is critical to patient care. Prognosis strongly depends on tumor size and the presence of metastatic disease at initial presentation. To put this into perspective, the 5-year survival decreases drastically from 70.1% in

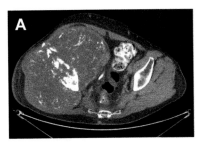
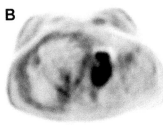
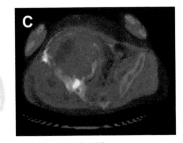

Fig. 3. A 72-year-old man with history of pathologically proven chondrosarcoma presented with recurrent mass at the right iliac fossa. Computed tomography scanning demonstrated a large heterogeneous mass with chondroid matrix, concerning for recurrent chondrosarcoma (A). On PET with fludeoxyglucose F 18, a 19.4 × 13.3 × 17.6 cm heterogeneous destructive mass centered at the right iliac bone was identified, demonstrating peripheral hypermetabolism and central hypometabolism, representing large central necrosis. The maximum standardized uptake value was 9.4 (B, C).

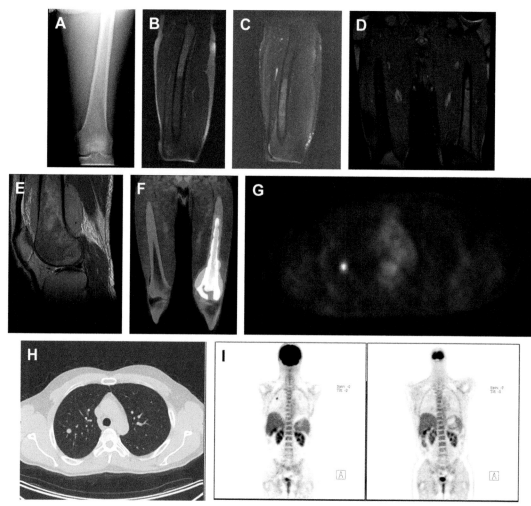

Fig. 4. A 40-year-old man with left knee pain demonstrated a permeative osteolytic lesion of the distal left femur (*A*). On MRI, a large marrow-replacing lesion was identified, which shows decreased T1-weighted uptake (*B*) and heterogeneously increased short tau inversion recovery (*C*) hypersignal intensity with heterogeneous postcontrast enhancement (*D, E*). The lesion is intensely hypermetabolic on PET with maximum standardized uptake value of 17.3 (*F*). The lesion was pathologically diagnosed as T-cell lymphoma. There is a small, metabolically active soft tissue density pulmonary nodule within the right lobe with maximum standardized uptake value of 3.7 (*G, H*), concerning for a metastatic lesion. The pulmonary lesion was completely resolved on postchemotherapy PET (*I*).

localized disease to 31.6% in the presence of metastasis.[20–24] Response to preoperative neoadjuvant chemotherapy is also a very important prognostic factor for disease-free survival.[25,26]

Imaging plays a key role in the management of osteosarcoma, with the initial diagnosis frequently made with conventional radiography, and with local staging performed with MRI to assess local soft tissue extension, bone marrow infiltration, and the presence of osseous skip lesions.[20,21] FDG PET scanning has a promising role in the management of osteosarcoma given its ability to help distinguish viable primary and recurrent

neoplasm from successfully treated disease and benign entities.

Like most other malignant tumors, osteosarcoma has an increased rate of glycolysis and consequently demonstrates increased uptake of FDG.[4] Therefore, FDG PET readily demonstrates local and systemic sites of activity that correlate well with disease severity.[27,28] FDG PET/CT scanning is highly useful for the evaluation of osteosarcoma, with a sensitivity of nearly 100% in initial staging, 85.7% in locally recurrent disease, and 95% in identifying distant metastasis.[29,30] Although PET/CT scanning has some limitations

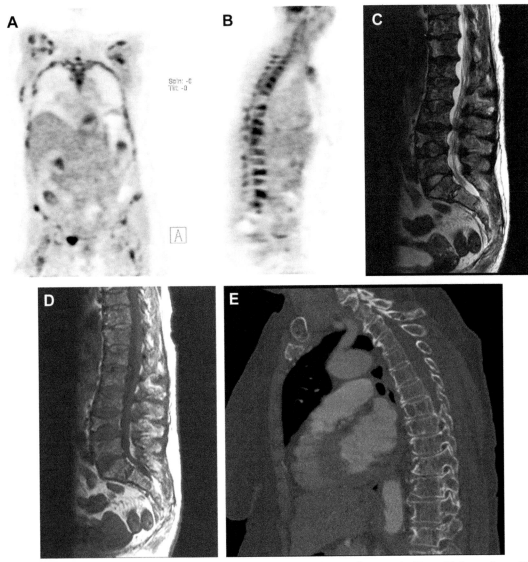

Fig. 5. A 65-year-old woman with generalized bone pain and anemia was diagnosed with multiple myeloma. PET-computed tomography (CT) scans revealed widespread osseous (*A*) myelomatous lesions with several infiltrative lesions of the spine (*B*) and superimposed pathologic fractures, as confirmed on MRI (*C*, *D*) and CT (*E*). The maximum standardized uptake value of the lesions in the lumbar spine was up to 17.2.

in the evaluation of pulmonary and lymph node metastases, it has been shown to have superior accuracy over bone scans in the detection of osseous dissemination.[29,30]

One of the main strengths of FDG PET scanning in osteosarcoma is in determining the metabolic response to treatment. SUV measurements have been found to parallel histopathologic findings, with high SUV values correlating with increased mitotic counts and lower values corresponding with areas of tumor necrosis. For example, Cheon and colleagues[25] and Ye and colleagues[26] demonstrated that a reduction in

SUV_{max} after chemotherapy correlates well with degree of tumor necrosis and subsequent patient outcome. In a recent study, Davis and colleagues[27] followed 34 patients with osteosarcoma and surveyed SUV_{max} on routine posttreatment surveillance for up to 10 weeks. The percent change of SUV_{max} from baseline to week 10 served as a metabolic predictor that correlated well with histologic response to therapy. A separate metaanalysis of 8 studies comprising 178 patients with osteosarcoma found that a postchemotherapy SUV_{max} of 2.5 or less and a ratio of SUV_{max} posttherapy to

SUV$_{max}$ pretherapy of 0.5 or less was a valuable predictor of histologic response to chemotherapy.[31] In another prospective study assessing therapeutic response in pediatric osteosarcomas, FDG PET scanning was also able to help discriminate responders from nonresponders.[31] Hence, PET/CT scanning may play an important role in the early identification of patients who are not responding to treatment and may benefit from a change in therapy.

FDG PET scanning also holds promise in its ability to distinguish posttherapy changes from disease recurrence, a challenging but important task. Studies have shown that FDG-PET can differentiate posttreatment changes from disease recurrence with greater sensitivity and specificity than other imaging modalities.[32] In particular, the degree of FDG uptake as calculated by SUV$_{max}$ may be helpful in distinguishing viable osteosarcoma from treated disease.[24] Although there remain some overlap in ranges of SUV values between malignant and nonmalignant processes, work continues to refine measurement techniques and guidelines to improve the specificity of FDG PET scanning.[28,33]

Although the value of PET/MRI for the staging and follow-up of osteosarcoma has not yet been well-established, some promising early results have been observed.[34,35] A study by Eiber and colleagues[36] compared the performance of PET/MRI and PET/CT scanning for the detection of bone lesions. These investigators found that anatomic localization and allocation of PET-positive lesions was superior on PET/MRI compared with PET/CT scanning, whereas detection and characterization was found to be on par with PET/CT scanning, possibly owing to inclusion of primarily FDG-avid lesions. The SUV$_{mean}$ in bone lesions was on average 12.4% ± 15.5% lower for PET/MRI than for PET/CT scanning, although this difference between modalities was not statistically significant.

At present, MRI is the preferred imaging modality for local tumor staging of osteosarcoma. PET scanning lends itself well to nodal staging, whereas PET scanning and MRI together are highly accurate for the detection of metastases.[34] Hence, whole body PET/MRI with concurrent diagnostic MRI imaging of the primary site of osteosarcoma can allow for complete TNM staging in a single session, providing convenience and resource savings as well as decreasing radiation exposure. In addition, the PET component can guide diagnostic biopsies and in turn allow for correct staging and grading, with subsequent impact on treatment selection and outcome.[16,34]

Ewing's Sarcoma

Ewing's sarcoma is the second most common primary malignancy of bone, with a peak incidence in children and adolescents aged 4 to 15 years. FDG PET/CT scanning has become a valuable imaging modality in staging, restaging, and assessment of treatment response in patients with Ewing's sarcoma, largely owing to its ability to provide metabolic information that is, not feasible with other modalities.[37–39]

Similar to the case with osteosarcoma, MRI is mainstay imaging in staging of Ewing's sarcoma. However, both MRI and CT imaging are limited in distinguishing viable from nonviable neoplastic tissues.[38,40] FDG PET scanning has been shown to detect tumor progression and regression even before morphologic alterations are seen on conventional imaging modalities, based on differences in intensity of FDG uptake.[35,37,41] PET/CT scanning in particular is already in use for this purpose in Ewing's sarcoma, and is able to differentiate viable from nonviable tumor with high sensitivity and specificity.[42] Typical viable Ewing's sarcoma demonstrates SUVs ranging from 3 to 10, with higher values correlating well with higher tumor grade. PET/CT scanning is also highly efficacious in detecting lymph node and bone metastases, with sensitivity values of 90% to 98% compared with 25% to 83% for conventional imaging methods, with good specificity as well (97% for PET/CT scanning vs 78% for conventional imaging).[41,43] The exception was in the detection of lung metastases, which was more accurate with CT scanning.[41]

Besides providing prognostic data, findings on PET/CT scanning during and after treatment can also guide decision making about continuing or altering therapy in patients with Ewing's sarcoma. For example, a study by Bredella and colleagues[44] demonstrated that a 30% decrease or increase in SUV reliably distinguished between adequate response to therapy and progression of disease, respectively. In addition, Hawkins and colleagues[45] showed that patients with tumors displaying a SUV$_{max}$ of less than 2.5 after neoadjuvant chemotherapy demonstrated an improvement in 4-year progression-free survival compared with those with higher SUV$_{max}$ (72% vs 27%, respectively) and that this effect was independent of initial disease stage.

A major limitation of PET/CT scanning in the pediatric population predominantly affected by Ewing's sarcoma is the relatively high radiation dose, particularly compared with whole body MRI, which does not involve ionizing radiation.[39] The introduction of whole-body PET/MRI allows for simultaneous regional staging and whole body evaluation for metastatic disease.[6,12] PET/MRI is especially helpful in overcoming some of the limitations of PET/CT scanning, specifically in the evaluation of disease in organs with relatively high background activity such as the brain, liver, kidney, and spinal canal.[7,13,14] PET/MRI may soon become the imaging modality of choice for staging of Ewing's sarcoma.

Chondrosarcoma

The diagnosis of chondrosarcoma can be challenging owing to the diverse nature of chondral neoplasms, the significant overlap with benign entities on conventional imaging, and difficulties in accurate sampling on tissue biopsy owing to tumor heterogeneity. FDG PET scanning was initially dismissed as an unreliable modality in the evaluation of chondroid neoplasms, but recent literature has demonstrated promising results. Generally, benign chondroid lesions such as enchondromas and osteochondromas are not FDG avid (SUV_{max} < 2). In contrast, most chondrosarcomas demonstrate low-grade FDG avidity (SUV_{max} > 2), with variable metabolic activity seen ranging from SUV_{max} of 1.3 to 12.4. SUV_{max} has been shown to correlate with tumor grade.[46–49] Unfortunately, there is significant overlap in SUV_{max} values between benign and malignant chondroid lesions, with SUV_{max} values between 2.0 and 4.5 having particularly poor specificity, and with up to 46% of lesions reported in a recent metaanalysis having SUV_{max} values in this range. However, recent large studies have demonstrated that, overall, when using an SUV_{max} threshold of 2.2 to 2.3, the sensitivity and specificity exceeds 90% in differentiating between benign/low-grade lesions from high-grade chondroid neoplasms.[46–51] Classifying lesions between benign/low-grade lesions and high-grade neoplasms helps clinicians to decide whether observation or active treatment is the optimal treatment strategy.[47,48]

The heterogeneity of chondroid tumors poses an ever-present risk of undersampling during biopsy and difficulty in obtaining appropriate excisional margins. FDG PET scanning ameliorates this problem by providing direct visual and quantitative assessment of tumor metabolic activity and extent. By targeting regions for biopsy with the greatest metabolic activity, radiologists and surgeons can reduce core needle biopsy sampling error, and consequently, the rate of false-negative biopsies. Subsequent correlation of imaging findings with histopathology also helps eliminate the potential error of undersampling.[46,50,51] In addition, as in other sarcomas, whole body imaging in PET/CT scanning can be used for initial staging

of chondrosarcoma and as an adjunct in postoperative imaging surveillance.[52]

There is a paucity of data on the use of PET/MRI in chondrosarcoma. One study by Purohit and colleagues[53] assessed laryngeal chondrosarcomas using PET/MRI, showing that PET/MRI successfully highlights regions of hypermetabolic dedifferentiated neoplasm (with concurrent low apparent diffusion coefficient values on diffusion-weighted imaging MRI sequences) in a background of hypometabolic, low-grade chondroid tissue. These investigators concluded that PET/MRI can provide additional functional information to supplement the morphologic mapping and histopathology of these tumors. Given the importance of accurate characterization of these heterogeneous lesions, it is expected that future research will highlight a potential role for PET/MRI in the management of chondrosarcoma.

Primary Bone Lymphoma

Primary bone lymphoma is an extranodal lymphoma that arises from the medullary cavity and manifests as a localized solitary lesion. Primary bone lymphoma is relatively uncommon, representing only 1% of all malignant lymphomas.[54,55,56] The tumor favors sites of persistent bone marrow formation, such as the femur, pelvis, tibia, fibula, and humerus.[54,56,57]

The role of FDG PET/CT scanning in the diagnosis, staging, and restaging of Hodgkin disease and non-Hodgkin lymphoma is well-established.[58,59] Accurate staging is essential for treatment planning and provides important prognostic information. PET/CT scanning can detect lymphoma with 90% sensitivity and 91% specificity, although overall positive predictive value is low, especially for disease progression.[59]

The usual appearance of primary bone lymphoma on FDG PET scanning is as a focal hypermetabolic lesion. There are few reports on the initial diagnosis of primary bone lymphomas using FDG PET or PET/CT scanning.[56,60,61] However, studies have demonstrated PET/CT scanning to be an effective modality for evaluation after therapy, particularly in documenting treatment response. In patients who respond successfully to treatment, FDG PET scanning will show a rapid decline in FDG uptake compared with baseline imaging. Similarly, any newly identified FDG-avid lesions are deemed to be recurrences. Hence, PET/CT scanning has the potential to assist in the management of patients with primary bone lymphoma.[62,63]

PET/MRI has shown encouraging results in early studies.[64,65] Sensitivity for assessment of disease burden is similar in PET/MRI and PET/CT scanning. In addition, the added information from diagnostic MRI sequences can help to characterize changes in the cellular content of lesions, particularly using diffusion-weighted imaging sequences and MRI spectroscopy.[64,66]

Multiple Myeloma

Multiple myeloma (MM) is a debilitating malignancy that is part of a spectrum of diseases ranging from monoclonal gammopathy of unknown significance to plasma cell leukemia.[67] The use of conventional radiography has traditionally been used in cases of newly diagnosed or relapsed myeloma, with the whole body skeletal survey used to assess extent of disease.[68] Radiographs typically demonstrate focal osteolytic lesions, but have a lower sensitivity in diffuse osseous involvement. They also do not provide any indication of disease activity except by monitoring changes over time.

FDG PET/CT scanning has been shown to have high sensitivity, specificity, and prognostic value in patients with MM, superior to conventional radiographs and comparable with MRI, providing valuable prognostic and therapy assessment information for the management of patients.[69] In a systematic review consisting of almost 800 patients with MM, FDG PET/CT scanning had a sensitivity and specificity of 80% to 90% and 80% to 100%, respectively, in the detection of osteolytic lesions.[70] Clinical use of FDG PET/CT scanning in myeloma has been validated in recent years with the revised Durie/Salmon PLUS staging system.[71] PET also has the advantage of identifying the degree of metabolic activity associated with focal lesions, which has been found to correlate with disease activity.[72,73] Solitary plasma cell neoplasms (plasmacytomas) are also FDG avid.[72,73] However, FDG PET scanning is somewhat less reliable when evaluating more diffuse or heterogeneous marrow involvement, with variable SUV measurements.[7] In addition, differentiating myelomatous lesions from background marrow FDG uptake can be difficult, particularly in the setting of diffuse marrow involvement.[7]

MRI in myeloma demonstrates T2 hyperintensity and T1 hypointensity in involved areas of bone, with variable contrast enhancement seen. The overall MRI pattern may be described as normal, focal, diffuse (change of signal of the entire fatty bone marrow), or a variegated/salt-and-pepper pattern (heterogeneous appearance of the entire bone marrow).[7]

Zamagni and colleagues[74] prospectively compared FDG PET/CT scanning, MRI, and whole body planar radiographs in the assessment of bone disease in 23 patients with newly diagnosed MM. PET/CT scanning was superior to plain radiographs, and highly sensitive to lesions out of the field of view of MRI, for both intramedullary and extramedullary disease. However, PET/CT scanning failed to depict some spine and pelvic lesions detected on MRI. A study by Shortt and colleagues[75] showed that a combination of data acquired from PET and whole body MRI improved specificity and positive predictive value. Bartel and colleagues[69] performed FDG PET/CT scanning in 239 patients at baseline and after neoadjuvant therapy, but before stem cell transplantation. Better overall and event-free survivals were correlated with complete normalization of FDG PET uptake before autologous stem cell transplantation.

Most studies and review articles pertaining to PET scanning and MRI have examined the 2 modalities separately.[76] However, preliminary reports suggest a role for combined PET/MRI in MM and other plasma cell dyscrasias. With the ability to image the whole body using both PET scanning and MRI, each of which can assess lesion distribution and characteristics, PET/MRI offers unique opportunities for assessing disease burden, monitoring for progression, and assessing response to treatment. For example, recent studies have demonstrated that PET/MRI can be effective in high-risk patients for initial staging and can serve as a baseline to assess treatment response as well as relapse of disease. If a patient's biochemical marker levels are increasing after therapy, PET/MRI can be used to assess for the presence of new lesions or an increase in size, avidity, or number of lesions on PET scanning.[7,76]

Giant Cell Tumor

Giant cell tumor of bone (GCT) is an uncommon primary intramedullary neoplasm, most prevalent in young adults. GCT is generally considered to be benign. However, these lesions are variable in behavior and can be locally aggressive, have a high local recurrence rate after treatment (up to 40%), and may even produce pulmonary metastases.[77,78] The management of GCT can be challenging and sometimes controversial.

On radiography and CT scanning, GCT typically manifests as an eccentric lytic lesion centered in the epiphysis of a long bone that extends to the articular surface and usually has a well-defined nonsclerotic margin. On MRI, GCT is hypointense on T1-weighted sequences, and heterogeneously intermediate to hypointense on T2-weighted sequences related to hemosiderin deposition within the tumor.[77]

On PET scanning, GCT tends to have an unusually high FDG uptake compared with other benign neoplasms of bone, and may be misdiagnosed as a malignant lesion.[51,78–81] A recent study by Muheremu and colleagues[82] demonstrated a mean lesional SUV_{max} of 9.2 ± 3.8 in 20 patients with proven GCT. Therefore, it is important to consider the diagnosis of GCT as well as soft tissue sarcomas in solitary musculoskeletal lesions with high FDG uptake.

Evaluation for pulmonary metastases of GCT can be challenging on PET. When lesions are small, they resemble pulmonary nodules, whose characterization is limited by their small size and limited spatial resolution of PET. In addition, over time these metastases can grow and show significant FDG uptake, mimicking primary malignant pulmonary lesions.[83] PET/CT scanning has been recognized as a valuable tool for early response evaluation of GCTs to new treatment options, such as denosumab.[84–87]

SUMMARY

The hybrid modalities of FDG PET/CT scanning and PET/MRI have transformed oncologic imaging by providing whole body scans that combine the sensitivity of metabolic imaging with the specificity of anatomic imaging. FDG PET/CT scanning has usefulness in the diagnosis, staging, and assessment of therapeutic response to treatment of several primary musculoskeletal malignancies. Although data on PET/MRI are limited at present, emerging studies demonstrate potentially promising applications, which allows for detailed local staging and tissue characterization, all while reducing patient's exposure to radiation.

REFERENCES

1. Hilner BE, Siegel BA, Liu D, et al. Impact of positron emission tomography/computed tomography and positron emission tomography (PET) alone on expected management of patients with cancer: initial results from the National Oncologic PET Registry. J Clin Oncol 2008;26:2155–61.

2. Lakkaraju A, Patel CN, Bradley KM, et al. PET/CT in primary musculoskeletal tumours: a step forward. Eur Radiol 2010;20(12):2959–72.

3. Blodgett TM, Meltzer CC, Townsend DW. PET/CT: form and function. Radiology 2008;242:360–85.

4. Choi YY, Kim JY, Yang SO. PET/CT in benign and malignant musculoskeletal tumors and tumor-like conditions [review]. Semin Musculoskelet Radiol 2014;18(2):133–48.

5. Watabe T, Shimosegawa E, Kato H, et al. Paradoxical reduction of cerebral blood flow after acetazolamide loading: a hemodynamic and metabolic study with (15)O PET. Neurosci Bull 2014;30: 845–56.

6. Disselhorst JA, Bezrukov I, Kolb A, et al. Principles of PET/MR imaging. J Nucl Med 2014;55:2S–10S.

7. Chaudhry AA, Gul M, Gould E, et al. Utility of positron emission tomography-magnetic resonance imaging in musculoskeletal imaging [review]. World J Radiol 2016;8(3):268–74.

8. Aoki J, Watanabe H, Shinozaki T, et al. FDG PET of primary benign and malignant bone tumors: standardized uptake value in 52 lesions. Radiology 2001;219:774–7.

9. Tian R, Su M, Tian Y, et al. Dualtime point PET/CT with F-18 FDG for the differentiation of malignant and benign bone lesions. Skeletal Radiol 2009;38: 451–8.

10. Zhuang H, Pourdehnad M, Lambright ES, et al. Dual time point 18FFDG PET imaging for differentiating malignant from inflammatory processes. J Nucl Med 2001;42:1412–7.

11. Hogendoorn PC, Athanasou N, Bielack S, et al, ESMO/EUROBONET Working Group. Bone sarcomas: ESMO clinical practice guidelines for diagnosis, treatment and follow-up. Ann Oncol 2010;21(Suppl 5):v204–13.

12. Werner MK, Schmidt H, Schwenzer NF. MR/PET: a new challenge in hybrid imaging. AJR Am J Roentgenol 2012;199:272–7.

13. Partovi S, Kohan AA, Zipp L, et al. Hybrid PET/MR imaging in two sarcoma patients - clinical benefits and implications for future trials. Int J Clin Exp Med 2014;7:640–8.

14. Fahey FH, Treves ST, Adelstein SJ. Minimizing and communicating radiation risk in pediatric nuclear medicine. J Nucl Med Technol 2012;40:13–24.

15. Hirsch FW, Sattler B, Sorge I, et al. PET/MR in children. Initial clinical experience in paediatric oncology using an integrated PET/MR scanner. Pediatr Radiol 2013;43:860–75.

16. Dehdashti F, Siegel BA, Griffeth LK, et al. Benign versus malignant intraosseous lesions: discrimination by means of PET with 2-[F-18] flouro-2- deoxy-D-glucose. Radiology 1996;200:243–7.

17. Costelloe CM, Chuang HH, Madewell JE. FDG PET/CT of primary bone tumors [review]. AJR Am J Roentgenol 2014;202(6):W521–31.

18. Strobel K, Exner UE, Stumpe KD, et al. The additional value of CT images interpretation in the differential diagnosis of benign vs. malignant primary bone lesions with 18F-FDGPET/CT. Eur J Nucl Med Mol Imaging 2008;35:2000–8.

19. Marulanda GA, Henderson ER, Johnson DA, et al. Orthopedic surgery options for the treatment of primary osteosarcoma. Cancer Control 2008;15(1): 13–20.

20. Vander Griend RA. Osteosarcoma and its variants. Orthop Clin North Am 1996;27(3):575–81.

21. Franzius C, Sciuk J, Daldrup-Link HE, et al. FDG PET for detection of osseous metastases from malignant primary bone tumours: comparison with bone scintigraphy. Eur J Nucl Med 2000;27:1305–11.

22. Daldrup-Link HE, Franzius C, Link TM, et al. Whole-body MR imaging for detection of bone metastases in children and young adults: comparison with skeletal scintigraphy and FDG PET. Am J Roentgenol 2001;177:229–36.

23. Even-Sapir E, Metser U, Flusser G, et al. Assessment of malignant skeletal disease: initial experience with 18F-fluoride PET/CT and comparison between 18F-fluoride PET and 18Ffluoride PET/CT. J Nucl Med 2004;45:272–8.

24. Meyers PA, Schwartz CL, Krailo M, et al. Osteosarcoma: a randomized, prospective trial of the addition of ifosfamide and/or muramyl tripeptide to cisplatin, doxorubicin, and high-dose methotrexate. J Clin Oncol 2005;23(9):2004–11.

25. Cheon GJ, Kim MS, Lee JA, et al. Prediction model of chemotherapy response in osteosarcoma by 18F-FDG PET and MRI. J Nucl Med 2009;50:1435–40.

26. Ye Z, Zhu J, Tian M, et al. Response of osteogenic sarcoma to neoadjuvant therapy: evaluated by 18FFDG- PET. Ann Nucl Med 2008;22:475–80.

27. Davis JC, Daw NC, Navid F, et al. ^{18}F-FDG uptake during early adjuvant chemotherapy predicts histologic response in pediatric and young adult patients with osteosarcoma. J Nucl Med 2018;59(1):25–30.

28. Brenner W, Bohuslavizki KH, Eary JF. PET imaging of osteosarcoma. J Nucl Med 2003;44:930–42.

29. Charest M, Hickeson M, Lisbona R, et al. FDG PET/CT imaging in primary osseous and soft tissue sarcomas: a retrospective review of 212 cases. Eur J Nucl Med Mol Imaging 2009;36(12):1944–51.

30. Fuglø HM, Jørgensen SM, Loft A, et al. The diagnostic and prognostic value of 18F-FDG PET/CT in the initial assessment of high-grade bone and soft tissue sarcoma. A retrospective study of 89 patients. Eur J Nucl Med Mol Imaging 2012;39(9):1416–24.

31. Hongtao L, Hui Z, Bingshun W, et al. 18F-FDG positron emission tomography for the assessment of histological response to neoadjuvant chemotherapy in osteosarcomas: a meta-analysis. Surg Oncol 2012;21(4):e165–70.

32. Franzius C, Daldrup-Link HE, Wagner-Bohn A, et al. FDG-PET for detection of recurrences from malignant primary bone tumors: comparison with conventional imaging. Ann Oncol 2002;13:157–60.

33. Rakheja R, Makis W, Skamene S, et al. Correlating metabolic activity on 18F-FDG PET/CT with histopathologic characteristics of osseous and soft-tissue sarcomas: a retrospective review of 136 patients. AJR Am J Roentgenol 2012;198(6):1409–16.

34. Buchbender C, Heusner TA, Lauenstein TC, et al. Oncologic PET/MRI, part 2: bone tumors, soft tissue tumors, melanoma, and lymphoma. J Nucl Med 2012;53:1244–52.

35. Purz S, Sabri O, Viehweger A. Potential pediatric applications of PET/MR. J Nucl Med 2014;55(Supplement 2):32S–9S.

36. Eiber M, Takei T, Souvatzoglou M, et al. Performance of whole-body integrated 18F-FDG PET/MR in comparison to PET/CT for evaluation of malignant bone lesions. J Nucl Med 2014;55:191–7.

37. Denecke T, Hundsdörfer P, Misch D, et al. Assessment of histological response of paediatric bone sarcomas using FDG PET in comparison to morphological volume measurement and standardized MRI parameters. Eur J Nucl Med Mol Imaging 2010;37:1842–53.

38. Ludwig JA. Ewing sarcoma: historical perspectives, current state of the art, and opportunities for targeted therapy in the future. Curr Opin Oncol 2008;20:412–8.

39. Kleis M, Daldrup-link H, Matthay K, et al. Diagnostic value of PET-CT for the staging and restaging of pediatric tumors. Eur J Nucl Med Mol Imaging 2009;36:23–36.

40. Guimarães JB, Rigo L, Lewin F, et al. The importance of PET/CT in the evaluation of patients with Ewing tumors. Radiol Bras 2015;48(3):175–80.

41. London K, Stege C, Cross S, et al. 18F-FDG PET/CT compared to conventional imaging modalities in pediatric primary bone tumors. Pediatr Radiol 2012;42:418–30.

42. Bestic JM, Peterson JJ, Bancroft LW. Pediatric FDG PET/CT: physiologic uptake, normal variants, and benign conditions. Radiographics 2009;29(5):1487–500.

43. Arush MW, Israel O, Postovsky S, et al. Positron emission tomography/computed tomography with 18-fluorodeoxyglucose in the detection of local recurrence and distant metastases of pediatric sarcoma. Pediatr Blood Cancer 2007;49:901–5.

44. Bredella MA, Caputo GR, Steinbach LS. Value of FDG positron emission tomography in conjunction with MR imaging for evaluating therapy response in patients with musculoskeletal sarcomas. AJR Am J Roentgenol 2002;179:1145–50.

45. Hawkins DS, Schuetze SM, Butrynski JE, et al. [18F] Fluorodeoxyglucose positron emission tomography predicts outcome for Ewing sarcoma family of tumors. J Clin Oncol 2005;23:8828–34.

46. Feldman F, Van Heertum R, Saxena C, et al. 18FDG-PET applications for cartilage neoplasms. Skeletal Radiol 2005;34(7):367–74.

47. Jesus-Garcia R, Osawa A, Filippi RZ, et al. Is PET-CT an accurate method for the differential diagnosis between chondroma and chondrosarcoma? Springerplus 2016;5:236.

48. Brenner W, Conrad EU, Eary JF. FDG PET imaging for grading and prediction of outcome in

chondrosarcoma patients. Eur J Nucl Med Mol Imaging 2004;31:189–95.

49. Subhawong TK, Winn A, Shemesh SS. F-18 FDG PET differentiation of benign from malignant chondroid neoplasms: a systematic review of the literature. Skeletal Radiol 2017;46(9):1233–9.

50. Lee FY-I, Yu J, Chang S-S, et al. Diagnostic value and limitations of fluorine-18 fluorodeoxyglucose positron emission tomography for cartilaginous tumors of bone. J Bone Joint Surg am 2004;86–A(12):2677–85.

51. Costelloe CM, Chuang HH, Chasen BA, et al. Bone windows for distinguishing malignant from benign primary bone tumors on FDG PET/CT. J Cancer 2013;4(7):524–30.

52. Sheikhbahaei S, Marcus C, Hafezi-Nejad N, et al. Value of FDG PET/CT in patient management and outcome of skeletal and soft tissue sarcomas. PET Clin 2015;10(3):375–93.

53. Purohit BS, Dulguerov P, Burkhardt K, et al. Dedifferentiated laryngeal chondrosarcoma: combined morphologic and functional imaging with positron-emission tomography/magnetic resonance imaging. Laryngoscope 2014;124(7):E274–7.

54. Singh T, Satheesh CT, Lakshmaiah KC, et al. Primary bone lymphoma: a report of two cases and review of the literature. J Cancer Res Ther 2010;6(3):296–8.

55. Kitsoulis P, Vlychou M, Papoudou-Bai A, et al. Primary lymphomas of bone. Anticancer Res 2006;26(1A):325–37.

56. Bosch-Barrera J, Arbea L, García-Velloso MJ, et al. Primary bone lymphoma of mandible and thyroid incidentaloma identified by FDG PET/CT: a case report. Cases J 2009;2:6384.

57. Kwee TC, Kwee RM, Nievelstein RA. Imaging in staging of malignant lymphoma: a systematic review. Blood 2008;111:504–16.

58. Hutchings M, Barrington SF. PET/CT for therapy response assessment in lymphoma. J Nucl Med 2009;50(Suppl 1):21S–30S.

59. Catlett JP, Williams SA, O'Connor SC, et al. Primary lymphoma of bone: an institutional experience. Leuk Lymphoma 2008;49:2125–32.

60. Breiback F, Julian A, Laurent C, et al. Contribution of the 2-[18F]- fluoro-s-deoxy-D-glucose positron emission tomography/computed tomography to the diagnosis of primary osseous Hodgkin lymphoma. BMJ Case Rep 2009;2009. Available at: http://www.ncbi.nlm.nih.gov/pubmed/21686679. Accessed January 14, 2014.

61. Lin EC. FDG PET/CT flip flop phenomenon in treated lymphoma of bone. Clin Nucl Med 2006;31(12):803–5.

62. Park YH, Kim S, Choi SJ, et al. Clinical impact of whole-body FDGPET for evaluation of response and therapeutic decision-making of primary

lymphoma of bone. Ann Oncol 2005;16(8):1401–2.

63. Huan Y, Qi Y, Zhang W, et al. Primary bone lymphoma of radius and tibia: a case report and review of literature. Medicine (Baltimore) 2017;96(15):e6603.

64. Rakheja R, Chandarana H, DeMello L, et al. Correlation between standardized uptake value and apparent diffusion coefficient of neoplastic lesions evaluated with whole-body simultaneous hybrid PET/MRI. AJR Am J Roentgenol 2013;201:1115–9.

65. Wu X, Korkola P, Pertovaara H, et al. No correlation between glucose metabolism and apparent diffusion coefficient in diffuse large B-cell lymphoma: a PET/CT and DW-MRI study. Eur J Radiol 2011;79:e117–21.

66. Hagtvedt T, Seierstad T, Lund KV, et al. Diffusion weighted MRI compared to FDG PET/CT for assessment of early treatment response in lymphoma. Acta Radiol 2015;56(2):152–8.

67. International Myeloma Working Group. Criteria for the classification of monoclonal gammopathies, multiple myeloma and related disorders: a report of the International Myeloma Working Group. Br J Haematol 2003;121(5):749–57.

68. Dimopoulos M, Terpos E, Comenzo RL, et al. International Myeloma Working Group consensus statement and guidelines regarding the current role of imaging techniques in the diagnosis and monitoring of multiple myeloma. Leukemia 2009;23:1545–56.

69. Bartel TB, Haessler J, Brown TL, et al. F18-fluorodeoxyglucose positron emission tomography in the context of other imaging techniques and prognostic factors in multiple myeloma. Blood 2009;114(10):2068–76.

70. Dammacco F, Rubini G, Ferrari C, et al. (18)F-FDG PET/CT: a review of diagnostic and prognostic features in multiple myeloma and related disorders. Clin Exp Med 2006;15(1):1–8.

71. Fechtner K, Hillengass J, Delorme S, et al. Staging monoclonal plasma cell disease: comparison of the Durie-Salmon and the Durie-Salmon plus staging systems. Radiology 2010;257(1):195–204.

72. Breyer RJ, Mulligan ME, Smith SE, et al. Comparison of imaging with FDG PET/CT with other imaging modalities in myeloma. Skeletal Radiol 2006;35:632–40.

73. Schirrmeister H, Bommer M, Buck AK, et al. Initial results in the assessment of multiple myeloma using 18F-FDG PET. Eur J Nucl Med Mol Imaging 2002;29:361–6.

74. Zamagni E, Nanni C, Gay F, et al. 18F-FDG PET/CT focal, but not osteolytic, lesions predict the progression of smoldering myeloma to active disease. Leukemia 2016;30(2):417–22.

75. Shortt CP, Gleeson TG, Breen KA, et al. Whole-Body MRI versus PET in assessment of multiple myeloma

disease activity. AJR Am J Roentgenol 2009;192: 980–6.

76. Shah SN, Oldan JD. PET/MR imaging of multiple myeloma. Magn Reson Imaging Clin N Am 2017; 25(2):351–65.

77. Purohit S, Pardiwala D. Imaging of giant cell tumor of bone. Indian J Orthop 2007;41(2):91–6.

78. Gong L, Liu W, Sun X, et al. Histological and clinical characteristics of malignant giant cell tumor of bone. Virchows Arch 2012;460:327–34.

79. Feigenberg SJ, Marcus RB Jr, Zlotecki RA, et al. Whole-lung radiotherapy for giant cell tumors of bone with pulmonary metastases. Clin Orthop Relat Res 2002;(401):202–8.

80. Park HL, Yoo IR, Lee Y, et al. Giant Cell tumor of the rib: two cases of F-18 FDG PET/CT findings. Nucl Med Mol Imaging 2017;51(2):182–5.

81. Hoshi M, Takada J, Oebisu N, et al. Overexpression of hexokinase-2 in giant cell tumor of bone is associated with false positive in bone tumor on FDG-PET/CT. Arch Orthop Trauma Surg 2012;132: 1561–8.

82. Muheremu A, Ma Y, Huang Z, et al. Diagnosing giant cell tumor of the bone using positron emission tomography/computed tomography: a retrospective study of 20 patients from a single center. Oncol Lett 2017;14(2):1985–8.

83. Makis W, Alabed YZ, Nahal A, et al. Giant cell tumor pulmonary 18 metastases mimic primary malignant pulmonary nodules on FFDGPET/CT. Nucl Med Mol Imaging 2012;46:134–7.

84. Gholamrezanezhad A, Chirindel A, Subramaniam R. Assessment of response to therapy. In: Peller P, Subramaniam R, Guermazi A, editors. PET-CT and PET-MRI in oncology. Medical radiology. Berlin (Germany): Springer; 2012. p. 279–322.

85. Boye K, Jebsen NL, Zaikova O, et al. Denosumab in patients with giant-cell tumor of bone in Norway: results from a nationwide cohort. Acta Oncol 2017; 56(3):479–83.

86. Gholamrezanezhad A, Basques K, Batouli A, et al. Applications of PET/CT and PET/MRI in Musculoskeletal, Orthopedic, and Rheumatologic Imaging. AJR Am J Roentgenol 2018;210(6):245–63.

87. Gholamrezanezhad A, Mehrkhani F, Olyaie M. Imaging approach in the evaluation of response to treatment of breast cancer. Nucl Med Commun 2018; 39(4):343–4.